Essentials of Emergency Surgery

Essentials of Emergency Surgery

Editor: Amy Walker

AMERICAN
MEDICAL PUBLISHERS
www.americanmedicalpublishers.com

AMERICAN
MEDICAL PUBLISHERS
www.americanmedicalpublishers.com

Cataloging-in-Publication Data

Essentials of emergency surgery / edited by Amy Walker.
p. cm.
Includes bibliographical references and index.
ISBN 978-1-63927-490-1
1. Surgical emergencies. 2. Medical emergencies. 3. Surgery. I. Walker, Amy.
RD93 .E77 2022
617.026--dc23

American Medical Publishers,
41 Flatbush Avenue,
1st Floor, New York,
NY 11217, USA

ISBN 978-1-63927-490-1 (Hardback)

Contents

Preface

Emergency surgery is performed on an acutely-ill patient who is at a high risk for death and other complications. Most surgically treatable emergencies fall within the purview of different specialties. Abdominal problems such as strangulated and incarcerated inguinal hernias, intestinal obstructions caused by volvulus, adhesions and worm infections, and appendicitis are certain abdominal conditions that require emergency surgery. Respiratory obstructions may arise due to trauma, tumors, head and neck infections, bleeding, etc. In cases where the obstruction is not resolved with change of position or insertion of a tube or an oral airway into the trachea, procedures such as tracheostomy or cricothyroidotomy may be required. Another condition that may require emergency surgery is urinary obstruction caused due to stones in the bladder obstructing the outlet, scarring of the urethra or an enlarged prostate compressing the urethra. In such cases, an emergency procedure called suprapubic cystostomy may be performed. This book contains some path-breaking studies in the field of emergency surgery. It outlines the procedures and practices that are the mainstay of modern emergency surgery in detail. This book includes contributions of experts and scientists which will provide innovative insights into this field.

The researches compiled throughout the book are authentic and of high quality, combining several disciplines and from very diverse regions from around the world. Drawing on the contributions of many researchers from diverse countries, the book's objective is to provide the readers with the latest achievements in the area of research. This book will surely be a source of knowledge to all interested and researching the field.

In the end, I would like to express my deep sense of gratitude to all the authors for meeting the set deadlines in completing and submitting their research chapters. I would also like to thank the publisher for the support offered to us throughout the course of the book. Finally, I extend my sincere thanks to my family for being a constant source of inspiration and encouragement.

Editor

1

Treatment of burns in the first 24 hours: simple and practical guide by answering 10 questions in a step-by-step form

Ziyad Alharbi[1*†], Andrzej Piatkowski[1,2†], Rolf Dembinski[3], Sven Reckort[1,4], Gerrit Grieb[1], Jens Kauczok[1] and Norbert Pallua[1]

Abstract

Residents in training, medical students and other staff in surgical sector, emergency room (ER) and intensive care unit (ICU) or Burn Unit face a multitude of questions regarding burn care. Treatment of burns is not always straightforward. Furthermore, National and International guidelines differ from one region to another. On one hand, it is important to understand pathophysiology, classification of burns, surgical treatment, and the latest updates in burn science. On the other hand, the clinical situation for treating these cases needs clear guidelines to cover every single aspect during the treatment procedure. Thus, 10 questions have been organised and discussed in a step-by-step form in order to achieve the excellence of education and the optimal treatment of burn injuries in the first 24 hours. These 10 questions will clearly discuss referral criteria to the burn unit, primary and secondary survey, estimation of the total burned surface area (%TBSA) and the degree of burns as well as resuscitation process, routine interventions, laboratory tests, indications of Bronchoscopy and special considerations for Inhalation trauma, immediate consultations and referrals, emergency surgery and admission orders. Understanding and answering the 10 questions will not only cover the management process of Burns during the first 24 hours but also seems to be an interactive clear guide for education purpose.

Keywords: Burn care, Burn surgery, Burn unit, Burn resuscitation, Burn care guidelines

Introduction

During a rotation to the emergency room (ER), surgical sector or burn unit, residents under training should pay attention to the pathophysiology and classification of burns, treatment, and the latest updates in burn science including burn injury prognosis [1]. Managing burn cases in the first 24 hours represents one of the biggest challenges in burn care and will indeed reflect the degree of morbidity and mortality. Therefore, a guide for treatment during the first 24 hours can be very helpful. A lot of trusted guidelines exist regarding this point such as the American Burn Association guidelines for referral criteria to burn centres and also operation guidelines in the burn unit. Furthermore, it should be noted that the International society for Burn injuries (ISBI) served a good purpose regarding the education and set several guidelines with the World Health Organisations and many European organisations including the European Burn Association, German Society for Burn Treatment and British Burn Association for the treatment of Burn injuries.

This practical guide is drawn to make it easy for any trainee, medical students and staff to understand the basic principles of management that should be carried out in each burn case during the first 24 hours. Any trainee should understand indeed his/her responsibility for these unique patients and should identify the management process in comprehensive way. This does not only mean covering of all wounds but also to bring the patient to his or her normal status including the psychological, social and of course the physical aspect.

* Correspondence: zalharbi@ukaachen.de
†Equal contributors
[1]Department of Plastic and Hand Surgery, Burn Centre Medical Faculty, RWTH Aachen University Hospital, Pauwelsstr 30, Aachen 52074, Germany

Objective

This article has been primarily written for education purposes. We believe that good and clear information will indeed enhance the quality of treatment even without big facilities. The target group is any physician, surgeon, trainee in training, interns, medical students and personnel who are responsible for burn patients in surgical sector, emergency room (ER) and intensive care unit (ICU) or Burn Unit.

Methods

A clear guide has been structured for the above target group, which includes 10 questions that should be asked and well answered to cover the treatment of burn patients in the first 24 hours. Herein, the following questions should be taken in consideration:

1. Does the patient meet the criteria for injuries requiring referral to the Burn Unit?
2. How to perform the Primary Survey and Secondary Survey?
3. How to estimate the total burned surface area (%TBSA) and the degree of burns?
4. What are the main aspects of Resuscitation?
5. What are the routine interventions that should be performed for each case of burn injury during admission to the Burn Unit?
6. What kind of laboratory tests should be done?
7. Does the patient have Inhalation Injury and is Bronchoscopy indicated for all patients?
8. What kind of consultations should be carried out immediately?
9. Does the patient need Emergency Surgery or not?
10. What kind of admission orders should be written?

Furthermore, this paper does not only state a guideline to be followed but also explains every point and takes in consideration that many hospitals around the world do not have a specialised burn unit and, thus most of the treatment process occurs in the emergency room (ER). Furthermore, international guidelines regarding burn treatment have been also reviewed in the literature.

10 questions as practical guide:

1. *Does the patient meet the criteria for injuries requiring referral to the Burn Unit?*
A clear answer should be given in the pre-hospital setting. This must be well performed by the referral person or the transporting physician. It is not meant that a patient with burn injury should immediately be moved to a burn unit. In the case of a burn centre not being able to accept a patient, the initial treatment process can also be conducted in the emergency room (ER) until the transport to the burn unit takes place.
The main criteria for referral to a burn unit include the following [2]:

- Second and third degree burns greater than 10% TBSA in patients younger than 10 years and older than 50 years.
- Second and third degree burns greater than 20%.
- Third degree burns greater than 5%.
- Burns to face, hands, feet, genitalia, perineum and major joints.
- Electrical burns (including lightning injury)
- Chemical burns
- Inhalation injury
- Patients with pre-existing conditions
- Circumferential third degree burns to extremity or chest
- Burns involving concomitant trauma with a great risk of morbidity and mortality (i.e. explosion trauma).

2. *How to perform the Primary Survey and Secondary Survey?*
The burn injury itself has a secondary role in the moment of *primary survey*. Directly on admission Advanced Trauma Life Support (ATLS) guidelines must be performed and the following points must be checked:

Airway: Early recognition of airway compromise followed by prompt intubation can be live saving [3]. If there is soot in the mouth consider early intubation even if the patient is breathing normally.
Breathing: Determine if the patient is moving air or not.
Circulation: Obtain appropriate vascular access and a monitor device to control heart rate and blood pressure.
Disability: Detect if there are any other manifestations including fractures and deformities, abdominal injury or neurological deficit.
Exposure: The patient should be completely exposed and should be out of clothes. Exposure of all orifices must be conducted in this part.
Fluid resuscitation: A mainstay in the treatment. This point is discussed in the third question after the calculation of the total burned surface area (%TBSA) but the guidelines of Acute Trauma Life Support (ATLS) should be followed in order to maintain the circulation process.
Note that a child is prone to hypothermia due to its high surface to volume ratio and low fat mass. Ambient temperature should be from 28° to 32°C

(82° to 90°F). The patient's core temperature must be kept at least above 34°C.
Secondary survey is designed as a burn-specific survey. It is performed during admission to the burn unit. Full history should be approached including:

- Detection of the mechanism of injury.
- Time of injury.
- Consideration of abuse [4].
- Height and weight.
- Possibility of carbon monoxide intoxication based on the history of burns in a closed area as well as the presence of soot in mouth and nose [5].
- Facial burns.

Examination of the cornea is important as well as the ear in case of explosion trauma. A systemic overview should be performed in this phase including a fast run on the *abdomen, genital region, lower and upper limbs* (think: X-Ray C-Spine, Thorax, and Pelvic). If the patient is a child, look for signs of abuse.

3. *How to estimate the total burned surface area (%TBSA) and the degree of burns?*
   Total body surface area (TBSA) is an assessment measure of skin burns. As shown in Figure 1, in adults the "*rule of nines*" is used to determine the total percentage of the burned area for each major section of the body [6,7].However, this rule cannot be used in pediatric burns. The *Lund-Browder chart* is one of the most accurate methods to estimate not only the size of the burn area but also the burn degree in each part. The use of this chart has shown an easy access and fast readability in the clinical practice as well as its use in pediatric burns [7]. It is available in many centres and also available online. Note that an internet address has been added at the end of this article to make it accessible for education purposes. Accurate estimation must be performed in order to estimate the amount of intravenous fluids, referral indications to the burn unit and indication of surgery as well as the estimation of prognosis.
   The degree of burns is calculated to estimate the prognosis as well as the type of treatment and consequently the type of surgery that should be conducted. Burns are classified to:

   First degree burns: typical redness and pain of the affected skin. Minor epithelial damage occurs without formation of blisters. Typically occurs with sunburns.
   Superficial second degree burns: complete epithelial damage and only papillary dermal damage occurs. This degree leaves no neurovascular damage. Thus,

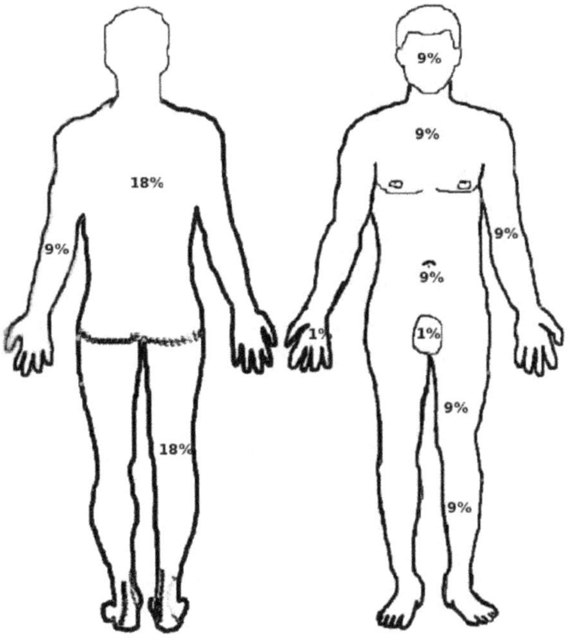

Figure 1 Rule of nines: This figure shows the different parts of the body that equal 9% of the body surface area (i.e. complete upper thigh = 9%, complete lower thigh = 9%, complete leg = 18%).

it causes pain, bleeds and presents with blisters. Epithelial repair occurs within 14 days. It mostly leaves no scars after healing. Sometimes discoloration stays.
Deep second degree burns: complete epithelial damage and damage of the reticular dermis present. It results in neurovascular damage. Thus, it generally presents without bleeding or sensation and appears white in colour. Blisters can also be present but are bigger than in superficial second degree burns. Healing can occur but takes longer than 14 days and results in scars.
Third degree burns: involving the epidermis, dermis and subcutaneous tissue. The skin appears leathery consisting of thrombotic vessels (Figure 2).
Forth degree burns (*debatable*): it is a third degree burn with involvement of the underlying fascia, muscles and even bones.

- Superficial burn injury (First degree).
- Superficial partial-thickness burns (Superficial second degree).
- Deep partial-thickness burns (Deep second degree).
- Full-thickness burns (Third degree).
- Fourth degree burns (debatable classification as some references do not support this degree [1]).

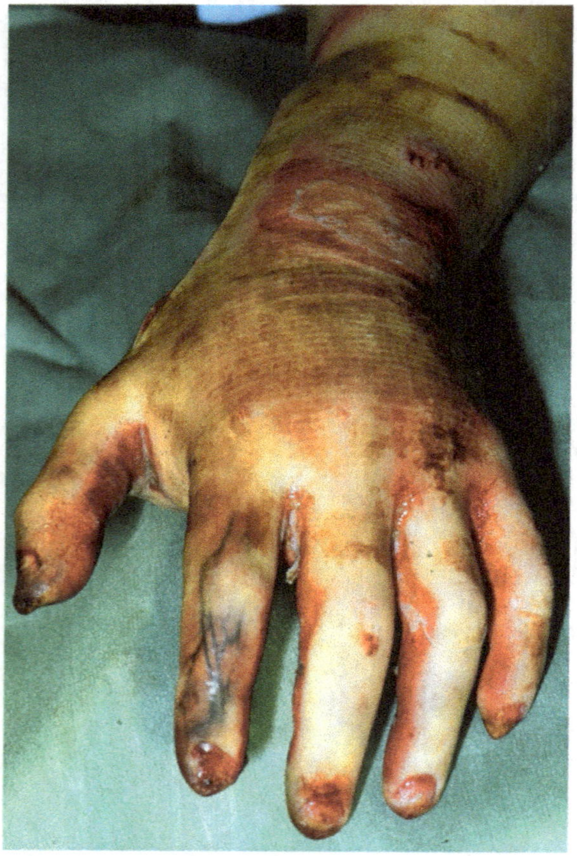

Figure 2 Third degree burns (Note the thrombotic vessels formation).

4. *What are the main aspects of Resuscitation?* Calculation of the total burned surface (% TBSA) area is essential in this part. Charles Baxter, MD, at Parkland Hospital, Southwestern University Medical Centre, designed in the 1960s [8,9] the *Parkland formula* to calculate the fluid needs for the first 24 hours. Although many modifications of this formula have been proposed this formula is still one of the easiest ways to calculate the fluid volume for burn patients.

$$4\text{ mL} \times \text{Patient's body weight} \times \text{TBSA} = \text{Volume to be given in the first 24 hours}$$

50% of this volume is infused in the first 8 hours, starting from the time of injury, and the other 50% is infused during the last 16 hours of the first day. The type of fluid administration is a debatable question. Lactated Ringer has been commonly used and is even used up to date. On the other hand, many centres suggest balanced electrolyte solutions like Ringer-acetate to prevent the high dose administration of lactate. According to our experience and to the best of our knowledge, we believe that balanced electrolyte solutions are a safe option and therefore they are recommended in our centre. Furthermore, specific burn populations usually require higher resuscitation volumes sometimes as much as 30-40% higher (close to 5.7 mL/kg/%TBSA) than predicted by the Parkland formula [10,11]. Klein et al have suggested that patients today are receiving more fluid than in the past. Their purpose was to find significant predictors of negative outcomes after resuscitation. They concluded that higher volumes equalled a higher risk for complications, i.e. lung-complications [12,13]. These results support that fluid overload in the critical hours of early burn management may lead to unnecessary oedema [14]. Overall, the use of Parkland formula is just a process of estimation. Clinically, fluid needs of an individual, after the use of any suggested formula, should be at least monitored by several important factors such urine output, blood pressure and central venous pressure. An important point and considered to be the goal in fluid resuscitation is to maintain a urine output of approximately 0.5 ml/kg/

h in adults and between 0.5 and 1.0 ml/kg/h in patients weighing less than 30 kg [15]. Failure to meet these goals should be addressed with gentle upward corrections in the rate of fluid administration by approximately 25% [16].
Due to the capillary leak, most burn centres advise not to use colloids and other blood products within the first 24 hours [17]. If used in the early phase (up to 12 h), it can lead to a prolonged tissue oedema and consecutive lung complications. Furthermore colloids are not associated with an improvement in survival, and are therefore more expensive than crystalloids [18]. Liberati et al advocated that there is no evidence that blood products (including human albumin) reduce mortality when compared with cheaper alternatives such as saline [19].
Maintenance dose is provided after the first 24 hours. It can be calculated as follows [1,20]:

100 ml/kg : for the first 10 kg
50 ml/kg : for the second 10 kg
20 ml/kg : every kilogram above 20 kg

Special considerations for children:
Modified Parkland Formula is used for this category of patients as follows [1,21]:

$$4\ \text{mL} \times \text{Patient's body weight} \times \text{TBSA} \times \text{Maintenance fluid} = \text{Volume to be given in the first 24 hours}$$

5. *What kind of routine interventions should be performed for each case of burns during admission to the Burn Unit?*
Injured patients differ in term of burns size and depth. Pre-existing conditions play an important role in this phase. *Central venous catheter* and *arterial line* are indicated if the patient is hemodynamically unstable or if frequent blood gas analysis is required. Furthermore, *nasogastric tube* and *urinary catheter* are indicated in patients with 20% TBSA or more. Nasogastric tube will initiate immediate feeding and decrease the possibility of ileus or aspiration. Urinary catheter that is equipped with a temperature probe is preferred.
Before washing the patients, *swabs for microbiological examination* should be taken from different areas including burn areas, mouth, nose and the inguinal area. It should be made clear that *the patient is washed* properly with warm water and then re-evaluated regarding the total burned surface area (TBSA) as well as the degree of burns. A definite evaluation of the total burned surface area (TBSA) can only be made when the patient is washed completely and the wounds can be judged properly. In this phase, indication for surgery is made including escharotomy, debridement and in certain situations skin grafting. This point will be discussed in the 9th question.
6. *What kind of laboratory tests should be done?*
Basic laboratory tests include the following:

- Complete blood count (CBC) and Arterial blood gas (ABG) analysis,
- Urea and Electrolytes (U&E),
- Prothrombin time (PT) / Partial thrombin time (PTT) and International Normalized Ration (INR),
- Sputum Culture and Sensitivity,
- Creatine Kinase (CK) and C-reactive protine (CRP),
- Blood glucose,
- Urine drug test,
- Human chorionic gonadotropin (B-HCG): if the patient is female,
- Albumin test.
- Thyroid values and myoglobin measures.

7. *Does the patient have Inhalation Injury and is Bronchoscopy indicated for all patients?*
Burns occurring in closed areas and all burns that are affecting the head are subjected to inhalation injury [22,23]. If Carbon monoxide (CO) intoxication is suspected, perform arterial blood gas (ABG) analysis to detect carboxyhemoglobin (COHb), immediate supply of 100% oxygen, chest X-Ray and discuss the possibility of hyperbaric oxygen (HBO) therapy. COHb higher than 20% or cases presented with neurological deficits are absolute indications for HBO, whereas COHb amounts of 10% and higher are seen as relative indications for HBO [24]. Overall, intubated burn patients provide a good access for bronchoscopy. In this case, fiberoptic bronchoscopy can be used to evaluate the extent of airway oedema and the inflammatory process that is caused by any form of inhalation injury including the carbon monoxide (CO) intoxication [22,23]. On the other hand, the role of bronchoscopy is debatable in terms of the therapeutic aspect as well as its invasive procedure.
8. *What kind of consultations should be carried out immediately?*
Depending on the secondary survey, several consultations may be necessary. In case of facial burns, consult:

- Otolaryngology (ENT) department: to exclude burns of the upper airway, laryngeal oedema or in case of explosion rupture of the tympanic membrane.
- Ophthalmology: to exclude erosion or ulceration of the cornea.

Follow the same procedure as performed in the primary survey. As guided by the Advance Trauma Life Support (ATLS), consult or re-consult if already performed:

- Trauma surgery,
- Abdominal surgery and
- Neurosurgery.

9. *Does the patient need Emergency Surgery or not?* *Debridement:*
The term "Debridement" is not merely a surgical procedure. Debridement can be performed by surgical, chemical, mechanical, or autolytic procedures. Surgical modalities including early tangential excision (*necrectomy*) of the burned tissue and early wound closure primarily by skin grafts has led to significant improvement in mortality rates and substantially lower costs in these patients [25,26]. Furthermore, in some circumstances, *escharotomy* or even *fasciotomy* should be performed.
Indications of surgical debridement:

1. Deep second degree burns.
2. Burns of any type, that are heavily contaminated
3. Third degree circumferential burns with suspected compartment syndrome (think of: *Escharotomy*)
4. Circumferential burns around the wrist (think of: *Carpal tunnel release*)

Benefits of surgical debridement:

1. To reduce the amount of necrotic tissue (beneficial for prognosis)
2. To get a sample for diagnostic purposes (if needed).

Complications of debridement:

1. Pain.
2. Bleeding.
3. Infection.
4. Risk of removal of healthy tissue.

Contraindications:

1. Low body core temperature below 34°C.
2. Cardiovascular and respiratory system instability.

Any trainee should be aware of the following terms:

- Tangential excision: Tangential excision of the superficial (burned) parts of the skin
- Epifascial excision: This technique is reserved for burns extending at least to the subcuticular level.
- Subfascial excision: indicated when burns extend vey deep and reach the fascia and muscles. It is needed only in special cases.
- Escharotomy: Indicated for third-degree and second degree deep dermal circumferential burns. This is used to prevent a soft tissue compartment syndrome, due to swelling after deep burn. An escharotomy is performed by making an incision through the eschar to expose the fatty tissue below. This can be illustrated in Figure 3. Note that escharotomy lines on the thumb and little finger, as an international standard, should be always performed on the radial side and not on the ulnar side. Escharotomy incisions for the index finger, middle finger and ring finger are performed along the ulnar side.
- Fasciotomy: Fasciotomy is a limb-saving procedure when used to treat acute compartment syndrome. An incision is made in the skin that extends into the fascia where it will relieve pressure. Note that Carpal Tunnel Syndrome (CTS) can result from the circumferential burns around the wrist by consecutive swelling.
  After any selected procedure from the above category, the resulted wound should be covered. Autografts, i.e. *split thickness skin grafts* (autologous skin transfer), remain the mainstay of treatment for many patients (Figure 4a-d and 5).

Dermal substitutes or matrices can be used if a large burn area exists. Here are some examples:

Biobrane: Biosynthetic wound dressing constructed of a silicone film with a nylon fabric.
Suprathel: Innovative skin substitute made of polylactide for the treatment of superficial dermal wounds especially the superficial second degree burns.
Alloderm: Cultured and processed dermis used under skin graft to reproduce the layered structure of dermis and epidermis in a graft
Integra: Bilayer wound matrix comprised of porous matrix of cross-linked bovine tendon collagen and glycosaminoglycan and a semi-permeable polysiloxane (silicone) layer. Must be used in a two-step-procedure [27].
Matriderm: Three dimensional matrix consisting of collagen and elastin. Its use guides autologous cells for the construction of a "neo-dermis" [28,29]. Can be used in a single-step as well as in a two-step-procedure.

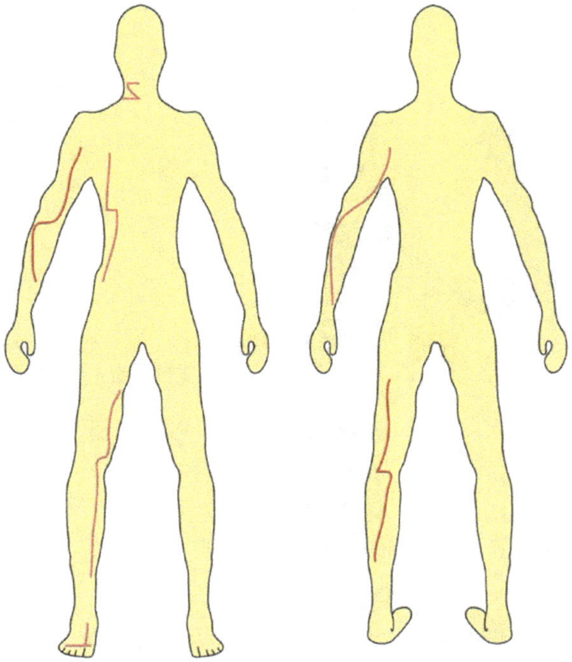

Figure 3 Escharotomy lines: Example of typical ways to incise the eschar. Note that the incisions should be made horizontally when crossing a joint.

Note that in many occasions, an immediate coverage of wounds cannot be achieved. In this case, a temporary coverage is favoured. After stabilization of patient and wound bed, a planned reconstruction takes place to close wounds permanently. In this point, some methods can be performed including:

Allografts: Cadaver Skin used for temporary cover.
Xenografts: Graft taken from other species (bovine of swine) can be used as temporary cover.

10. *What kind of admission orders should be written?* Routine admission orders include:

- Vital signs: Continuous monitoring of Heart rate, Blood pressure, Pulse pressure, Respiratory rate, Temperature and Central venous pressure.
- Documentation of allergies
- Diet: Nil per os (NPO) if burn more than 30% during the first 24 hours. Nasogastric tube will initiate immediate feeding and decrease the possibility of ileus or aspiration.
- I.V. fluids: follow the Parkland formula.
- Decubitus precautions.
- Consultation: Psychiatry or Psychology (only if patient is awake).
- Multivitamins and Traces: Vitamine C, ZnSo4, Selenium and Vitamine E.
- Tetanus prophylaxis.
- Ulcer prophylaxis.

Analgesia: the choice is dependent on burn size, depth, age and other trauma factor such as blunt trauma and fractures.

- Additional medications (for mechanically ventilated adults with smoke inhalation injury): nebulized heparin sulfate mixed in 3 ml normal saline every 4 hours and 3 ml 20% nebulized N-acetylcysteine plus 0.5 ml albuterol sulfate every 4 hours for 7 days [30].

Discussion

Several guidelines regarding burn management exist. This includes those guidelines setup by organisations and by clinicians or researchers in the field. Kis et al searched the literature between 1990 and 2008 and retrieved 546 citations, of which 24 were clinical practice guidelines on the general and intensive care of burn patients. All major burn topics were covered by at least one guideline, but no single guideline addressed all areas important in terms of outcomes [31]. For example, Alsbjoern B et al structured a guideline for treatment but that was mainly concentrating on wound treatment rather than the comprehensive way [32].

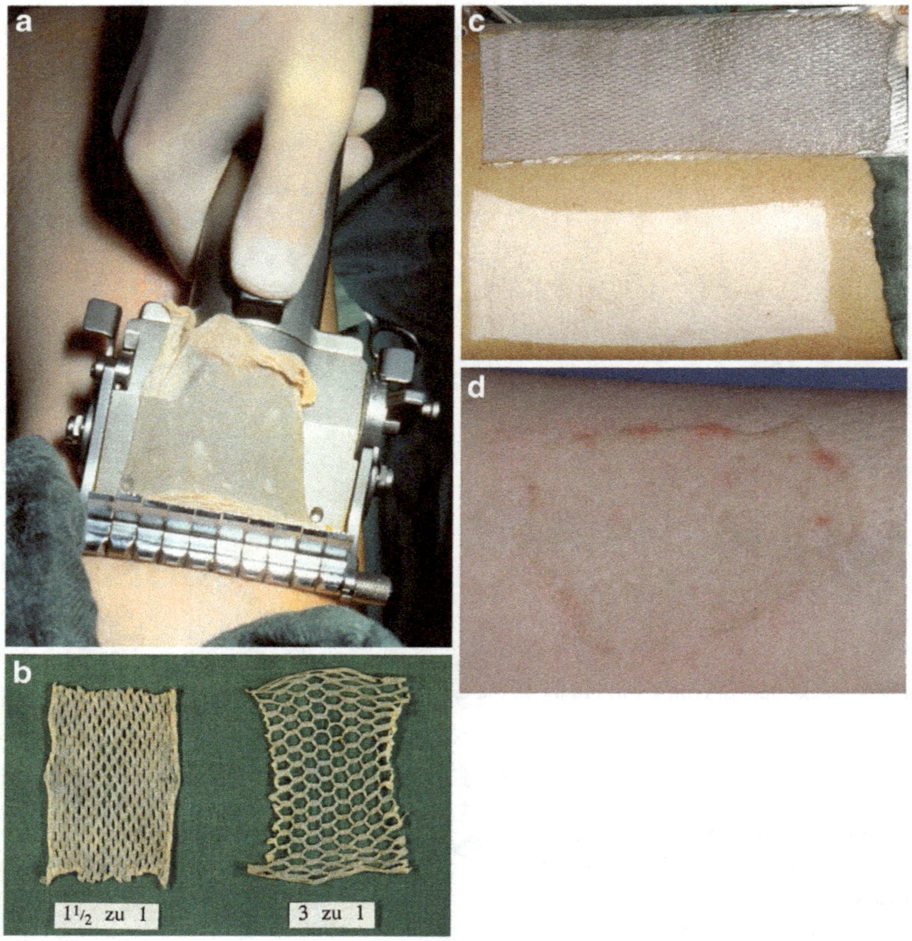

Figure 4 **a: Harvesting a skin graft with a dermatome, b: MESH skin graft with different sizes, c: the donor site after harvesting the skin graft, d: the appearance of the skin graft after its attachment to the Recipient area (3 Weeks later).**

One of the most renown and used guidelines have been set up by the International Society for Burn Injuries (ISBI) and the American Burns Association. The IBSI works together with the World Health Organisation and, thus enhances the education process concerning burn injury treatment in the developing world. The American Burn Association guidelines are considered one of the most reliable guidelines and are even followed and trusted by other big associations and societies like the South African Burn Society or the Australian and New Zealand Burn Association.

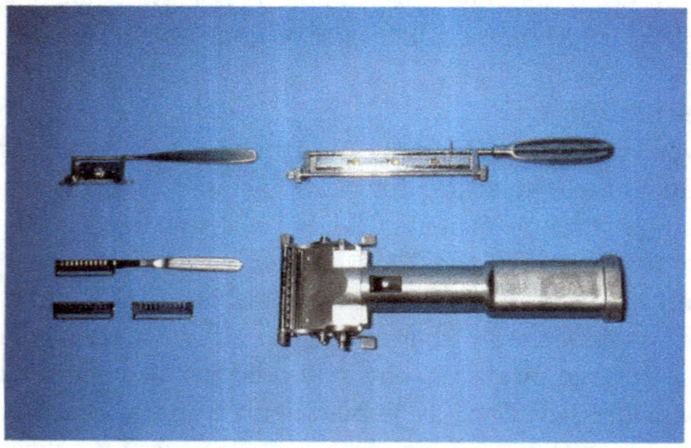

Figure 5 **This figure shows the most widely used instruments for skin debridement and harvesting of the graft.**

The criteria for transfer to a burn centre may differ between the above stated organisations. However, the criteria setup by the American Burn association represents the most widespread so far and are also fully supported by the American College of Surgeons [33-36]. In Europe, a workgroup of burn centres in German speaking countries (DAV) developed very well established guidelines for the treatment as well as the referral to a burn unit, which are accepted by the German Society for Burn Treatment (DGV), as well as the Austrian and the Swiss Burn Societies [37]. On the other hand, these guidelines don't discuss all aspects of treatment in the acute phase. There is no doubt that these guidelines and other factors including the development of advanced technologies in burn care enhanced the quality of treatment for burn patients in the last decades. However, many of these guidelines are made primarily for plastic surgeons and represent too much information regarding wound management and long term planning of surgical reconstruction.

In contrast to the above stated guidelines this paper discusses the first 24 hours in Burns and includes not only the surgical treatment but also a polytrauma protocol as well as a basic intensive care treatment plan for those patients.

This paper is written without intention to cover the therapy of electrical and chemical burns. We believe that electrical and chemical burns need a special evaluation and treatment that differs from thermal burns. Overall, thermal burns are common if compared to the last 2 types and, thus this guide concentrates on thermal burns. Furthermore, this paper takes in consideration that the information must be simple but also effective with good explanation just to be easily reached in a time frame as short as possible.

Conclusion

Understanding and answering the above stated 10 questions will not only cover the management process of Burns during the first 24 hours but also should be an interactive clear guide for education purpose. Burn cases can extremely differ and, thus trainee, medical students and personnel in surgical sector, emergency room (ER) and intensive care unit (ICU) or Burn Unit face a multitude of questions regarding these critically ill patients. We found that this method serves good purposes and increases not merely the quality of treatment but also enhances education. Therfore it was good reason and positive motivation for us to structure another 10 questions as a clear guide that cover the treatment of burns after the first 24 hours until discharge.

Recommendations

Advanced Burn Life Support (ABLS) Course by American Burn Association provides guidelines in the assessment and management of the burn patient during the first 24 hours post injury. To date, this course is of great importance like the **Advanced Trauma Life Support (ATLS)** course, which is provided by the American College of Surgeons and many centres around the world. We should declare that there is no financial or commercial relationship between authors and those organisations providing these types of courses.

Recommendation of further sources for education purpose

- *Abbreviated burn severity index (ABSI) / Belgian outcome in burn injury (BOBI)*
- *Lund and Browder chart for calculating the percentage of total body surface area burnt: http://www.tg.org.au/etg_demo/etg-lund-and-browder.pdf*
- *internet-based burns chart: www.burnschart.com*
- *Harris Benedict Equation / Curreri Formula for calorie needs.*

Competing interests
Authors declare that they have no competing interests.

Authors' contributions
ZA carried out the design of the review, participated in literature review and prepared the manuscript. AP participated in the preparation of illustrations and figures of the review, preparation of the manuscript and literature review. SR, GG and JK participated in preparation of the draft and manuscript review. RD and NP contributed to critical discussion of the draft, preparation of the draft and manuscript review. All authors read and approved the final manuscript.

Author details
[1]Department of Plastic and Hand Surgery, Burn Centre Medical Faculty, RWTH Aachen University Hospital, Pauwelsstr 30, Aachen 52074, Germany. [2]Department of Plastic and Reconstructive Surgery, azM University Hospital, Maastricht, Netherland. [3]Department of Operative Intensive Care, Medical Faculty, RWTH Aachen University, Aachen, Germany. [4]Department of Anaesthesia and Intensive Medicine, St. Elisabeth Hospital Geilenkirchen, Geilenkirchen, Germany.

References

1. Roth JJ, Hughes WB: In *The Essential Burn unit Handbook*. QMP Clinical Handbooks; 2004:P10–P121.
2. Guidelines for the Operations of Burn Units: *Resources for Optimal Care of the Injured Patient* Committee on Trauma, American College of Surgeons; 1999:55–62.
3. Silver GM, Freiburg C, Halerz M, Tojong J, Supple K, Gamelli RL: **A survey of airway and ventilator management strategies in North American pediatric burn units.** *J Burn Care Rehabil* 2004, **25**(5):435–440.
4. Patel BC: **Emergency eye care in the accident and emergency department.** *Arch Emerg Med* 1993, **10**(4):387–388.
5. Becker DG, Himel HN, Nicholson WD, Edlich RF: **Salvage of a patient with burn inhalation injury and pancreatitis.** *Burns* 1993, **19**(5):444–446.
6. O'Sullivan, Susan B, Schmitz, Thomas J: *Physical Rehabilitation*. 5th edition. Philadelphia: FA Davis Company; 2007:1098.
7. Hettiaratchy S, Papini R: **Initial management of a major burn: II–assessment and resuscitation.** *BMJ* 2004, **329**(7457):101–103.
8. Holm C, Mayr M, Tegeler J, *et al*: **A clinical randomized study on the effects of invasive monitoring on burn shock resuscitation.** *Burns* 2004, **30**(8):798–807.
9. Tricklebank S: **Modern trends in fluid therapy for burns.** *Burns* 2009.
10. Navar PD, Saffle JR, Warden GD: **Effect of inhalation injury on fluid resuscitation requirements after thermal injury.** *Am J Surg* 1985, **150** (6):716–720.
11. Darling GE, Keresteci MA, Ibanez D, Pugash RA, Peters WJ, Neligan PC: **Pulmonary complications in inhalation injuries with associated cutaneous burn.** *Journal of Trauma-Injury Infection & Critical Care* 1996, **40** (1):83–89.
12. Klein MB: **Overview of day 2: burn rehabilitation.** *J Burn Care Res* 2007, **28** (4):586.

13. Klein MB, Hayden D, Elson C, Nathens AB, Gamelli RL, Gibran NS, *et al*: **The association between fluid administration and outcome following major burn: A multicenterstudy.** *Ann Surg* 2007, **245**(4):622–628.
14. Molyneux Kate: **"Fluid Resuscitation in Burn Patients: Above and Beyond Baxter".** *School of Physician Assistant Studies* 2008:Paper 182.
15. Baxter CR, Shires T: **Physiological response to crystalloid resuscitation of severe burns.** *Ann NY Acad Sci* 1968, **150**(3):874–894.
16. Pham TN, Cancio LC, Gibran NS, American Burn A: **American burn association practice guidelines burn shock resuscitation.** *J Burn Care Res* 2008, **29**(1):257–266.
17. Pruitt BA Jr, Mason AD Jr, Moncrief JA: **Hemodynamic changes in the early postburn patient: the influence of fluid administration and of a vasodilator (hydralazine).** *J Trauma* 1971, **11**(1):36–46.
18. Perel P, Roberts I: **Colloids versus crystalloids for fluid resuscitation in critically ill patients.** *Cochrane Database Syst Rev* 2011, **Issue 3. Art. No:** CD000567. doi:10.1002/14651858.CD000567.pub4.
19. Liberati A, Moja L, Moschetti I, Gensini GF, Gusinu R: **Human albumin solution for resuscitation and volume expansion in critically ill patients.** *Intern Emerg Med* 2006, **1**(3):243–5.
20. **Burn Transfer Guidelines**. 2nd edition. NSW Severe Burn Injury Service; [http://www.health.nsw.gov.au/policies/gl/2008/pdf/GL2008_012.pdf]
21. Klein MB: **Thermal, chemical and electrical injuries**. In *Grabb and smith's Plastic surgery*. 6th edition. Edited by Thorne CH. New York: Lippincott Williams and Wilkins; 1997:132–149.
22. Tan WC, Lee ST, Lee CN, Wong S: **The role of fibreoptic bronchoscopy in the management of respiratory burns.** *Ann Acad Med Singapore* 1985, **14** (3):430–4.
23. Marek K, Piotr W, Stanisław S, Stefan G, Justyna G, Mariusz N, Andriessen A: **Fibreoptic bronchoscopy in routine clinical practice in confirming the diagnosis and treatment of inhalation burns.** *Burns* 2007, **33**(5):554–60. Epub 2007 Mar 21.
24. Alharbi Z, Grieb G, Pallua N: **Carbon Monoxide Intoxication in Burns**. In *Burns: Prevention, Causes and Treatment*. Edited by McLaughlin ES, Paterson AO. New York: Nova Science Publishers [in press].
25. Atiyeh BS, Dham R, Kadry M, *et al*: **Benefit-cost analysis of moist exposed burn ointment.** *Burns* 2002, **28**(7):659–663.
26. Alharbi Z, Grieb G, Pallua N: **Carbon Monoxide Intoxication in Burns.** In *Burns: Prevention, Causes and Treatment*. Edited by McLaughlin ES, Paterson AO. New York: Nova Science Publishers; 2012: 171-180.
27. Kahn SA, Beers RJ, Lentz CW: **Use of acellular dermal replacement in reconstruction of nonhealing lower extremity wounds.** *J Burn Care Res* 2011, **32**(1):124–8.
28. Haslik W, Kamolz L-P, Nathschläger G, Andel H, Meissl G, Frey M: **First experiences with the collagen-elastin matrix Matriderm as a dermal substitute in severe burn injuries of the hand.** *Burns* 2007, **33**(3):364–368.
29. Ryssel H, Gazyakan E, Germann G, Öhlbauer M: **The use of Matriderm in early excision and simultaneous autologous skin grafting in burns- A pilot study.** *Burns* 2008, **34**(1):93–97.
30. Elamin E, Miller A: **Impact of nebulized unfractionated heparin and *N*-acetylcysteine in management of smoke inhalation injury.** *Critical Care* 2009, **13**(Suppl 1):P438.
31. Kis E, Szegesdi I, Dobos E, Nagy E, Boda K, Kemény L, Horvath AR: **Quality assessment of clinical practice guidelines for adaptation in burn injury.** *Burns* 2010, **36**(5):606–15. Epub 2009 Dec 22.
32. Alsbjörn B, Gilbert P, Hartmann B, Kaźmierski M, Monstrey S, Palao R, Roberto MA, Van Trier A, Voinchet V: **Guidelines for the management of partial-thickness burns in a general hospital or community setting–recommendations of a European working party.** *Burns* 2007, **33**(2):155–60.
33. Karpelowsky J, Wallis L, Madaree A, Rode H: **South African burn society burn stabilisation protocol.** *South African Medical Journal* 2007, **97**(8):574–577.
34. Guidelines for the operations of Burns Centres, American Burn Association [http://www.ameriburn.org/Chapter14.pdf?PHPSESSID=dcf54e247df6fbfcb5dc61209913e773/]
35. Australian and New Zealand Burn Association [http://www.anzba.org.au/index.php?option=com_content&view=frontpage&Itemid=1/]
36. Stander M, Wallis LA: **The emergency management and treatment of severe burns.** *Emerg Med Int* 2011, **2011**:161375. Epub 2011 Sep 4.
37. Vogt PM, Busche MN: **Evaluation of infrastructure, equipment and training of 28 burn units/burn centers in Germany, Austria and Switzerland.** *Burns* 2011, **37**(2):257–64. Epub 2010 Nov 17.

2

One year experience of swine dermal non-crosslinked collagen prostheses for abdominal wall repairs in elective and emergency surgery

Giulia Montori[1*], Federico Coccolini[1], Roberto Manfredi[1], Marco Ceresoli[1], Luca Campanati[1], Stefano Magnone[1], Michele Pisano[1], Elia Poiasina[1], Gabriela Nita[1], Fausto Catena[2] and Luca Ansaloni[1]

Abstract

Introduction: The approach to the abdominal wall surgical repair is dramatically changed in the last years. This study evaluates our institutional outcomes about the usage of biological meshes for abdominal wall repair in different setting: in elective surgery, in emergency surgery and in abdominal wall repair following open abdomen (OA) procedure.

Methods: A database was prospectively conducted (January–December 2014) and data were reviewed for patients who underwent to an abdominal wall reconstruction with swine dermal non-cross linked collagens prostheses either in elective or emergency setting, and following OA/laparostomy procedure. Demographic data, co-morbidities, indications for surgery, intra-operative details, post-operative complications and outcome (peri-operative, 3, 6, 9-months) were analyzed.

Results: A total of 30 cases were reported: 9 in elective surgery (Group 1), 4 in emergency surgery (Group 2) and 17 with abdominal wall closure following OA management (Group 3). Two meshes were removed: 1 in the Group 1 and 1 in the Group 3. During follow-up only one patient in the Group 3 had a recurrence of the incisional hernia. Mortality rate was 11.1 % at 3 months in Group 1, 0 % in the Group 2, and 29.4 % in peri-operative period in the Group 3.

Conclusions: The use of non-cross linked biological meshes can be safe and versatile in different situations from elective to emergency surgery, and also for the reconstruction of the abdominal wall after OA procedure, with an acceptable recurrence and mortality rate.

Keywords: Biological mesh, Ventral hernia, Abdominal wall repair, Swine dermal collagen, Open abdomen, Laparostomy, Emergency surgery

Background

Abdominal wall hernia is one of the most common conditions encountered by general surgeons. Procedures to repair abdominal wall defects are more than 990.000 each year in USA, with an estimated 567.000 of them performed in emergency [1, 2]. Similar data are reported in other Western countries [3]. In most cases emergency hernia repair are performed in adults over 65 years old [2]. These age-related increasing rates of emergency hernia repair are associated with increased morbidity and mortality risks [2]. In these particular situations the use of biological materials can be safer than synthetic meshes [4]. Actually in the late 1990s, biologic materials for hernia repair were introduced as a possible biocompatible material to support "in vivo" tissue regeneration to restore the physiological function of the abdominal wall [4, 5]. Although these biomaterials enacted a new conceptual approach in abdominal wall reconstruction [5, 6], the main reported problems related with the use of biological meshes are: wound infections, seromas, fistula formation, recurrence of the defect (25–28 % in grade 3–4 of the Ventral Hernia Working Group (VHWG) classification [4]) and costs [7, 8]. Nevertheless definitive conclusions about the use of these biological

* Correspondence: giulia.montori@gmail.com
[1]Unit of General and Emergency Surgery, Papa Giovanni XXIII Hospital, P.zza OMS 1, 24128 Bergamo, Italy

materials are difficult to drawn due to: lack of adequate follow-up, use either of different surgical techniques and/or different types of biological meshes and absence of high levels of evidence studies [7, 8]. However there are many advantages in using biological meshes compared to the synthetic prostheses: less prosthetic erosions and/or fistulization, less chronic pain, and minor risk of infection [9].

Porcine dermal prostheses are manufactured by collagenic tissue harvesting, followed by a variety of patented chemical treatments and delipidation processes [10]. Although natural cross-links exist in native collagen and function to stabilize the structure of the collagenic proteins, giving mechanical strength and protection from collagenase [10], however some prostheses undergo to an additional phase chemical cross-linking process to increase the collagen strength [10]. The addition of chemical cross-linking between the collagen chains seems to further reduce the bacterial and host collagenase enzymes activity, slowing the degradation process of the prostheses. For this reason the indications report in literature suggest a use of cross-linked mesh in more contaminated field [11]. However some authors reports that porcine biologic non-cross-linked mesh has been used to support the repair of abdomen wall with a hernia recurrence rates of 7 % in case of underlay position, while in the cross-linked porcine mesh group infection and explantation rates were relatively higher [9]. These data indicate that there is currently no ideal biologic mesh for complex hernia repair and the candidate for biologic mesh implantation has not been clearly defined yet. A Randomized Control Trial (SIMBIOSE study: use of biological mesh versus standard wound care in infected incisional ventral hernias) is ongoing to evaluate the efficacy of biologic mesh in infected field [12].

This study evaluates our institutional outcomes about the usage of biological meshes for abdominal wall repair in three different setting: in elective surgery, in emergency surgery and following open abdomen (OA)/laparostomy procedure.

Methods

An analysis was performed on a prospectively maintained database from January 1st, 2014 to December 31st, 2014 of all patients who underwent primary or recurrent hernia repair with the usage of swine dermal collagens prostheses at Papa Giovanni XXIII Hospital (Bergamo, Italy). Enclosed patients were divided into 3 groups: abdominal wall reconstruction in elective surgery (Group 1), in emergency surgery (Group 2) and following OA/laparostomy management (Group 3). In all patients were used 1.4 mm thick, non-cross linked swine dermal collagen prostheses, with different dimensions (8*14, 10*20, 25*18, 20*30) (Protexa™, Tecnoss, Giaveno, Italy), fixed to the fascia with resorbable PDS 1 or 0. In case of elective surgery and in clean field the antibiotic prophylaxis used was Cefazolin 2 g, in the dirty and contaminated field the antibiotic theraphy was accord to the WSES guideline for the management of the intra-abdominal infection (IAI) [13]. Patients data were collected and analyzed evaluating demographic characteristics, co-morbidities, surgical indications, intra-operative details, complications (according to the Dindo-Clavien classification [14]) and outcome (peri-operative, at 3, 6, 9 months). Incisional hernia was classified according to the VHWG classification [4]. In case of septic implant, the peritonitis severity was evaluated according to the Mannheim Peritonitis Index (MPI) at the first laparotomy and at every subsequent abdominal exploration if indicated [15]. The severity of the trauma was calculated according to the Injury Severity Score (ISS) [16]. Balthazar score was used to evaluate the severity of pancreatitis [17]. The OA was classified according to the Björck classification [18].

Results

Thirty patients undergoing abdominal wall reconstruction with indication for biologic mesh placement and with swine dermal non-crosslinked collagen prostheses implant were enrolled in the study period. Of these patients, 9 were in Group 1 (Table 1), 4 in Group 2 (Table 2), and 17 in Group 3 (Table 3). According to the Hernia Grading System [4] 5 of the 30 patients presents a clean surgical site but high comorbidities, 21 patients have a contaminated field, and four patients have a dirty surgical site.

Demographics characteristics

In Group 1, nine patients were enrolled: four of them were female. The mean age was 68.3 years (range 53–83). In all patients the surgical indication was incisional hernia repair. The use of the biological mesh was imposed due to the co-morbidities of the patients (grade 2 VHWG classification) and due to the presence of a previous wound infection and/or gastrointestinal tract resection (grade 3 VHWG classification). In six patients one or more co-morbidities were present and listed as follows: immunodepression, a concomitant malignancy, abdominal aortic aneurism, diabetes, cardiopathy, bronchopneumopathy chronic obstructive. The others 3 patients have no comorbidity. However all these nine patients presented an intra-operative condition requiring the placement of a biological prosthesis: six patients underwent to colic anastomosis for colic resection, one patient had a prosthetic infection, and two patients had intra-abdominal infections (abscess from acute appendicitis and a ischemic small bowel).

In Group 2, four patients were enclosed (2 were female), with a mean age of 76.5 years (range 66–89). In this group the surgical indications were the following:

Table 1 Patients characteristics underwent to abdominal wall repair in elective surgery

Characteristics (*N* = 9)	Value	*N* (%)
Gender	Male	5 (55.6)
	Female	4 (44.4)
Age	Mean (SD), yrs	68.3 (±9.3)
	Median (range), yrs	68 (53–83)
Surgical indications	Incisional hernia	9 (100)
Comorbidities[a]	Immunodepression	4
	Abdominal aortic aneurism	1
	Diabetes	1
	Malignancy	3
	Cardiopathy	2
	BPCO	2
	None	3
Indications for the positioning of the prostheses	Colic anastomosis	6 (66.7)
	Previous prosthetic infection	1 (11.1)
	Intraabdominal infection	2 (22.2)
Prosthetic position	Onlay	0 (0)
	Inlay	0 (0)
	Retromuscolar	6 (66.7)
	Preperitoneal	0 (0)
	Intraperitoneal	3 (33.3)
Hospital stay	Mean (SD), dys	21 (±21)
	Median (range), dys	14 (7–70)
Mortality rates	At 1 month	0
	At 3 months	1 (11.1)
	At 6 months	0
	At 9 months	0

(*SD* standard deviation; *pts* patients, *yrs* years, *BPCO* bronchopneumopathy chronic obstructive)
[a]More than one patient has more than one comorbidity

Table 2 Patients characteristics underwent to abdominal wall repair in emergency surgery

Characteristics (*N* = 4)	Value	*N* (%)
Gender	Male	2 (50)
	Female	2 (50)
Age	Mean (SD), yrs	76.5 (±9.4)
	Median (range), yrs	75.5 (66–89)
Surgical indications	Complicated incisional hernia	1 (25)
	Diverticular perforation and incisional hernia	1 (25)
	Eventration and ileo anastomosis	1 (25)
	Recto-vaginal fistula and incisional hernia	1 (25)
Comorbidities[a]	Corticosteroid therapy	2
	Cardiovascular disease	2
	Inflammatory bowel disease	1
	Cerebrovascular disease	1
	None	2
Prothetic position	Onlay	1 (25)
	Inlay	1 (25)
	Retromuscolar	2 (50)
	Preperitoneal	0 (0)
	Intraperitoneal	0 (0)
Hospital stay	Mean (SD), dys	21.5 (±16.8)
	Median (range), dys	16.5 (7–45)
Mortality rates	At 1 month	0 (0)
	At 3 months	0 (0)
	At 6 months	0 (0)
	At 9 months	0 (0)

(*SD* standard deviation, *pts* patients, *dys* days, *yrs* years)
[a]More than one patient has more than one comorbidity

abdominal hernia complicated with an enterocutaneous fistula, a diverticular perforation with a large incisional hernia, an eventration complicating a previous surgery with a small bowel resection and anastomoses, and an incisional hernia with a recto-vaginal fistula in Crohn disease. Two patients presented more than one comorbidity: corticosteroid therapy, cardio-vascular disease, inflammatory bowel disease, and cerebrovascular disease. The other two patients had no previous diseases.

In Group 3, 17 patients were analyzed (9 patients were female). The mean age was 62.6 years (range 18–79). The main frequent comorbidities were: presence of cardiopathy and vasculopathy, the malignancy (gastric and colic cancer), and an immunosuppressed status. The others comorbidities present were the following: abdominal aortic aneurism, hemodialysis, and diabetes. Only three patients had no comorbidity. Seven patients (41.2 %) underwent to an OA procedure for intra-abdominal sepsis (anastomotic leak, appendicular peritonitis, biliary peritonitis), four patients (23.6 %) for intestinal ischemia, three patients (17.6 %) for trauma, two patients (11.8 %) after vascular surgery complications (duodenal perforation after exclusion of aortic aneurism), one patient (5.8 %) for severe acute pancreatitis. In 12 patients (70.6 %) the choice for the OA was to prevent the abdominal compartment syndrome; in 5 cases (29.4 %) the OA was performed to treat an increase of intra-abdominal pressure. In all patients the abdominal closure was planned at the first laparotomy and the decision of the biological prostheses usage was related to the intra-operative condition at the moment of the abdominal wall reconstruction. Eight patients (47 %) were from the Intensive Care Unit (ICU). For the three trauma patients the mean and median ISS were 38.3 (SD ± 14.3)

Table 3 Patients characteristics underwent to abdominal wall repair in open abdomen

Characteristics (*N* = 17)	Value	*N* (%)
Gender	Male	8 (47)
	Female	9 (53)
Age	Mean (SD), yrs	62.6 (±18.6)
	Median (range), yrs	72 (18–79)
Surgical indications to open abdomen	Intra-abdominal sepsis and/or post-operative complications	7 (41.2)
	Pancreatitis	1 (5.8)
	Trauma	3 (17.6)
	Vascular complications	2 (11.8)
	Intestinal ischemia	4 (23.6)
Comorbidities[a]	Corticosteroid therapy	2
	Cardiopathy and vasculopathy	9
	Malignancy	6
	Infectious diseases, immunodepression	5
	Abdominal aortic aneurism	4
	Hemodialisis	1
	Diabetes	1
	None	3
Provenience of the pts	ICU	8 (47)
	Ward	5 (29.5)
	Emergency department	4 (23.5)
ISS (*N* = 3)	ISS mean (SD)	38.3 (±14.3)
	ISS median (range)	35 (26–54)
Bathazar score (*N* = 1)	E	
MPI (*N* = 14)	MPI mean (SD)	26.6 (±8.8)
	MPI median (range)	26 (15–43)
	<21	4 (28.6)
	21–29	5 (35.7)
	>29	5 (35.7)
Bjorck classification at the first laparotomy	Ia	7 (41.4)
	Ib	4 (23.5)
	IIa	0 (0)
	IIb	6 (35.1)
	III	0 (0)
	IV	0 (0)
Bjorck classification at the closure	Ia	13 (76.6)
	Ib	0 (0)
	IIa	3 (17.6)
	IIb	0 (0)
	III	0 (0)
	IV	1 (5.8)
Causes of OA	Prevention of ACS	12 (70.6)
	Treatment of ACS	5 (29.4)
Type of OA	NPWT	16 (94.2)
	Skin closure	1 (5.8)
Closure abdominal wall	Mean (SD), dys	6.1 (±3.5)
	Median (range), dys	6 (1–15)
Stoma	Yes	4 (23.5)
	- colostomy	2 (50)
	- ileostomy	1 (25)
	- urostomy	1 (25)
	No	13 (76.5)
Intestinal anastomosis	Yes	11 (64.7)
	No	6 (35.3)
Enterocutaneous fistula	Yes	1 (5.8)
	No	16 (94.2)
Fascia closure	Yes	9 (53)
	No	8 (47)
Prothetic position	Onlay	2 (11.8)
	Inlay	1 (5.8)
	Retromuscolar	9 (52.8)
	Preperitoneal	0 (0)
	Intraperitoneal	5 (29.6)
Hospital stay	ICU	
	Mean (SD), dys	23.9 (±18.2)
	Median (range), dys	20 (2–71)
	Ward	
	Mean (SD), dys	28.4 (±21.2)
	Median (range), dys	23 (0–70)
Mortality rates	Peri-operative	5 (29.4)
	At 3 months	0 (0)
	At 6 months	0 (0)
	At 9 months	0 (0)

(*NPWT* negative pressure wound therapy, *pts* patients, *dys* days, *yrs* years, *SD* standard deviation, *ISS* Injury Severity Score, *MPI* Mannheim Peritoneal Index, *OA* Open Abdomen)
[a]More than one patient has more than one comorbidity

and 35 (range 26–54) respectively. For the patient with pancreatitis the Balthazar score before surgery was E.

Intraoperative details

In Group 1, the mesh was placed intra-peritoneally in three patients and in the retromuscolar plane in six patients.

In Group 2, the mesh was placed inlay (as a bridge between the medial edges) and onlay (in the subcutaneous space) in one patient each, and in the retromuscolar plane in two patients.

In Group 3, in 14 patients (the three trauma patients were excluded) the mean MPI was 26.6 (range 15–43). Four patients had a MPI < 21, five patients had a MPI between 21 to 29 and five patients had a MPI up to 29. According to the Björck score the majority of the patients (7 patients) had a grade Ia at the first laparotomy. Four patients had a grade Ib, and six patients had a grade IIb. At the closure, the rate of grade Björck Ia was in 13 patients (3 patients had a Björck IIa, and 1 patient a Björck IV). In 16 patients the OA was managed with a negative pressure wound therapy (NPWT) technique, and in 1 case the skin closure technique was performed. At the definitive intervention, the fascial closure was performed in nine patients (53 %), in the others eight patients only the posterior fascia was closed. In all 17 patients the abdominal wall was reinforced with a biological mesh: in nine patients the mesh was placed in the retromuscolar plane (sublay), in five patients intraperitoneally, in two patients onlay, and in 1 pt it was placed inlay. The time to definitive abdominal closure after OA was 6.1 days, with a range of 1–15. In four patients (25 %) a stoma was performed, meanwhile 11 patients (70.6 %) had an intestinal resection and anastomoses during the abdomen revision.

Outcome

In two patients the mesh was removed: in the first case (Group 1) because the patient was re-operated for an intestinal ischemia, in the other patient (Group 3) for a duodenal fistula. In the last case the patient was left open and the wound was treated with a Vacuum Assisted Therapy (VAC).

In Group 1 the mean hospital stay was 21 days (range 7–70). The follow up at 3-months was completed for 9 patients: 2 patients has a grade I complication (wound infection), 1 patient had a grade IVb (re-operated for a small bowel ischemia), 1 patient died for a septic shock in a leucopenia, 4 patients were free from complications. One patient was lost at the follow-up. Four patients completed the follow-up at 6 months: 3 patients were free from complications, one patient died for a septic shock in leucopenia for the important lymphoproliferative disorder associated with recent chemotherapy regimen. One patient was lost at the follow-up. No patients completed the 9-months follow-up. One patient (11.1 %) died (septic shock in leucopenia).

In Group 2 the mean hospital stay was 21.5 days (range 7–45). One patient presented a grade I complication (wound infections), one patient presented a grade II complication (wound dehiscence) requires a vacuum-assisted closure technique. Two patients had no complications. One patient was lost to follow-up. The overall mortality was 0 %.

In the Group 3 the mean and median ICU stay was 23.9 days (range 2–71), and the mean ward stay was 28.4 days (range 0–70). In peri-operative time: 4 patients presented a grade I complication (wound infection), 1 patient presented a IIIb complications (a duodenal fistula due to a dehiscence of the duodenal perforation that required another surgical intervention and a VAC therapy to manage the fistula) and the patient is still hospitalized. Seven patients were free from complications. Five patients died (2 for aortic rupture, 2 for septic shock, and 1 for respiratory insufficiency and septic shock). Twelve patients completed the follow-up at 3 months: 1 patient presented a Grade II complication (incisional hernia non complicated), 1 patient require the pursuit of the VAC therapy to manage the duodenal fistula. Seven patients are free of complications. Three patients were lost to follow-up. No patients died at 3 months follow-up. Six patients completed the follow-up at 6 months: 1 patient presented a Grade II complication (incisional hernia non complicated). Two patients were healthy. Three patients were lost to follow-up. No patients died at 6 months follow-up. Two patients completed the follow-up at 9 months: 1 patient had no complications. One patient was lost to follow-up. No patients died at 9 months follow-up. The overall peri-operative mortality was 29.4 % (5 patients).

Discussion

Incisional hernia remains a common complication in abdominal surgery and occurs after elective laparotomy with an incidence from 2 to 20 % or more [7, 19, 20]. However, these rates can increase (as high as 50 %) after abdominal closure in emergency surgery and in the abdominal repair following OA procedure [21–23]. The approach to the abdominal wall surgical repair is dramatically changed in the last years due to the availability of new repair materials, like biologic prostheses. Although in last years many studies tried to find an agreement about specific technique and materials that should be applied to repair of complex ventral hernia, at present, no strong consensus has been found yet [4, 24]. However the use of biologic prostheses is actually accepted by the medical community for addressing abdominal wall defects, particularly in contaminated and potentially contaminated fields [11, 25]. Despite this, the numerous advantages of biologic materials have been proven [11, 26, 27].

The present study reports a one-year experience about the usage of biological prostheses in different fields from elective surgery to emergency surgery and OA procedure. We analyze our surgical indications to the usage of biological meshes to evaluate the outcomes and the feasibility in these fields.

In the first group we considered only the patients underwent to ventral hernia repair in elective surgery. In all patients the abdominal wall defect was associated with high risk of contamination or an already existing infection imposed the positioning of a biological prostheses.

The decision of the positioning of the prosthesis was based on the VHWG and the Italian Biological Prostheses work-group recommendations [4, 11], according to the degree of contamination potential or effective, and according to co-morbidities of the patient. In literature also others studies confirmed and supported these recommendations [7, 28, 29]. In our study, more than half of the patients of this group had more than one comorbidity (in particular immunosuppression and malignancy), that associated with a local wound infection or intra-abdominal infection have prevented the use of a synthetic mesh. In two third of patients the mesh was placed in the retromuscolar space, in line with the literature [9, 30]. The "sublay" position (posterior to the rectus muscle) has been the most used, in fact it allows for better tissue incorporation and lower chance of bacterial contamination, increases neo-angiogenesis and avoids the direct contact with intra-abdominal viscera [1, 9]. In this group only one patient died at three months for a septic shock, and in one case we had to remove the mesh because the patient was re-operated for an intestinal ischemia.

At the analysis of the second group (patients underwent to ventral hernia repair in emergency conditions) we found that the presence of wound infection or intra-abdominal infection are the main indication requiring a biological mesh positioning. This decision was also dictated by the important comorbidities present in half of patients. The other important point has been the age of patients (older than patients in others group, with a median age of 75.5 years). In last year the number of elderly patients (>65 years) underwent to ventral hernia repair in emergency setting is increasing [2]. A recent study reports that the risk of operative factors associated with the risk of surgical site infection were open procedures, incisional/ventral repairs, and hernia repairs with bowel obstruction/necrosis [2]. Into account of these data and according to the VHWG recommendations [4] we decided to repair the abdominal wall defect with a biological mesh, with favorable outcomes and with an acceptable hospital stay (median 16.5 days).

The third group was the largest group. The problem of abdomen closure after OA procedure remains the most critical point for these patients [21–23]. Data about long-terms outcome after repair of abdominal wall in OA procedure are still lacking and the durability of the different biologic meshes has not been clinically proved [26, 31]. Our surgical indications for an OA procedure requiring a biological prostheses positioning were the difficulty to close the abdominal wall (the anterior and the posterior fascia) or to reinforce the closure of the posterior fascia (when the anterior fascia was impossible to close). The main causes for a laparostomy were secondary peritonitis, intestinal ischemia and trauma. The conditions that required leaving the abdomen open remains the abdominal compartment syndrome (ACS) or the conditions that promote an intra-abdominal hypertension (IAH) (intestinal ischemia, acute severe pancreatitis, vascular complications), or in case of damage control surgery (trauma) [13, 26, 32–34]. Recently the approach to the intra-abdominal sepsis was changed and leaving the abdomen open in that condition has been proven to reduce mortality and post-operative complications [31, 35]. The primary goal remains the source control and a temporary abdominal closure was considered a valid instrument to manage severe abdominal sepsis [35]. In our series the traumatized patients undergone to OA had severe trauma (ISS > 25). In the two-third of cases we have proceed to OA management to prevent an ACS; in only one-third OA procedure was considered as treatment of the IAH or of the ACS. In patients with intra-abdominal sepsis the scoring system to estimate the severity and prognosis of secondary peritonitis we used was the MPI [15]. Literature reports that a MPI greater that 29 relates with high mortality rates (100 % vs 0–2.3 % in patients with MPI < 21) [15]. In our series one–third of patients have severe peritonitis (MPI > of 29), and these MPI values associated with the important comorbidities may be the responsible for the high peri-operative mortality rate (29.4 % at our analysis). In the present series the status of the OA has been evaluated at the first laparotomy and at the last one according to the Björck classification [18]. Data reported an increased number of patients presenting a Grade 1A (clean OA without adherence between bowel and abdominal wall or fixity) at the abdomen closure (from 41.4 %, at the first laparotomy, to 76.6 %, at the last laparotomy). These results showed the efficacy of the OA treatment in reducing the intra-abdominal contamination. Regarding to the technique used for temporary abdominal closure we used the NPWT in almost all cases. This strategy seems to be the best in preventing evisceration, actively remove any infected or toxic fluid from the peritoneal cavity, prevent the formation of entero-atmospheric fistulas, preserve the fascia and the abdominal wall domain, make reoperation easy and safe, and achieve early definitive closure [23, 26, 36]. Our goals were to close the abdomen wall as soon as possible (within 5–7 days) [26, 27, 37] to reduce the OA complications. A recent prospective controlled trial and a systematic review suggested that use of a dynamic fascial sutures combined with NPWT in the treatment of OA for intra-abdominal sepsis is safe and associated to a low rate of incisional hernias and entero-atmospheric fistula [22, 23]. However in our series almost all patients despite the NPWT alone, the closure of the abdominal wall happened in an average of 6.1 days, but in 53 % of cases the fascia was closed with a mesh in the retromuscolar space [9, 30]. The main complications after OA remain the enterocutenaous fistula and the long-term ventral hernia, in addition to the high rate of morbidity and mortality associated with the procedure [8, 26, 38]. A recent meta-analysis about OA and temporary abdominal closure techniques in non-trauma patients (4358 patients) reported a mortality rate near to 30 %, with an overall rate of fistula of 12.1 %, with a 14.6 % in series applying NPWT without fascial traction, and of 5.7 % after NPTW with fascial traction [38]. Others studies reported a high delayed facial closure rate ranging from 34 % and 73.6 % in septic patients, with lower rates in trauma patients due to the more frequent early abdominal closure [23]. In our study only one patient had a duodenal fistula and required the removal of the prostheses (being managed with a VAC therapy to control the spillage of duodenal contents [38]) and only one patient presented an incisional hernia without complications. These low rates of incisional hernia are probably due to the lack of a long-term follow-up. The other complications in present study were related wound infection or dehiscence that were managed with local wound dressing. Also in our data the rate of perioperative mortality remains high (29.4 %), similar with the data find in the literature (30 %), however this is probably due to the extremely compromised conditions of the patients and the paucity of cases [2, 38].

Despite the limitations present study showed that the use of non-cross-linked porcine dermal meshes in different surgical setting, particularly in elderly and septic patients is safe and effective, without worsening morbidity and mortality.

Conclusions

The present one-year prospective analysis shows that the use of swine dermal non cross-linked collagen prostheses for abdominal wall repair is safe and effective in general and emergency surgery, particularly in elderly and in immune-compromised patients. However more data are necessary. For this reason the development of big prospective studies are mandatory.

Competing interest
The authors declare that they have no competing interests.

Authors' contributions
GM and FeCo collected data and wrote the manuscript. LA did the statistical analysis and reviewed the manuscript. All authors read and approved the final manuscript.

Author details
[1]Unit of General and Emergency Surgery, Papa Giovanni XXIII Hospital, P.zza OMS 1, 24128 Bergamo, Italy. [2]General surgery department, Ospedale Maggiore, Parma, Italy.

References

1. Coccolini F, Poiasina E, Bertoli P, Gossetti F, Agresta F, Dassatti MR, et al. The Italian register of biological prostheses. Eur Surg Res. 2013;50(3–4):262–72.
2. Beadles CA, Meagher AD, Charles AG. Trends in emergent hernia repair in the United States. JAMA Surg. 2015;150:194–200.
3. Ansaloni L, Coccolini F, Fortuna D, Catena F, Di Saverio S, Belotti LM, et al. Assessment of 126,913 inguinal hernia repairs in the Emilia-Romagna region of Italy: analysis of 10 years. Hernia. 2014;18(2):261–7.
4. Ventral Hernia Working Group, Breuing K, Butler CE, Ferzoco S, Franz M, Hultman CS, et al. Incisional ventral hernias: review of the literature and recommendations regarding the grading and the technique of repair. Surgery. 2010;148(3):544.
5. Coccolini F, Catena F, Catena F, Poiasina E, Poletti E, Ansaloni L. Biomaterials in abdominal wall surgery: change your mind! Ann Surg. 2014; [Epub ahead of print].
6. Sipe JD. Tissue engineering and reparative medicine. Ann NY Acad Sci. 2002;961:1–9.
7. Kissane NA, Itani KMF. A decade of ventral incisional hernia repairs with biologic acellular dermal matrix: what have we learned? PRSJ. 2012;130;5S-2:194S–2.
8. Peralta R, Latifi R. Long-Term outcomes of abdominal wall reconstruction. What are the real numbers? World J Surg. 2012;36:534–8.
9. Diaz Jr JJ, Cullinane DC, Khwaja KA, Tyson GH, Ott M, Jerome R, et al. Eastern Association for the Surgery of Trauma: management of the open abdomen, part III-review of abdominal wall reconstruction. J Trauma Acute Care Surg. 2013;75(3):376–86.
10. Smart NJ, Bryan N, Hunt JA, Daniels IR. Porcine dermis implants in soft-tissue reconstruction: current status. Biologics Target and Therapy. 2014;8:83–90.
11. Coccolini F, Agresta F, Bassi A, Catena F, Crovella F, Ferrara R, et al. Italian Biological Prosthesis Work-Group (IBPWG): proposal for a decisional model in using biological prosthesis. World J Emerg Surg. 2012;7(1):34.
12. Biological Meshes in Infected Fields: a Randomized Controlled Trial (SIMBIOSE). https://clinicaltrials.gov/ct2/show/NCT01594450.
13. Sartelli M, Viale P, Catena F, Ansaloni L, Moore E, Malangoni M, et al. 2013 WSES guidelines for management of intra-abdominal infections. World J Emerg Surg. 2013;8(1):3.
14. Dindo D, Demartines N, Clavien PA. Classification of surgical complications: a new proposal with evaluation in a cohort of 6336 patients and results of a survey. Ann Surg. 2004;240(2):205–13.
15. Mishra SP, Tiwary SK, Mishra M, Gupta SK. An introduction of tertiary peritonitis. J Emerg Trauma Shock. 2014;7(2):121–3.
16. Baker SP, O'Neill B, Haddon Jr W, Long WB. The injury severity score: a method for describing patients with multiple injuries and evaluating emergency care. J Trauma. 1974;14(3):187–96.
17. Chatzicostas C, Roussomoustakaki M, Vardas E, Romanos J, Kouroumalis EA. Balthazar computed tomography severity index is superior to Ranson criteria and APACHE II and III scoring systems in predicting acute pancreatitis outcome. J Clin Gastroenterol. 2003;36(3):253–60.
18. Björck M, Bruhin A, Cheatham M, Hinck D, Kaplan M, Manca G, et al. Classification–important step to improve management of patients with an open abdomen. World J Surg. 2009;33(6):1154–7.
19. Le Huu NR, Mege D, Ouaïssi M, Sielezneff I, Sastre B. Incidence and prevention of ventral incisional hernia. J Visc Surg. 2012;149:e3–14.
20. Sbitany H, Know E, Chern H, Finlayson E, Varma MG, Hansen SL. Outcomes analysis of biological mesh use for abdominal wall reconstruction in clean-contaminated and contaminated ventral hernia repair. Ann Pl Surg. 2013; [Epub ahead of print].
21. Kaoutzanis C, Lichtle SW, Mouawad NJ, Welch KB, Lampman RM, Wahl WL, et al. Risk factors for postoperative wound infections and prolonged hospitalization after ventral/incisional hernia repair. Hernia. 2013;19(1):113–23.
22. Fortelny RH, Hofmann A, Gruber-Blum S, Petter-Puchner AH, Glaser KS. Delayed closure of open abdomen in septic patients is facilitated by combined negative pressure wound therapy and dynamic fascial suture. Surg Endosc. 2014;28(3):735–40.
23. Atema JJ, Gans SL, Boermeester MA. Systematic review and meta-analysis of the open abdomen and temporary abdominal closure techniques in Non-trauma patients. World J Surg. 2015;39(4):912–25.
24. Latifi R, Leppaniemi A. Compelx andominal wall defects and enterocutaneous fistulae in the era of biological mesh: did we make any real progress? World J Surg. 2012;36:495–6.

25. Lee L, Mata J, Landry T, Khwaja KA, Vassiliou MC, Fried GM, et al. A systematic review of synthetic and biologic materials for abdominal wall reinforcement in contaminated fields. Surg Endosc. 2014;28:2531–46.
26. Demetriades D, Salim A. Management of the open abdomen. Surg Clin North Am. 2014;94(1):131–53.
27. Godat L, Kobayashi L, Costantini T, Coimbra R. Abdominal damage control surgery and reconstruction: world society of emergency surgery position paper. World J Emerg Surg. 2013;8(1):53.
28. Nieuwenhuizen J, Eker HH, Timmermans L, Hop WC, Kleinrensink GJ, Jeekel J, et al. A double blind randomized controlled trial comparing primary closure with mesh augmentes closure to reduce incisional hernia incidence. BMC Surg. 2013;13:48.
29. Butler CE, Baumann DP, Janis JE, Rosen MJ. Abdominal wall reconstruction. Curr Probl Surg. 2013;50:557–86.
30. Muysoms F, Campanelli G, Champault GG, DeBeaux AC, Dietz UA, Jeekel J, et al. EuraHS: the development of an international online platform for registration and outcome measurement of ventral abdominal wall hernia repair. Hernia. 2012;16(3):239–50.
31. Regner JL, Kobayashi L, Coimbra R. Surgical strategies for management of open abdomen. World J Surg. 2012;36:497–510.
32. Kirkpatrick AW, Roberts DJ, De Waele J, Jaeschke R, Malbrain ML, De Keulenaer B, et al. Intra-abdominal hypertension and the abdominal compartment syndrome: updated consensus definitions and clinical practice guidelines from the World Society of the Abdominal Compartment Syndrome. Intensive Care Med. 2013;39(7):1190–206.
33. Sartelli M, Catena F, Ansaloni L, Coccolini F, Corbella D, Moore EE, et al. Complicated intra-abdominal infections worldwide: the definitive data of the CIAOW Study. World J Emerg Surg. 2014;9:37.
34. Navsaria P, Nicol A, Hudson D, Cockwill J, Smith J. Negative pressure wound therapy management of the "open abdomen" following trauma: a prospective study and systematic review. World J Emerg Surg. 2013;8(1):4.
35. Dutton WD, Diaz JJ, Miller RS. Critical care issues in managing complex open abdominal wound. J Int Care Med. 2012;27(3):161–71.
36. Olona C, Caro A, Duque E, Moreno F, Vadillo J, Rueda JC, et al. Comparative study of open abdomen treatment: ABThera™ vs. abdominal dressing™. Hernia. 2015;19(2):323–8.
37. Sugrue M, D'Amours SK, Kolkman KA. Temporary abdominal closure. Acta Clin Belg. 2007;62 Suppl 1:210–4.
38. Demetriades D. Total management of the open abdomen. Int Wound J. 2012;9 Suppl 1:17–24.

3

Quality of life and long-term outcomes of octo- and nonagenarians following acute care surgery

Sayf Gazala[1], Yvonne Tul[1], Adrian Wagg[2], Sandy L Widder[1], Rachel G Khadaroo[1*] on behalf of the Acute Care and Emergency Surgery (ACES) Group

Abstract

Background: While advanced age is often associated with poorer surgical outcomes, long-term age-related health status following acute care surgery is unknown. The objective of our study was to assess post-operative cognitive impairment, functional status, and quality of life in elderly patients who underwent emergency surgery.

Methods: We identified 159 octo- and nonagenarians who underwent emergency surgery between 2008 and 2010 at a single tertiary hospital. Patients were grouped into three cohorts: 1, 2, and 3 years post-operative. We conducted a survey in 2011, with octo- and nonagenarians regarding the impact of emergency surgical procedures. Consenting participants responded to four survey questionnaires: (1) Abbreviated Mental Test Score-4, (2) Barthel Index, (3) Vulnerable Elders Survey, and (4) EuroQol-5 Dimensional Scale.

Results: Of the 159 octo- and nonagenarians, 88 (55.3%) patients were alive at the time of survey conduction, and 55 (62.5%) of the surviving patients consented to participate. At 1, 2, and 3 years post-surgery, mortality rates were 38.5%, 44.7%, and 50.0%, respectively. More patients had cognitive impairments at 3 years (33.3%) than at 1 (9.5%) and 2 years (9.1%) post-operatively. No statistical difference in the ability to carry out activities of daily living or functional decline with increasing time post-operatively. However, patients perceived a significant health decline with the greater time that passed following surgery.

Conclusions: Our study showed that half of the patients over the age of 80 are surviving up to 3 years post-operatively. While post-operative functional status appears to be stable across the 3 cohorts of patients, perceived health status declines over time. Understanding the long-term post-operative impact on cognitive impairment, functional status, and quality of life in elderly patients who undergo acute care surgery allows health care professionals to predict their patients' likely post-operative needs.

Keywords: Elderly, Emergency Surgery, Health Outcomes

Background

By 2040, 1 in 4 American and Canadians will be over age 65, nearly double today's senior population, with about 19 millions over the age of 85 years in the United States [1-3]. In the developed regions of the world life expectancy is projected to increase and reach on average about 80 years [4]. These older patients are presenting for surgical evaluation of acute illness in increasing numbers [5]. Acute diseases requiring emergency surgical intervention are more risky than elective procedures given individuals' age, comorbidities, as well as their acute physiological changes [6]. Many of these elderly patients therefore present unique medical challenges, often with a significant burden of pre-existing illness, poly-pharmacy, frailty, as well as limited social support. Acute surgical services, designed to address acute problems with rapid diagnosis and turnover, may fail older people who require longer-term support, restorative care and follow-up, even from so-called "minor" surgical procedures.

* Correspondence: khadaroo@ualberta.ca
[1]Department of Surgery, University of Alberta, 2D WMC, 8440-112 St NW, Edmonton, AB, Canada T6G 2B7

Assessment of function and frailty in the elderly is gaining popularity as a predictor of outcomes in older patients undergoing surgery [7,8]. Functional capacity indicates a person's ability to carry out everyday tasks [9]. It provides a measure of independence, which is of particular concern to seniors' health related quality of life (HRQOL). Functional capacity takes into account both basic activities of daily living (ADLs) – eating, bathing, dressing, toileting, walking – and instrumental activities of daily living (IADLs) – shopping, banking, housekeeping [10]. Unfortunately, it is not always possible to perform a comprehensive pre-surgical assessment in the emergency setting. Frail elderly patients are often associated with poorer surgical outcomes and increased morbidity (surgical site infections, end organ dysfunction, anastomosis leakage, and sepsis), post-operative delirium and in-hospital falls [11,12], however long term age-related health status following acute care surgery (ACS) is unknown. To date there has been limited published reports of post-operative outcomes following ACS in older patients. We conducted a cross sectional study in an older cohort to provide quantitative data regarding the long-term impact of emergency procedures. We wanted to assess the presence of cognitive impairment; functional status, frailty and health related quality of life in elderly patients who underwent ACS.

Methods

We retrospectively identified 159 octo- and nonagenarians who underwent emergency surgeries between 2008 and 2010 under a specialized emergency service at a single tertiary center (University of Alberta Hospital's Acute Care Emergency Surgery (ACES) service, Edmonton, Alberta). The service is unique in that there is a fully functional theatre and team dedicated to emergency general surgery cases exclusively during day time hours, in addition to the emergency after hours. Older patients (≥65) comprise a significant proportion of those admitted to our ACES service with up to one third of these patients being greater than the age of 80 and account for 25% of annual operations. Typical surgical procedures include: colonic surgery- resection and diversion (23%), small bowel surgery- adhesions and resection (20%), exploratory and trauma laparotomy (16%). cholecystectomy (10%), Hernia surgery- incarceration and strangulation (9%), duodenal ulcer surgery-bleeding and perforation (5%), and other less commonly performed procedures (17%)

A cross sectional study design was implemented based on the year the surgical procedure was performed. Patients were then grouped into three groups based on the duration since the surgery: *Group 1* included patients who had an emergency procedure in 2010 and were contacted 1 year post-op; *Group 2* included patients who had an emergency procedure in 2009 and were contacted 2 years post-op; *Group 3* included patients who had an emergency procedure in 2008 and were contacted 3 years post-op.

After identifying those patients who are still alive, the three cohorts of patients were contacted by telephone to conduct the survey (up to three attempts). Follow-up calls were completed between November 2011 and January 2012. Participants who were hard-of-hearing were mailed surveys and asked to return them in pre-paid envelopes. In some instances, a surrogate (spouse or relative) was used if the patient was unable to respond (demented or no English).

Consented participants, or their surrogates, responded to the following four survey questionnaires: (1) Abbreviated Mental Test Score-4 (AMTS-4), a brief 4-item survey that screens for cognitive impairment. Patients are considered cognitively impaired if they fail to answer any of the four questions [13]. (2) Barthel Index, a 10-item questionnaire with three levels of answers, which assesses the level of independence with activities of daily living [14,15]. (3) Vulnerable Elders Survey (VES-13), is a 13-item questionnaire that measures frailty in older persons. It has a maximum score of 10 (high score indicates worse health state). The VES-13 has been validated in elderly patients to predict death and decline in function [6,16,17]. (4) EuroQol-5 Dimensional Scale (EQ-5D), a health utility measure that has five questions with three levels of answers for each question, and can yield a health state between 0 and 1 (where 0 is death and 1 is the best health state a person can have). The EQ-5D is a valid and reliable tool for the measurement of health related quality of life [18]. The four questionnaires have been used and are reliable in this patient population group. The results will give a clear indication on cognitive function, independence, activity of daily living, and health related quality of life in general. In addition, participants were asked whether they currently live alone, and whether their place of residence had changed since the time of their surgery.

The study received ethical committee approval from the HREB at the University of Alberta. STATA data analysis and statistical software, version 12, was used for the statistical analysis. ANOVA was used to assess the difference between the three groups for each of the questionnaires. A p value of <0.05 was used to assign statistical significance for comparisons.

Results

A total of 159 octo- and nonagenarians were operated on under the ACES service during the study period (approximately 7% of the total volume). 88 (55.3%) patients were alive at the time of follow-up. For those patients contacted at 1 year following surgery (group 1) (N=52), there was a 38.5% mortality rate. At 2 years post-surgery, group 2, (N=47), there was a 44.7% mortality rate, and at 3 years

Table 1 The three cohorts included in the analysis

	No. death (%)	No. alive (%)	No. included (%)	No. excluded (%)	Reasons for exclusion
Group 1	20 (38.5)	32 (61.5)	23 (71.9%)	9 (28.1)	-Loss to follow up
					-Dementia
					-Refusal
Group 2	21 (44.7)	26 (55.3)	16 (61.5)	10 (38.5)	-Loss to follow up
					-Dementia
					-Refusal
Group 3	30 (50)	30 (50)	16 (53.3)	14 (46.7)	-Loss to follow up
					-Dementia
					-No English
					-Refusal

post-surgery, group 3, (N=60), there was a 50.0% mortality rate. Fifty-seven (64.8%) of the surviving patients consented to participate in the follow-up survey, 23 (71.9%) from Group 1, and 16 (61.3%) from Group 2 and 16 (53.3%) from Group 3 (Table 1). Fifteen were excluded because of dementia and/or institutionalization, refusal to participate, or an inability to speak English and lack of access to an interpreter. Seven were lost to follow up.

Demographics and geographical location

In Group 1, there were 7 females (mean age 83.4, SD 1.7) and 9 males (mean age 81.3, SD 1.2). More than half of the respondents (60.9%) were living with someone, usually a spouse or a family member. In Group 2, there were 8 females (mean age 83.1, SD 2.6) and 8 males (mean age 83.2, SD 3.1). Less than half of the respondents (43.8%) were living with someone. In Group 3, there were 13 females (mean age 83.4, SD 2.7) and 10 males (mean age 83.4, SD 2.3). Half of them were living with someone. Demographic characteristics of the groups are shown in Table 2.

Table 2 Demographic characteristics of the three groups

	Sex (M:F)	Age (mean, (SD))	Living alone (%)
Group 1	Male 9	81.3 (1.2)	(60.9)
	Female 7	83.4 (1.7)	
Group 2	Male 8	83.2 (3.1)	(43.8)
	Female 8	83.1 (2.6)	
Group 3	Male 10	83.4 (2.3)	(50.0)
	Female 13	83.4 (2.7)	

Cognitive status

Data from the abbreviated mental test score-4 (AMTS-4) indicate that more patients had cognitive impairments at 3 years (33.3%) than at 1 (9.5%) and 2 years (9.1%) following ACS (See Figure 1). There is a statistically significant difference between the proportion of those with cognitive impairment at 3 years post-operatively and that at 1 and 2 years after surgery (p value =0.05). We found no statistically significant difference comparing the proportion of men and women with cognitive impairment combining the three groups, Odds Ratio of 1.3 (p = 0.18).

Functional status

There was no statistical difference among the three groups in their ability to carry out activities of daily living or functional decline post-operatively. There were no statistically significant differences in functional status between females and males comparing either the Barthel Index score or the VES-13 over the three years following ACS.

Health related quality of life

The mean (SD) EQ-5D for the three groups was 0.83 (0.2) for Group 1, 0.77 (0.17) for Group 2, and 0.82 (0.2) for Group 3. There was no statistical significance between scores in the three groups. Figure 2 describes the patients who reported problems with each of the five dimensions of the EQ-5D (moderate and severe problems). Perceived health state of the patients from the visual analogue scale (VAS) of the EQ-5D, was higher in patients who had more recent surgery (Group 1) than the other groups, but the difference was not statistically significant (See Figure 3).

Discussion

Investigating ways to optimize health care for elders is important to maximize quality of life and reduce the burden of comorbid disease, functional and cognitive impairment on society. In the next 35 years, 1 in 4 North Americans and Europeans will be over the age of 65 years. These changing demographics need to alter the way we think

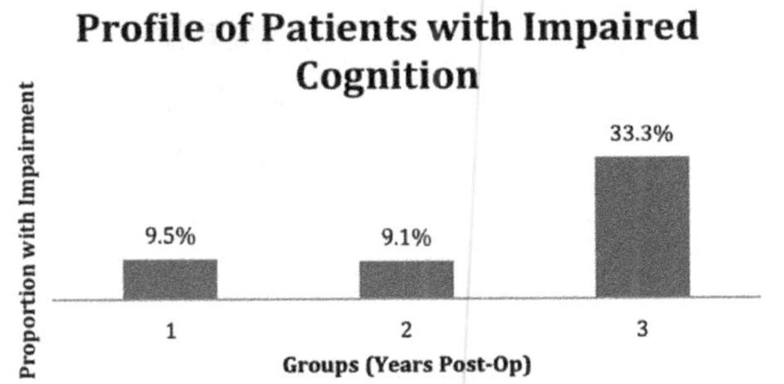

Figure 1 Using the AMTS-4, a score between 0–3 indicates impaired cognition; a score of 4 indicates normal cognition.

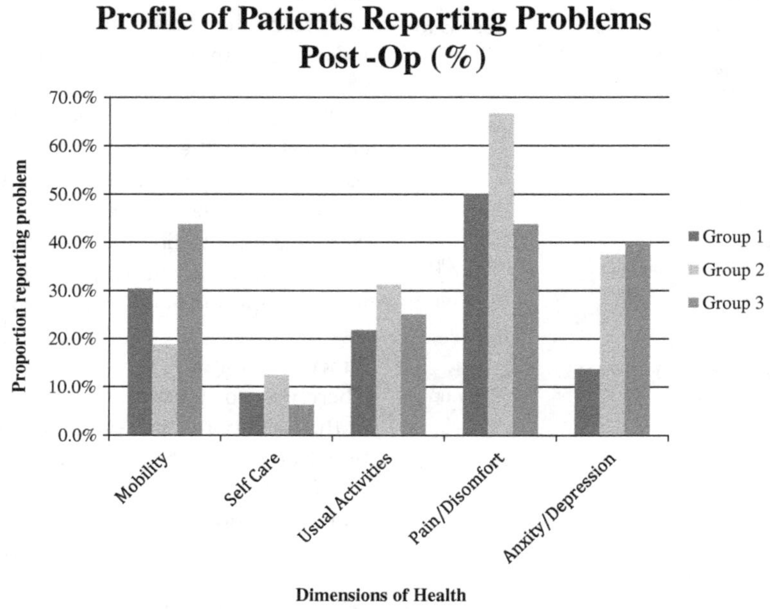

Figure 2 **Quality of Life as measured by the EQ-5D questionnaire for the three groups.**

about and how we deliver healthcare. There are an increasing proportion of elderly patients presenting to our acute care hospitals who often also have multiple comorbidities; unfortunately most current models of health care delivery do not take into account the aforementioned. In order to provide health care specific to the elderly, accurate data on outcomes from acute emergency surgical interventions is needed. There has to date been limited attempts to measure change in the quality of life of the elderly following surgery and few reports that considers return to home and normal function following acute surgical intervention [19,20]. These factors are probably the most important to consider in this group. How early patients return home, their level of physical and cognitive function, the amount of support they need and their discharge destination are of critical importance to healthcare planners who need to allocate resources in a political and social environment where expectations are high and where costs and resource limitations need to be taken into consideration.

Results from our mid-term follow-up revealed that greater than half of patients greater than 80 years who underwent emergency surgery survived up to 3 years post-operatively. Post-operative functional status appeared to be stable across the 3 cohorts of patients, regardless of time of assessment post surgery. This evidence supports that good surgical outcomes is possible even in the elderly, and that much more

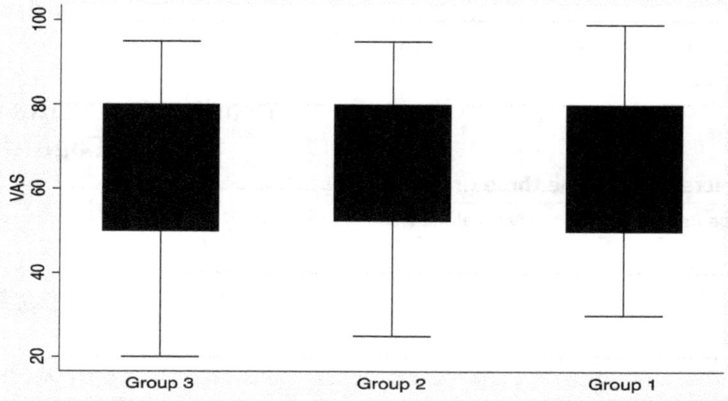

Figure 3 **EQ-5D Visual Analogue Scale comparing the three cohorts.**

must be considered than simply age alone. Although there was a cognitive decline at 3 years post-operatively compared to 1 and 2 years following surgery, this difference was not statistically significant.

Overall, there was moderate variability in the reported limitations in functional capacity of our sample of elderly patients, underlining the diversity of this acute care population. With age, losses in functional capacity become more common and are increasingly severe. Most people with a limitation in functional capacity, when younger than 85 years, report only mild limitations. However, 25% of seniors 85 years and over report a moderate (15%), severe (5%), or total (5%) limitation in functional capacity [1]. Our sample reported no decline in their HRQOL following surgery but also had a significantly better HRQOL compared to the general elderly population of Alberta (greater than75 years), this most likely can be explained by multiple factors. One of the most important being, patients with better HRQOL are more likely to undergo an emergency surgical intervention when compared to those with lower HRQOL at baseline. Additionally, patients with better HRQOL are more likely to respond to our study surveys.

There are several limitations to this study including the retrospective nature of the study that will limit the data available for analysis, the presence of selection and survivor biases. As well, we specifically only examined the outcomes of those elderly patients who had a surgical intervention. We did not include those patients with acute surgical conditions who were treated conservatively. Other factors such as socioeconomic status, type of residence (rural vs. urban), and professional background might have a confounding effect on the results of this analysis and were not accounted for in this analysis.

Our study also was not designed to measure pre- to post-acute care changes in cognitive impairment, functional status, or quality of life. Rather, the intent was to get a "snapshot" of how elderly patients fare after surgery and assess the feasibility of collecting data from this elderly, more vulnerable group. For this reason, it is not possible to assess what impact ACS might have had on our patients' level of independence and quality of life. We are currently undertaking a prospective study, which addresses these limitations in order to provide greater insight on the effects of ACS on this elderly population.

Conclusion

Our research demonstrates that acute care surgery patients over 80 years of age had a greater than fifty percent survival rate at 3 years post-operatively, and of those elderly patients who survived had a stable health related quality of life and functional status. Understanding the characteristics of the geriatric acute care surgery population allow health care professionals to deliver more effective services to older patients.

Competing interests
The authors declare that they have no competing interests.

Authors' contributions
SG: Study design, data analysis, data interpretation, and writing, YT: data collection, writing, AW: study design, data interpretation, and critical revision, SLW: Study design, data interpretation, and critical revision, RGK: Study design, data analysis, data interpretation, and critical revision. All authors read and approved the final manuscript.

Acknowledgments
*We gratefully thank the University of Alberta's ACES group for their support in this research. The ACES group includes: Drs. Ronald Brisebois, Klaus Buttenschoen, Kamran Fathimani, Stewart M Hamilton, Rachel G Khadaroo Gordon M Lees, Todd PW McMullen, William Patton, Marry Van Wijngaarden-Stephens, J Drew Sutherland, Sandy L Widder, and David C Williams. Funding for this study was from a University (Alberta) Hospital Foundation grant and the M.S.I. foundation (RGK).

Author details
[1]Department of Surgery, University of Alberta, 2D WMC, 8440-112 St NW, Edmonton, AB, Canada T6G 2B7. [2]Department of Medicine, University of Alberta, Edmonton, Alberta, Canada.

References
1. Canada, D.o.A.a.S.H: *Canada's aging population.* Ottawa, Canada: Minister of Public Works and Government Services; 2002.
2. Canadian Institute for Health Information, Health Care in Canada: *A Focus on Seniors and Aging.* Ottawa, Ont.: CIHI; 2011.
3. Jacobsen LA, Kent M, Lee M, Mather M: **America's Aging Population.** *Popul Ref Bureau* 2011, **66:**1.
4. Department of Economic and Social Affairs: *World population aging.* United Nation; 2009.
5. Etzioni DA, Liu JH, Maggard MA, Ko CY: **The aging population and its impact on the surgery workforce.** *Ann Surg* 2003, **238:**170–177.
6. Preston D, Southall A, Nel M, Das S: **Geriatric Surgery is about disease.** *Not age J R Soc Med* 2008 Aug, **101**(8)**:**409–415.
7. Ferrucci L, Guralink JM, Studenski S, Fried LP, Cutler GB Jr, Walston JD: **Designing randomized controlled trials aimed at preventing or delaying functional decline and disability in frail, older persons: A consensus report.** *J Am Geriatr Soc* 2004, **52:**625–634.
8. Fried LP, Tangen CM, Walston J, Newman AB, Hirsch C, Gottdiener J, *et al*: **Frailty in older adults: Evidence for a phenotype.** *J Gerontol Biol Med Sci* 2001, **56:**M146–M156.
9. Christensen K, Doblhammer G, Rau R, Vaupel JW: **Ageing populations: The challenges ahead.** *Lancet* 2009, **374:**1196–1208.
10. Applegate WB, Blass JP, Williams TF: **Instruments for the functional assessment of older patients. current concepts in geriatrics.** *N Engl J Med* 1990, **322**(17)**:**1207–1215.
11. Fukuda N, Wada J, Niki M, Sugiyama Y, Mushiake H: **Factors predicting mortality in emergency abdominal surgery in the elderly.** *World J Emerg Surg* 2012, **7**(12).
12. Farhat J, Velanovich V, Falvo A, Mathilda H, Swarts A, Patton J, *et al*: **Are the frail distained to fail? Frailty index as predictor of surgical morbidity and mortality in the elderly.** *J Trauma Acute Care Surg* 2012 June, **72**(6)**:**1526–1530.
13. Swain DG, O'Brien AG, Nightingale PG: **Cognitive assessment in elderly patients admitted to hospital: The relationship between the shortened version of the abbreviated mental test and the abbreviated mental test and mini-mental state examination.** *Clin Rehabil* 2000, **14:**608–610.
14. Sainsbury A, Seebass G, Bansal A, Young JB: **Reliability of the Barthel index when used with older people.** *Age Aging* 2005, **34**(3)**:**228–232.
15. Pietra G, Savio K, Oddone E: **Validity and reliability of barthel index administered by telephone.** *Stroke* 2011, **42:**2077–2079.

16. Saliba D, Elliott M, Rubenstein LZ, Solomon DH, Young RT, Kamberg CJ, *et al*: **The vulnerable elders survey: A tool for identifying vulnerable elders in the community.** *J Am Geriatr Soc* 2001, **49**(12):1691–1699.
17. Min LC, Elliott MN, Wenger NS, Saliba D: **Higher vulnerable elders survey scores predict death and functional decline in vulnerable older people.** *J Am Geriatr Soc* 2006, **54**(3):507–511.
18. Min L, Yoon W, Mariano J, Wenger NS, Elliott MN, Kamberg C, *et al*: **The vulnerable elders-13 survey predicts 5-year functional decline and mortality outcomes in older ambulatory care patients.** *J Am Geriatr Soc* 2009, **57**(11):2070–2076.
19. EuroQol group. Health policy: **A new facility for the measurement of health-related quality of life.** *Health Policy* 1990, **16**(3):199–208.
20. Deiner S, Silverstein J: **Long term outcomes in elderly surgical patients.** *Mt Sinai J Med* 2012, **79**(1):95–106.

4

A retrospective observational study comparing hair apposition technique, suturing and stapling for scalp lacerations

Derya Ozturk, Bedriye Müge Sonmez, Ertugrul Altinbilek, Cemil Kavalci*, Engin Deniz Arslan and Serhat Akay

Abstract

Aim: Scalp lacerations are commonly encountered in patients presenting to emergency department with trauma. Lacerations are repaired with suturing, stapling, adhesive tapes, and tissue adhesives. In this study, we aimed to compare the effectiveness of suturing, stapling, and hair apposition techniques used in repair of scalp lacerations in patients who presented to emergency department with scalp laceration.

Materials and method: After obtaining approval of local ethics committee, we examined the effects of the three technique used to repair scalp lacerations on wound healing, complication rate, and patient satisfaction by recording data. Categorical variables were expressed as n and %. X^2 test was used for statistical analysis. A p value less than 0.05 was accepted statistically significant.

Results: Our study included a total of 134 patients of whom were treated 37 (27.6%) with hair apposition technique 49, 48 (35.8%) with suturing, and (36.6%) with stapling. There was a significant difference between the scalp repair technique and 7th and 15th day patient satisfaction rates in favor of the hair apposition technique ($p < 0.05$). There was a significant difference between the scalp repair technique and cosmetic problems after 15 days ($p < 0.05$). Cosmetic problems 15 days after the procedure were significantly lower in the hair apposition technique.

Conclusion: In patients presenting to emergency departments with linear scalp laceration suturing, stapling, and hair apposition techniques can be safely applied. However, hair apposition technique has the advantages of being more satisfying, and having lower cosmetic problem and complication rates compared with other techniques.

Keywords: Scalp laceration, Suturing, Stapling, Hair apposition, Emergency

Introduction and objective

The main objective of wound repair is to restore skin integrity and, while doing this to reduce rate of infection, scarring, and functional impairment [1]. Lacerations are repaired with sutures, staples, adhesive tapes, and tissue adhesives. Each method has its own advantages and disadvantages [2]. Suturing is the most commonly used method in laceration repair [3]. It is the strongest of all wound closure materials and allows best approximation of wound edges irrespective of wound shape. However, it is also the most time-consuming and user-dependent among all techniques available. Repair via stapling is another method used for scalp lacerations. It is preferable to suturing in emergency services because it is a quicker and less painful procedure and associated with a lower cost and risk of needle stick injury to the operator. It is also preferred in pediatric age groups owing to the above-mentioned properties [4-6]. Hair apposition technique is an alternative technique in scalp lacerations. Hair apposition technique was first defined by Hock et al. in 2002. In this technique, 4–5 strands of hair are grasped on each side of the wound. These strands are crossed once and a drop of glue is placed where the strands cross to secure the wound [7]. In this study, we aimed to compare the effectiveness of suturing, stapling, and hair apposition techniques used in repair of scalp lacerations in patients who presented to emergency department with scalp laceration.

* Correspondence: cemkavalci@yahoo.com
Numune Training and Research Hospital, Emergency Department, Ankara, Turkey

Materials and method

This study was performed in a retrospectively at Numune Training and Research Hospital Emergency department between 01 January 2010 and 01 July 2010 after approval of the study by the local ethics committee (2010-33). Research carried out on humans must be in compliance with the Helsinki Declaration. Cosmetic problems, patient satisfaction, wound healing status, and complications were determined from the files of the patients who returned for follow-up examination on 7th and 15th days of suturing. After gathering data of the patients with scalp lacerations who were applied any of the hair apposition, suturing, or stapling methods. Method of wound closure was made to physician preference. Inclusion and exclusion criteria of the study given on Table 1. There was a used standart inclusion and exclusion criteria for three methods. Length and localization of the laceration, length of hair, the applied technique, satisfaction of the patient and complication parameters were recorded on study forms. Degree of pain in patients evaluated with visual analog scale (VAS). Infection was defined with redness and purulent wound drainage. Cosmetic problem defined according to doctor. The patients were divided into 3 groups as follows: Group 1, patients who were applied hair apposition technique; Group 2, patients who were applied suturing technique; and Group 3, patients who were applied stapling technique. Study data were analyzed using SPSS 15.00 software package. Categorical variables were expressed as n and %. X^2 test was used for statistical analysis. A p value less than 0.05 was accepted statistically significant.

Results

Our study included a total of 134 patients of whom were treated 37 (27.6%) with hair apposition technique, 48 (35.8%) with suturing, and49 (36.6%) with stapling. The distribution of the technique according to patient demographics is given on Table 2.

Table 1 Inclusion/ Exclusion criteria

Inclusion criteria	Exclusion criteria
Hair length of at least 1 cm	Nonlinear lacerations
Linear lacerations	Contaminated wounds
Laceration length shorter than 10 cm	Active arterial bleeding
Laceration repair carried out with the method of simple spaced percutaneous suturing using 4/0 monofilament polypropylene	Unstable vital signs or shock
Laceration repair carried out with stapling	Altered conscioussness
Laceration repair carried out with hair apposition and tissue adhesive	Irregular wound edges and associated tissue loss
	İmmunocompromised patient
	Comorbiditiy patient

Table 2 The distribution of the technique according to patient demografics

	Hair apposition	Suturing	Stapling	p value
Sex (Male/Female, n)	33/4	36/12	43/6	$X^2 = 4.04$, $p > 0.05$
Age (mean ± SD)	31.68 ± 8.7	32.35 ± 9.5	32.02 ± 9.1	$X^2 = 0.10$, $p > 0.05$

Distrubution of patient according to the technique and hair length was shown on the Table 3.

A crosstabulation between the techniques used and the percentage of satisfaction after 7 days revealed that the latter was higher in hair apposition technique as compared with the other techniques (Figure 1). There was a significant relationship between the technique and satisfaction level after 7 days ($X^2 = 6.13$, $p < 0.05$).

The most common complications after 7 days were redness and pain. These complications occurred most commonly in the suturing group (34.55% and 21.87%, respectively) followed by stapling technique (26.42% and 13.21%, respectively), and hair apposition technique (16.22% and 13.51%, respectively). The distribution of the complications 7 days after the procedure by the technique used is summarized on Table 4.

There was a significant relationship between the technique and the satisfaction level after 15 days ($X^2 = 6.75$, $p < 0.05$). According to this, satisfaction after 15 days depends on the technique used. The crosstabulation between the techniques used and satisfaction level after 15 days revealed that a stapling and suturing techniques were association with dissatisfaction whereas hair apposition technique was associated with much lower dissatisfaction rate (Figure 2).

The crosstabulation between the techniques used and the rate of cosmetic problems after 15 days revealed a higher rate of cosmetic problems in the suturing group than other groups ($X^2 = 8.81$, $p < 0.05$) (Figure 3).

Discussion

Emergency physicians can also employ hair apposition technique in addition to suturing and stapling in the treatment of scalp lacerations. In our study, hair apposition technique was associated with a higher rate of satisfaction

Table 3 Distrubution of the classified hair length and techniques used in the treatment of scalp laceration

Hair lenght	Hair apposition (n)	Suturing (n)	Stapling (n)	p value
Short (<3 cm)	12	20	25	$X^2 = 5.02$, $p > 0.05$
Medium (3–6 cm)	17	14	15	
Long (>6 cm)	8	14	9	

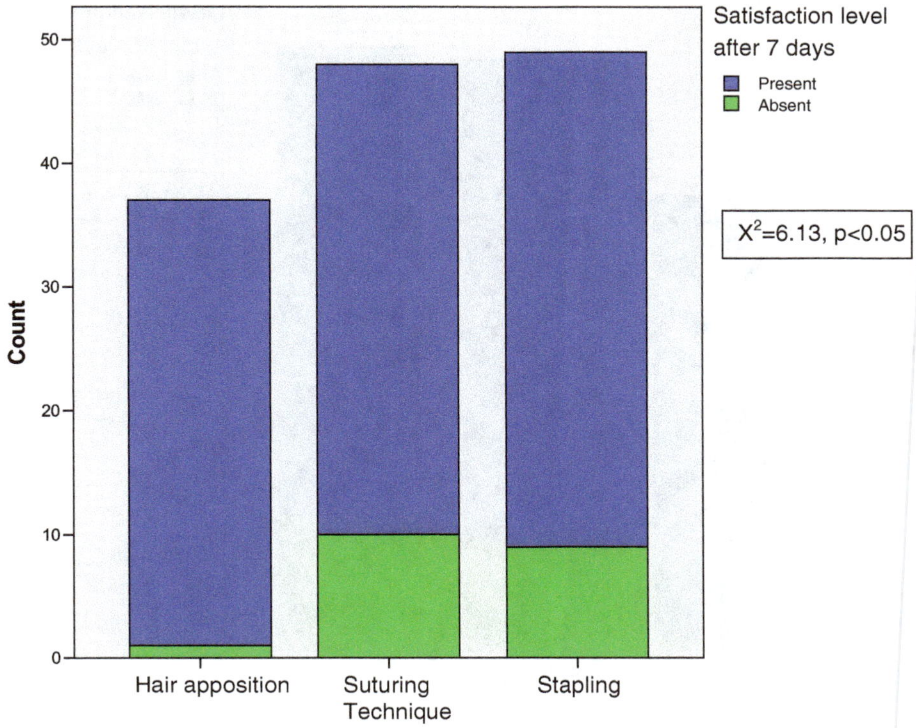

Figure 1 The graph of the relationship between the techniques and satisfaction level after 7 days.

than other techniques 7 days and 15 days after the procedure.

Hock et al., in a study where they used techniques of suturing and hair apposition in patients with scalp laceration, included lacerations up to 10 cm but did not mentioned about any relationship between the technique used and laceration length [7]. Both our study and previous studies suggested that a hair length of at least 1 cm is essential for application of hair apposition technique in scalp lacerations [7,8]. In our study there was no significant difference between the technique used and hair length.

Hock et al. compared complication and healing rates 7 days after treatment of scalp lacerations with suturing or hair apposition techniques and reported that wound healing and scar formation occurred more commonly in suturing whereas rates of infection or bleeding were not different in both groups [7]. Karaduman et al. used all three techniques in scalp lacerations and reported no cases of infection 7 days after the procedure. They reported abnormal hair growth in a patient who was treated with hair apposition, which was attributed by the authors to excess amount of glue used in the procedure, causing spread of glue in the wound [8]. Ong et al. used suturing or hair apposition in scalp lacerations and reported fewer complications 7 days after the procedure with the hair apposition technique [9]. Kanegaye et al., in a study on pediatric scalp lacerations, compared stapling and suturing with respect to complication rates 7 days after the procedure and reported fewer complications in stapling

Table 4 Distribution of the complications on 7th day by the techniques used

	Hair apposition		Suturing		Stapling		p value
Complications	n	%	n	%	n	%	
Pain	5	13.51	12	21.87	7	13.21	$X^2 = 2.56$, $p > 0.05$
Serous wound drainage	1	2.7	0	0	0	0	$X^2 = 2.61$, $p > 0.05$
Infection	0	0.0	3	5.45	1	1.89	$X^2 = 3.05$, $p > 0.05$
Redness	6	16.22	19	34.55	14	26.42	$X^2 = 5.54$, $p > 0.05$
Hair loss	0	0	5	9.093	2	3.77	$X^2 = 4.78$, $p > 0.05$
Wound dehiscence	1	2.7	0	0	3	5.66	$X^2 = 3.15$, $p > 0.05$

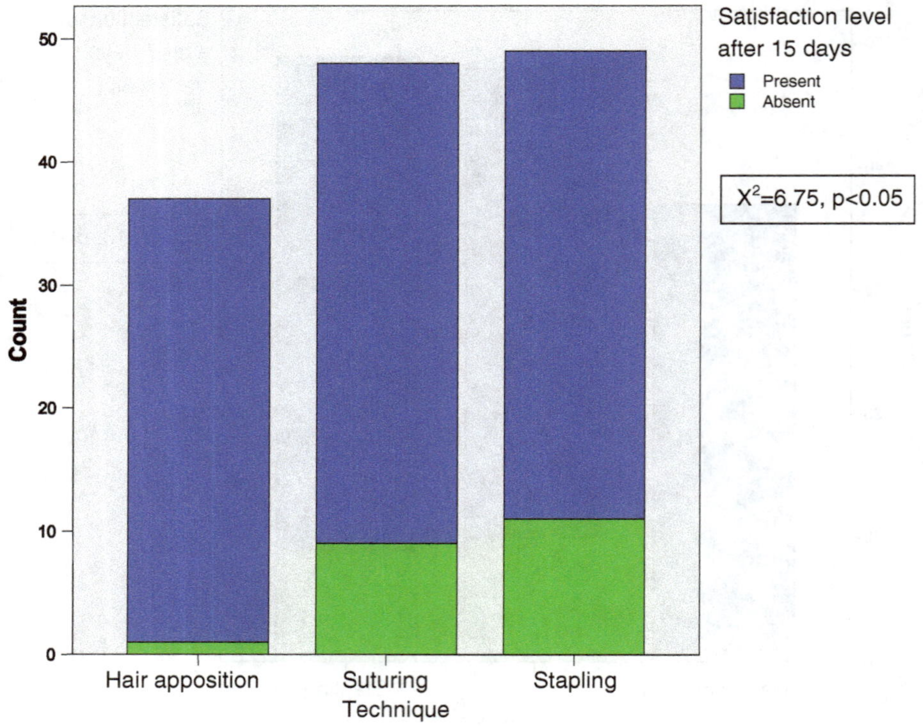

Figure 2 The graph of the relationship between the techniques and satisfaction level after 15 days.

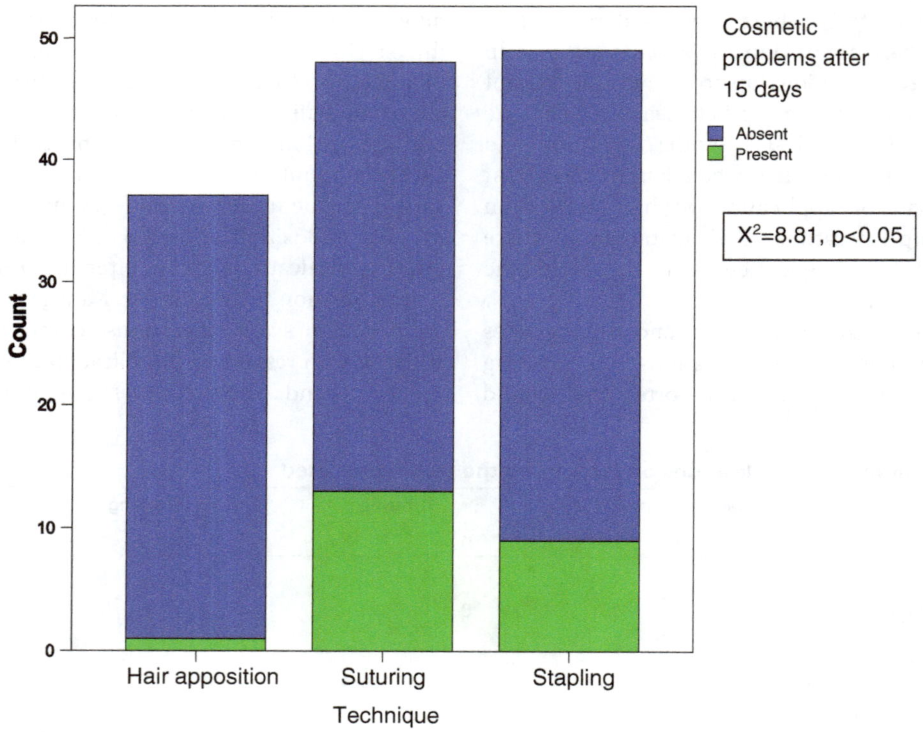

Figure 3 The graph of the relationship between the techniques and cosmetic problems.

group [10]. We also found that the highest complication rate was with suturing. The most common complications 7 days after the procedure included redness, pain, and hair loss, which occurred most commonly with suturing followed by stapling and hair apposition techniques. The highest rate of infection was associated with suturing technique followed by stapling technique. Hair loss, an important cosmetic problem, occurred most commonly with suturing followed by stapling technique whereas hair apposition technique was not associated with hair loss 7 days after the procedure. Hock et al. reported a higher rate of satisfaction in patients treated with hair apposition technique compared with those treated with suturing technique. This high rate of satisfaction was related by the authors to the properties of the technique including quick application, less painful nature due to absence of need for anesthesia, and absence of need for shaving and suture removal [7]. Karaduman et al. applied all three techniques to their patients with scalp laceration and looked at patient satisfaction on day 30th. They reported a high rate of satisfaction in those who were applied hair apposition technique and 97% of patients would prefer this method in the event they sustained a scalp laceration in the future [8]. The rate of satisfaction was related with the technique used, such that patients were dissatisfied with stapling and suturing while dissatisfaction rate was quite low. In our study, Assessment of 7th and 15th day satisfaction rates revealed significant differences in favor of hair apposition technique. The painless nature of the technique and absence of suture removal may have increased patient satisfaction. In our study there was a significant association between the technique used and emergence of cosmetic problems 15 days later. We found that cosmetic problems were most prevalent in patients treated with suturing while they were least common in those managed with hair apposition technique. We think that this is because there was no need to shave hairs in this technique and we carefully placed only one drop of glue on the crossed strands without bringing the glue into contact with the wound. Otherwise excessive amount of glue will result in hair knots, leading to haircut while contact of tissue adhesive with laceration will result in decreased hair growth [11]. Kanegaye et al. compared the cosmetic outcomes of stapling or suturing in pediatric scalp lacerations 1 week after the procedure when they removed suture materials. They reported no cosmetic problems in stapling group [10].

In literature there are plenty of studies on application time of these techniques. Hock et al. compared suturing and hair apposition techniques with respect to application time and found that hair apposition technique was applied in a shorter time than other technique [7]. Kanegaye et al. reported that stapling technique was applied in a shorter time compared to suturing in pediatric patients with scalp laceration [10]. In a surgical study stapling and suturing techniques used in the treatment of long lacerations were compared in terms of application times. Stapling technique was reported to be associated with five-to-seven times shorter times compared with the suturing technique [12-15]. Karaduman et al., in a study examining the hair apposition and suturing techniques in emergency department patients with scalp laceration in terms of application times, reported that hair apposition technique was associated with shorter procedure time [8]. As our study was retrospective, we could not gather any information on application times. However, experience from our daily practice suggests that stapling method can be performed in a relatively shorter time.

Ong et al. compared hair apposition and suturing techniques in terms of treatment cost in scalp lacerations and reported that hair apposition technique had a significantly lower cost. They related that result to a shorter time of the procedure, absence of need for anesthesia and suture removal, and low complication rates. They expressed that the rate of scalp lacerations in EDs remain high and this technique would provide considerable cost saving [11]. Orlinsky et al., in a general study on costs of treatment of scalp lacerations in emergency departments, found that stapling was considerably advantageous with respect to overall cost [16]. We did not perform a cost analysis.

Hair apposition technique may be used more commonly in daily practice by virtue of its low complication and cosmetic problem rate coupled with high patient satisfaction rate. Determination of the ideal wound closure technique requires more prospective, randomized controlled studies with larger sample size that investigate factors effective on wound healing and satisfaction level.

Limitations of the study

A major limitations of the study was a retrospectively of it. We could not gather any information on application times. As the social security institution of Turkey employs a per case payment system for suturing materials and procedure, no cost analysis was performed for any of the 3 groups.

Conclusion

Emergency departments are one of the leading clinics where patient crowding is greatest. Thus, time-consuming procedures such as laceration repair may be problematic for the operators. In our study all these criteria were met by the hair apposition technique. Considering its low cost in addition to all these positive results, we feel that this technique will be used or preferred more frequently by physicians and patients in our country as the rest of the world.

Competing interests
The authors declare that they have no competing interests.

Authors' contributions
DO: conception and design, or acquisition of data, or analysis and interpretation of data, have given final approval of the version to be published. BMS: acquisition of data, EA: revising it critically for important intellectual content; CK: analysis and interpretation of data or revising it critically for important intellectual content; EDA: have made substantial contributions to conception and design. SA: have made substantial contributions to conception and design. All authors read and approved the final manuscript.

References

1. Hollander JE, Singer AJ, Valentine S, Henry MC: **Wound registry: development and validation.** *Ann Emerg Med* 1995, **25:**675–685.
2. Turnage B, Maull KI: **Scalp laceration: an obvious 'occult' cause of shock.** *South Med J* 2000, **93:**265–266.
3. Baker MD, Lanuti M: **The management and outcome of lacerations in urban children.** *Ann Emerg Med* 1990, **19:**1001–1005.
4. Hollander JE, Singer AJ, Valentine SM, Shofer FS: **Risk factors for infection in patients with traumatic lacerations.** *Acad Emerg Med* 2001, **8:**716–720.
5. Berk WA, Osbourne DD, Taylor DD: **Evaluation of the "golden period" for wound repair: 204 cases from a third world emergency department.** *Ann Emerg Med* 1988, **17:**496–500.
6. Hollander JE, Richman PB, Werblud M, Miller T, Huggler J, Singer AJ: **Irrigation in facial and scalp lacerations: does it alter outcome?** *Ann Emerg Med* 1998, **31:**73–77.
7. Hock MO, Ooi SB, Saw SM, Lim SH: **A randomized controlled trial comparing the hair apposition technique with tissue glue to standard suturing in scalp lacerations (HAT study).** *Ann Emerg Med* 2002, **40:**19–26.
8. Karaduman S, Yürüktümen A, Güryay SM, Bengi F, Fowler JR: **Modified hair apposition technique as the primary closure method for scalp lacerations.** *Am J Emerg Med* 2009, **27:**1050–1055.
9. Ong ME, Chan YH, Teo J, Saroja S, Yap S, Ang PH, Lim SH: **Hair apposition technique for scalp laceration repair: a randomized controlled trial comparing physicians and nurses (HAT 2 study).** *Am J Emerg Med* 2008, **26:**433–438.
10. Kanegaye JT, Vance CW, Chan L, Schonfeld N: **Comparison of skin stapling devices and standard sutures for pediatric scalp lacerations: a randomized study of cost and time benefits.** *J Pediatr* 1997, **130:**808–813.
11. Ong M, Coyle D, Lim S, Stiell I: **Cost-effectiveness of hair apposition technique compared with standard suturing in scalp lacerations.** *Ann Emerg Med* 2005, **46:**237–242.
12. George TK, Simpson DC: **Skin wound closure with staples in the accident and emergency department.** *J Royal Coll Surg* 1985, **30:**54–56. Edinburgh.
13. MacGregor FB, McCombe AW, King PM, Macleod DAD: **Skin stapling of wounds in the accident department.** *Injury* 1989, **20:**347–348.
14. Kavalci C, Cevik Y, Durukan P, Sayhan MB: **Comparison of different suture techniques.** *JCAM*. doi: 10.4328/JCAM.1690 true.
15. Smith TO, Sexton D, Mann C, Donell S: **Sutures versus staples for skin closure in orthopaedic surgery: meta-analysis.** *BMJ* 2010, **340:**c1199. doi: 10.1136/bmj.c1199 true.
16. Orlinsky M, Goldberg RM, Chan L, Puertos A, Slajer HL: **Cost analysis of stapling versus suturing for skin closure.** *Am J Emerg Med* 1995, **13:**77–81.

5

Predictors of in-hospital mortality and complications in very elderly patients undergoing emergency surgery

Shaheed Merani[1], Judd Payne[1], Raj S Padwal[2], Darren Hudson[3], Sandy L Widder[1,3], Rachel G Khadaroo[1,3,4*]
on behalf of the Acute Care and Emergency Surgery (ACES) Group

Abstract

Introduction: With the increasing aging population demographics and life expectancies the number of very elderly patients (age ≥ 80) undergoing emergency surgery is expected to rise. This investigation examines the outcomes in very elderly patients undergoing emergency general surgery, including predictors of in-hospital mortality and morbidity.

Methods: A retrospective study of patients aged 80 and above undergoing emergency surgery between 2008 and 2010 at a tertiary care facility in Canada was conducted. Demographics, comorbidities, surgical indications, and perioperative risk assessment data were collected. Outcomes included length of hospitalization, discharge destination, and in-hospital mortality and morbidity. Multivariable logistic regression was used to identify predictors of in-hospital mortality and complications.

Results: Of the 170 patient admissions, the mean age was 84 years and the in-hospital mortality rate was 14.7%. Comorbidities were present in 91% of this older patient population. Over 60% of the patients required further services or alternate level of care on discharge. American Society of Anesthesiologist Physical Status (ASA) Classification (OR 5.30, 95% CI 1.774-15.817, $p = 0.003$) and the development of an in-hospital complications (OR 2.51, 95% CI 1.210-5.187, $p = 0.013$) were independent predictors of postoperative mortality. Chronological age or number of comorbidities was not predictive of surgical outcome.

Conclusions: Mortality, complication rates and post-discharge care requirements were high in very elderly patients undergoing emergency general surgery. Advanced age and medical comorbidities alone should not be the limiting factors for surgical referral or treatment. This study illustrates the importance of preventing an in-hospital complication in this very vulnerable population. ASA class is a robust tool which is predictive of mortality in the very elderly population and can be used to guide patient and family counseling in the emergency setting.

Keywords: Elderly, Acute care, Emergency, Surgery, Morbidity, Mortality

Introduction

It is estimated that the majority of people born in developed nations during the 21st century will live to their 100th birthdays [1]. Both the increased number of elderly and the inherent complexity of their health have resulted in increased demands on the health care system [1-5]. Comparative studies across nations have suggested that increased survival to the highest ages is associated with worse health [1]. Overall, the current population will be living longer with more health problems than in the past.

The very elderly (age ≥ 80 years) often suffer from frailty. Frailty is associated with advanced age, but is also influenced by comprehensive determinants including medical comorbidity, nutritional status, mental health, social support, and cognition [6]. Neither a single definition nor measure of frailty exists; however, there is consensus that very elderly individuals have an

* Correspondence: khadaroo@ualberta.ca
[1]Department of Surgery, Faculty of Medicine and Dentistry, University of Alberta, Edmonton, Alberta, Canada
[3]Division of Critical Care Medicine, Faculty of Medicine and Dentistry, University of Alberta, Edmonton, Alberta, Canada

increased risk of adverse outcomes from physiological stress and disease.

A growing body of evidence on the outcome of elective operative management of very elderly patients has become available over the last decade [6-12]. However, there are limited data on the outcome of very elderly patients undergoing emergency general surgical procedures [6,13-15]. While elective surgical care affords the benefit of comprehensive geriatric assessment and the pre-operative optimization of comorbid states, emergency surgery differs in that there is limited time for information collection (including goals of care). The baseline health, mental, and social status of elderly patients who present with acute surgical emergencies is often unknown and comorbidities under recognized. The absence of this information exacerbates the vulnerability of these patients to known insults which occur during hospitalization [16]. Post-operative care itself has traditionally been a source of such insults including fasting for gastrointestinal healing, polypharmacy, immobility, nasogastric tubes, and bladder catheterization. These, in turn, place surgical patients at higher risk of complications including delerium [8].

The purpose of this study is to characterize the very elderly population, who received emergency general surgery, and examine their surgical outcomes including identification of factors associated with in-hospital mortality and morbidity. We hypothesized that the number of medical comorbidities and American Society of Anesthesiologist Physical Status Classification (ASA class) would be the strongest predictors of poor outcomes.

Materials & methods

A retrospective cohort study was conducted on very elderly patients undergoing emergency general surgery at the University of Alberta Hospital, a tertiary care academic teaching hospital in Edmonton, Alberta, Canada between 2008 and 2010.

Inclusion criteria included patients who had an age of 80 years or older and at least one emergency general surgical procedure during admission. We defined emergency surgery as an operative procedure that was meant to prevent morbidity or mortality, not booked from an outpatient clinic (elective basis), and required an unplanned operation on their admission to hospital.

Patient demographics including age, sex, weight, height, pre-hospitalization medication use and comorbidities were collected. Additionally, operative data including anesthesiologist assigned ASA class, Comorbidity-Polypharmacy Score (CPS) (which combines the number of pre-illness medications with the number of comorbidities to estimate the severity of comorbid condition [17]), operative procedure performed, and surgical diagnoses were collected. Clinical outcomes measured included in-hospital complications, length of hospital stay, in-hospital mortality, and discharge location. The University of Alberta Human Research Ethics Board approved this research.

Data was collected using a Microsoft Access database, and statistical analysis was performed with SPSS 17.0. Frequencies and percentages were tabulated for categorical and ordinal variables; means and standard deviations calculated for continuous variables. The statistical association between categorical variables was studied with chi-square analysis. Binary logistic regression analysis was used to identify predictors of in-hospital mortality and complications. A multi-variate model was built using age, gender, BMI, number of pre-hospitalization medications and comorbidities, ASA class, and number of in-hospital complications as factors entered in a single step. A p-value of < 0.05 was considered evidence of an association not attributable to chance, and therefore of statistical significance.

Results

Patient demographics, diagnoses, and operative procedures

During three years studied (2008-2010) a total of 170 patients aged 80 or above were admitted for emergency general surgery. The mean age was 84.1 years, over half were male (51.2%), and the average BMI was 24.8 kg/m^2 (Table 1).

Comorbid illness was present in 91.2% of elderly patients in this cohort. The most common were hypertension, respiratory disease (including COPD), diabetes, hypothyroidism, and heart failure (Table 2).

Table 1 Patient admission characteristics and comorbidities

	n (%)
Age (years) Mean = 84.1 (SD = 3.6)	
80-84	105 (61.8%)
85-90	50 (29.4%)
≥ 90	15 (8.8%)
Sex	
Female	83 (48.8%)
BMI (kg/m^2) Mean = 24.8 (SD = 4.6)	
< 18.5 (Underweight)	13 (7.6%)
18.5-25 (Normal weight)	74 (43.5%)
25-30 (Overweight)	53 (31.2%)
> 30 (Obese)	19 (11.2%)
ASA class	
1E	1 (0.7%)
2E	11 (8.2%)
3E	78 (58.2%)
4E	44 (32.8%)

Table 2 Patient comorbidities: total comorbidity number, medication use, ASA class, and CPS

	n (%)
Comorbidity	
Hypertension	112 (65.9%)
Respiratory disease (including COPD)	44 (25.9%)
Diabetes	34 (20%)
Hypothyroid	33(19.4%)
Heart failure	29 (17.1%)
Osteoarthritis	26 (15.3%)
Osteoporosis	23 (13.5%)
Smoking history	19 (11.2%)
Stroke with residual deficit	7 (4.1%)
Myocardial infarction (within last 6 months)	7 (4.1%)
Total number of comorbidities	
None	15 (8.8%)
1-2	95 (55.9%)
3-5	58 (34.1%)
> 5	2 (1.2%)
Number of home medications	
None	19 (11.2%)
1-2	37 (21.8%)
3-5	81 (47.6%)
> 5	33 (19.4%)
Home medication use	
ACE inhibitor	73 (42.9%)
Anti-platelet agent	73 (42.9%)
Beta-blocker	66 (38.8%)
Statin	62 (36.5%)
Diuretics	54 (31.8%)
Calcium channel blocker	45 (26.5%)
Anti-coagulant	42 (24.7%)
CPS	
0-3	44 (25.9%)
4-7	80 (47.1%)
8-10	36 (21.2%)
> 10	10 (5.9%)

Correspondingly, 89% of patients were using at least one home medication prior to hospitalization. The most common medications used were angiotensin converting enzyme inhibitors, anti-platelet agents, beta-blockers, statins, and diuretics (Table 2). Median ASA class was 3E (58.2% of patients) (Table 1). Median CPS score was 6 (range of 0 to 14).

The majority of emergency general surgical procedures were for colon resection (22.9%), small bowel resection (19.4%) or laparotomy (15.9%) followed by cholecystectomy (10.6%) (Table 3).

In-hospital complication, mortality, and length of stay

In-hospital complications were experienced by over a fifth of patients (Table 4). The most common complications were pulmonary in nature (16.5% of patients) including respiratory failure (requiring intensive care unit support), pneumonia, and pulmonary embolism. Other common complications included both surgical (post-operative bleeding, wound infection and dehiscence), and medical (acute or acute-on-chronic renal failure).

A total of 25 of very elderly patients receiving emergency surgery died in the hospital (14.7% mortality). There was lower mortality in the octogenarian group (12.9%) compared with 33% in the nonagenarian group, while not statistical significant this may be reflective of the relatively small numbers in the groups (Table 1, p = 0.08).

The median length of stay was 14 days (range 1 to 164 days). Twenty one percent of patients remained in hospital for greater than 30 days (not including any post-discharge admission to a transition or rehabilitation facility). Of the patients who were discharged from hospital, 62% required residential health services beyond their admission (transfer to another hospital, assisted care facility, rehabilitation center, or home-care nursing). Over a third of patients were discharged home without services.

Table 3 Diagnoses and procedures performed

	n (%)
Operative procedure	
Colon (Laparotomy for resection or diversion)	39 (22.9%)
Small Bowel (Laparotomy for adhesions or resection)	33 (19.4%)
Laparotomy (other)	27 (15.9%)
Cholecystectomy	18 (10.6%)
Hernia – Incarcerated/Strangulation	15 (8.8%)
Duodenal Bleed/Perforation	9 (5.3%)
Primary diagnosis	
Small Bowel Obstruction	25 (14.7%)
Hernia	20 (11.8%)
Cholelithiasis (Complicated)	17 (10%)
Colon Cancer	14 (8.2%)
Duodenal Ulcer	13 (7.6%)
Appendicitis	9 (5.3%)
Bowel Ischemia	9 (5.3%)
Colon Obstruction	9 (5.3%)
Colon Perforation	8 (4.7%)
Gastrointestinal Bleed	6 (3.5%)

Common diagnoses and procedures performed on admitted patients.

Table 4 Complications, mortality, length of stay, and disposition following surgery

	n (%)
Complication	
Respiratory failure (requiring intubation)	12 (7.1%)
Bleeding	11 (6.5%)
Renal Failure	10 (5.9%)
Sepsis	9 (5.3%)
Wound Complication	8 (4.7%)
PE	3 (1.8%)
Stroke	2 (1.2%)
Total number of complications	
0	135 (79.4%)
1-2	30 (17.6%)
3-5	5 (2.9%)
Mortality	25 (14.7%)
Length of Stay (Median 14 days)	
< 7 days	36 (21.2%)
8-14 days	52 (30.6%)
15-30 days	45 (26.5%)
31-90 days	30 (17.6%)
> 90 days	6 (3.5%)
Disposition (n = 145)	
Home	78 (53.8%)
Without additional services	54 (37.2%)
With homecare services	24 (16.7%)
Rehabilitation/home hospital	54 (37.2%)
Assisted Living/long term care	9 (6.2%)
Other	4 (2.8%)

Predictors of in-hospital morbidity and complications

Multivariable logistic regression analysis was used to identify variables associated with in-hospital mortality (Table 5). Of these, ASA class (OR 5.30, 95% CI 1.774-15.817, p = 0.003) and in-hospital complications (OR 2.51, 95% CI 1.210-5.187, p = 0.013) were statistically significantly predictive of in-hospital mortality (Figure 1). Majority of the patients were ASA class 3 (n = 78, 58%). The death rate for each ASA class were 1 (0%), 2 (0%), 3 (7.7%) and 4 (31.8%). The number of comorbidites, age, or CPS score was not predictive of mortality. The regression model to identify those patients at higher risk of at least one in-hospital complication (Table 6) did not identify any statistically significant covariates.

Table 5 Factors associated with in-hospital mortality - multivariable logistic regression analysis

Factor	B	p-value	OR	95% CI for OR	
				Lower	Upper
Age	.061	.436	1.063	.912	1.239
Sex (Female)	.407	.488	1.502	.476	4.743
BMI	.019	.755	1.019	.904	1.150
Medications	-.118	.425	.889	.665	1.188
Comorbidities	.388	.093	1.474	.938	2.318
ASA class	1.667	.003*	5.297	1.774	15.817
Complications	.918	.013*	2.505	1.210	5.187

*p < 0.05.

Conclusion

By the year 2040 it is estimated that greater than 25% of the population will be seniors [18]. The rapid growth of the aging population has prompted the necessity for a better understanding of the needs and outcomes of elderly patients undergoing emergency surgery. The present study demonstrates that the majority of patients aged 80 or above admitted for emergency general surgery had pre-existing co-morbidity, were taking one or more medications, and had functional limitations of their illness (as demonstrated by an ASA class of 3E or above). Over sixty percent of the patients in this study required additional healthcare services beyond their admission. There is relatively good long-term survival in this very elderly population where we found fifty percent alive on our three years post-surgery follow-up [19]. From a system perspective, early resource utilization planning can occur if we better understand this population's predicted demand for acute care beds and longer term need for appropriate supportive care, alternate level of care, and rehabilitation or transition beds.

There is a paucity of studies examining emergency surgery in elderly patients, which makes it difficult to determine outcomes in this patient population. In ambulatory medical practice and elective surgery, adverse outcomes are associated with frailty measures including loneliness, cognitive impairment functional limitations, poor nutritional status, and depression [6,7]. In the Reported Edmonton Frail Scale (REFS) as well as other frailty scales, measures of general health (comorbidities and medications) constitute only a very small portion of the composite frailty [20], however, in the emergency setting, it is a challenge to perform a comprehensive geriatric assessment of frailty.

Other scoring systems to estimate outcomes and mortality in elderly surgical patients include the Acute Physiology and Chronic Health Evaluation II (APACHE II) score [21]. However, the APACHE II score can be difficult to apply to the typical emergency surgery patient since it is predictive only for patients in the critical care setting. As well, an arterial blood gas is not typically part of the pre-operative work-up. The APACHE II is a score that is applied within the first 24 hours to a critically ill patient; therefore, it also does not take into account the

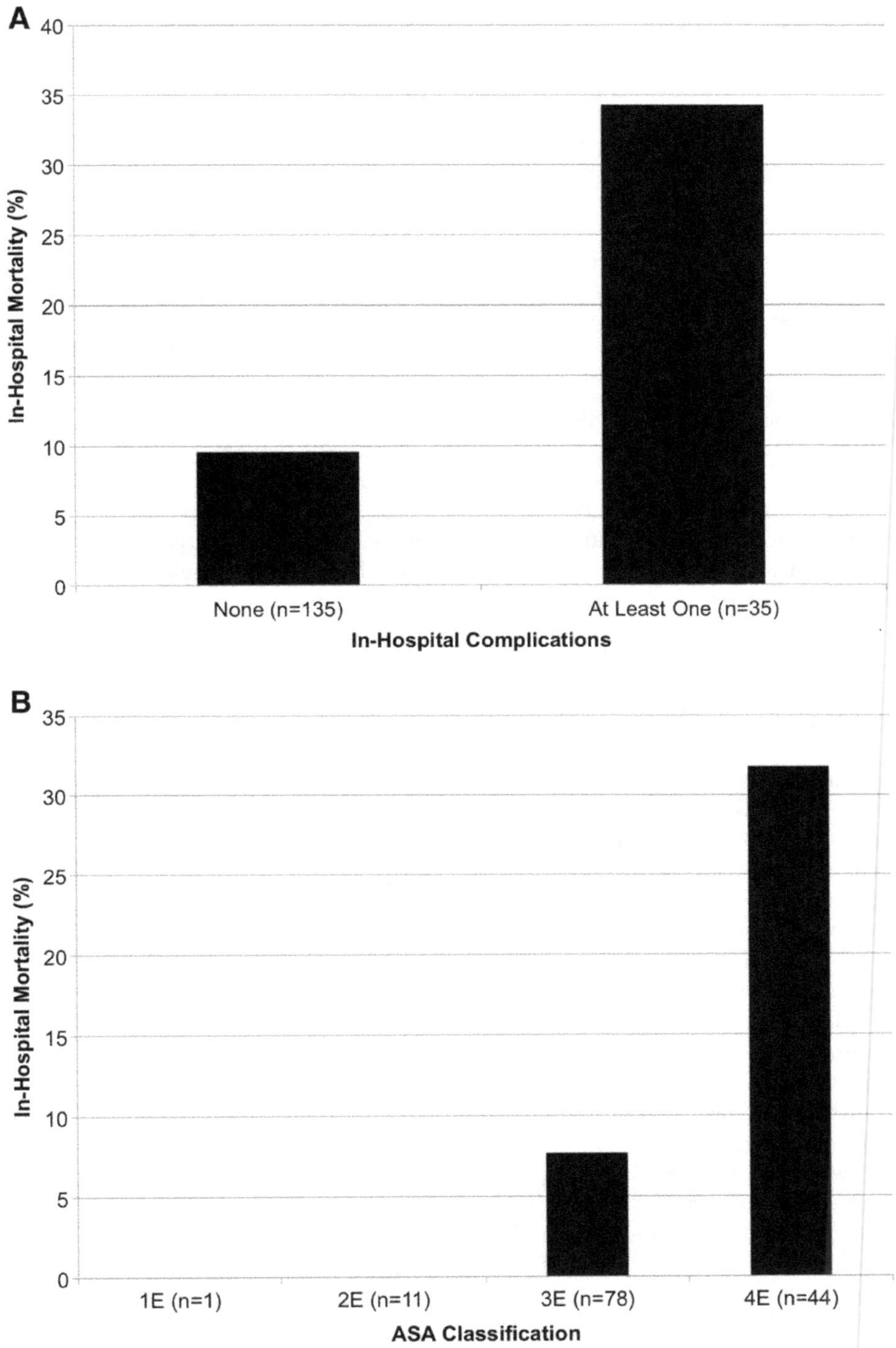

Figure 1 Multivariable Logistic regression analysis demonstrated statistically significant factors predictive of in-hospital mortality. Development of in-hospital complication is predictive of in-hospital mortality **(A)**, and increasing ASA class is predictive of in-hospital mortality **(B)**.

physiological insults and complications that an elderly patient may experience at a later time. By contrast the ASA classification, initially described by Saklad et al. 1941, can be quickly determined on admission [22]. It has been shown to be predictive of complications and mortality in a global surgical cohort [23]. Our study reinforces that higher ASA class is associated with mortality following emergency general surgery in the elderly. While anesthesia providers often use this score our study demonstrates the value for surgeons using the

Table 6 Factors associated with in-hospital morbidity - multivariable logistic regression analysis

Factor	B	p-value	OR	95% CI for OR	
				Lower	Upper
Age	-.096	.254	.908	.770	1.071
Sex (Female)	.051	.919	1.053	.392	2.828
BMI	.012	.826	1.013	.906	1.132
Medications	.118	.348	1.125	.879	1.440
Comorbidities	-.210	.304	.810	.543	1.210
ASA class	.409	.325	1.506	.667	3.399

ASA classification for preoperative risk stratification and discussions.

There may be reluctance by physicians to refer patients for surgical treatment due to advanced age and medical co-morbidities. However, our findings show there was no clear relationship between chronologic age or number of comorbidities with postoperative outcome (morbidity or mortality) after multivariable adjustment. Therefore, age or comorbidities alone should not be the limiting factors for surgical referral or treatment. For most of these surgically treated illnesses, withholding operative care will result in death. Our results indicate markedly higher mortality with rising ASA class. Specifically patients with ASA 4 (severe systemic disease that is a constant threat to life) had the highest risk of death at 33%. Which means surgeons can use this information preoperatively to give estimates of death and morbidity to patients and families.

Our analysis suggests that chronological age alone in the cohort of patients aged 80 and above is not a robust measure of outcome. This could be due to a lack of statistical power. However, it may also be that chronological age is not a major predictor of mortality once more important predictors, such as baseline physical health (ASA class), is accounted for. Or potentially there may even be a ceiling effect of age wherein age alone does not affect morality in the very elderly population.

Although it is always desirable to prevent complications, it is impossible to perform surgery that is complication free. Surgical complications in this group involve a complex interrelationship between baseline vulnerability and precipitating insults occurring during hospitalization [16]. Emergency abdominal surgery is accompanied by many such insults that place elders at particularly high risk for post-operative complications including fasting for gastrointestinal healing, addition of multiple drugs, immobility, nasogastric tubes, and bladder catheterization. Many of these are modifiable and attention to these risk factors should be assessed to prevent post-operative complications in this frail population. The results from this study underscore an important association between the development of complications and mortality. Therefore, this finding emphasizes the importance of implementing recommendations and best practices to prevent perioperative complications.

The present study is limited by its retrospective design, sample size, and recruitment from a single hospital. Understandably, only patients who could be included were those pre-selected by their surgeons for operative management, it is suspected that many elderly patients presenting to the emergency department with surgical disease that was managed non-operatively on non-surgical units or with end-of-life care goals.

Identifying patients at risk of developing in-hospital complications, and developing tailored preventative strategies, should be a focus to improve care for the elderly emergency general surgical patient. Age or number of comorbidies alone should not be the limiting factors for surgical referral or treatment. We advocate for the use of ASA class as both an available and robust tool for prediction of in-hospital mortality following emergency general surgery in very elderly patients. This information can be meaningful to patients and their families when used for perioperative counseling aimed at setting realistic expectations and assisting patients or surrogates decision makers to understand the goals of care and treatment.

Abbreviations

ASA: American Society of Anesthesiologist Physical Status; BMI: Body mass index; CPS: Comorbidity-Polypharmacy score.

Competing interests

The author(s) declare that they have no competing interests.

Authors' contributions

SM, RP, SW, RK contributed to study design. DH built a custom database for data acquisition. JP performed data acquisition, initial analysis, and wrote the initial draft manuscript. SM performed data analysis and wrote the final manuscript. All authors read and approved the final manuscript.

Acknowledgments

We gratefully thank the University of Alberta's ACES group for their support in this research. The ACES group includes: Drs. Ronald Brisebois, Klaus Buttenschoen, Kamran Fathimani, Stewart M Hamilton, Rachel G Khadaroo, Gordon M Lees, Todd PW McMullen, William Patton, Mary vanWijngaarden-Stephens, J Drew Sutherland, Sandy L Widder, and David C Williams. Thank you to Ms. Yvonne Tul for her editing of the paper. Funding for this study was from a University (Alberta) Hospital Foundation grant and the M.S.I. Foundation (RGK).

Author details

[1]Department of Surgery, Faculty of Medicine and Dentistry, University of Alberta, Edmonton, Alberta, Canada. [2]Department of Medicine, University of Alberta, Edmonton, Alberta, Canada. [3]Division of Critical Care Medicine, Faculty of Medicine and Dentistry, University of Alberta, Edmonton, Alberta,

Canada. [4]Department of Surgery, University of Alberta, 2D Walter Mackenzie Center, 8440-112 St. NW, Edmonton, Alberta T6G 2B7, Canada.

References

1. Christensen K, Doblhammer G, Rau R, Vaupel JW: **Ageing populations: the challenges ahead.** *Lancet* 2009, **374:**1196–1208.
2. Abbas S, Booth M: **Major abdominal surgery in octogenarians.** *N Z Med J* 2003, **116:**U402.
3. Rosenberg M, Moore E: **The health of Canada's elderly population: current status and future implications.** *Can Med Assoc J* 1997, **157:**1025–1032.
4. Canadian Institute for Health Information: *Health Care in Canada, 2011: A Focus on Seniors and Agingle*; 2011.
5. Statistics Canada: *Population Projections for Canada, Provinces and Territories, 2009 to 2036*; 2011.
6. Bettelli G: **Preoperative evaluation in geriatric surgery: comorbidity, functional status and pharmacological history.** *Minerva Anestesiol* 2011, **77:**637–646.
7. Dasgupta M, Rolfson DB, Stolee P, Borrie MJ, Speechley M: **Frailty is associated with postoperative complications in older adults with medical problems.** *Arch Gerontol Geriatr* 2009, **48:**78–83.
8. Turrentine FE, Wang H, Simpson VB, Jones RS: **Surgical risk factors, morbidity, and mortality in elderly patients.** *J Am Coll Surg* 2006, **203**(6):865–877.
9. Story DA, Finkf M, Myles KLPS, Yap SJ, Beavistt V, Kerridgeii R-K, Mcnicol PL: **Perioperative mortality risk score using pre- and postoperative risk factors in older patients.** *Anaesth Intensive Care.* 2009, **37**(3):392–398.
10. Robinson TN, Wallace JI, Wu DS, Wiktor A, Pointer LF, Pfister SM, Sharp TJ, Buckley MJ, Moss M: **Accumulated frailty characteristics predict postoperative discharge institutionalization in the geriatric patient.** *J Am Coll Surg* 2011, **213:**34–37.
11. Louis D, Hsu A, Brand M, Saclarides T: **Morbidity and Mortality in Octogenarians and Older Undergoing Major Intestinal Surgery.** *Dis Colon Rectum* 2009, **1:**59–63.
12. Devon KM, Urbach DR, McLeod RS: **Postoperative disposition and health services use in elderly patients undergoing colorectal cancer surgery: a population-based study.** *Surgery* 2011, **149:**705–712.
13. Akinbami F, Askari R, Steinberg J, Panizales M, Rogers SO: **Factors affecting morbidity in emergency general surgery.** *Am J Surg* 2011, **201:**456–462.
14. Pelavski AD, Lacasta A, Rochera MI, De Miguel M, Roige J: **Observational study of nonogenarians undergoing emergency, non-trauma surgery.** *Br J Anaesth* 2011, **106**(November 2010):189–193.
15. Alcock M, Chilvers CR: **Emergency surgery in the elderly: a retrospective observational study.** *Anaesth Intensive Care* 2012, **40:**90–94.
16. Inouye SK: **Prevention of delirium in hospitalized older patients: risk factors and targeted intervention strategies.** *Ann Med* 2000, **32:**257–263.
17. Evans DC, Cook CH, Christy JM, Murphy CV, Gerlach AT, Eiferman D, Lindsey DE, Whitmill ML, Papadimos TJ, Beery PR, Steinberg SM, Stawicki SP: **Comorbidity-Polypharmacy Scoring Facilitates Outcome Prediction in Older Trauma Patients.** *J Am Geriatr Soc* 2012, **60**(8):1465–1470.
18. Population Division US Census Bureau: *Projections of the Population by Age and Sex for the United States: 2010 to 2050 (NP2008-T12)*; 2008.
19. Gazala S, Tul Y, Wagg A, Widder S, Khadaroo RG: **Quality of life and long-term outcomes of octo- and nonagenarians following acute care surgery: a cross sectional study.** *World J Emerg Surg* 2013, **8:**23.
20. Hilmer SN, Perera V, Mitchell S, Murnion BP, Dent J, Bajorek B, Matthews S, Rolfson DB: **The assessment of frailty in older people in acute care.** *Australas J Ageing* 2009, **28:**182–188.
21. Minne L, Ludikhuize J, De Jonge E, De Rooij S, Abu-hanna A: **Prognostic models for predicting mortality in elderly ICU patients: a systematic review.** *Intensive Care Med* 2011, **37:**1258–1268.
22. Keats AS: **The ASA classification of physical status–a recapitulation.** *Anesthesiology* 1978, **49:**233–236.
23. Wolters U, Wolf T, Stützer H, Schröder T, Pichlmaier H: **Risk factors, complications, and outcome in surgery: a multivariate analysis.** *Eur J Surg* 1997, **163:**563–568.

6

Diaphragmatic rupture causing repeated vomiting in a combined abdominal and head injury patient

Dimitrios Symeonidis*, Michail Spyridakis, Georgios Koukoulis, Grigorios Christodoulidis, Ioannis Mamaloudis and Konstantinos Tepetes

Abstract

Background: Diaphragmatic rupture after blunt abdominal injury is a rare trauma condition. Delayed diagnosis is not uncommon especially in the emergency room setting. Associated injuries often shift diagnosis and treatment priorities towards other more life-threatening conditions.

Case presentation: We present a challenging case of a young male with combined abdominal and head trauma. Repeated episodes of vomiting dominated on clinical presentation that in the presence of a deep scalp laceration and facial bruising shifted differential diagnosis towards a traumatic brain injury. However, a computed tomography scan of the brain ruled out any intracranial pathology. Finally, a more meticulous investigation with additional imaging studies confirmed the presence of diaphragmatic rupture that justified the clinical symptoms.

Conclusions: The combination of diaphragmatic rupture with head injury creates a challenging trauma scenario. Increased level of suspicion is essential in order to diagnose timely diaphragmatic rupture in multiple trauma patients.

Keywords: Abdominal trauma, Diaphragmatic rupture, Multiple trauma, Motor vehicle accident, Emergency Surgery

Background

Diaphragmatic rupture (DR) after blunt abdominal trauma is a rare condition usually masked by multiple associated injuries [1,2]. The overall incidence of diaphragmatic injury is 2.5 - 5% in blunt abdominal trauma and 1.5% in blunt thoracic trauma [1]. Left sided injuries are substantially more frequent [1,2]. However, bilateral injuries have also been reported [2]. Delayed diagnosis is not uncommon especially in the emergency room (ER) setting. Despite improvement in investigative techniques a significant amount of these injuries are overlooked. Associated injuries often shift diagnosis and treatment priorities towards other more life-threatening conditions.

However, constant clinical surveillance and repeated evaluations of the patient are of paramount importance in order to minimize the likelihood of missing injuries with non-typical clinical presentation such as DR. Non-specific symptoms emanating from the respiratory system i.e. dyspnea often are the only clues for the diagnosis [3]. On the other hand, strangulation and perforation represent the final devastating consequences of the prolonged herniation of the abdominal organs into the chest [3]. Sometimes, a displaced nasogastric tube within the left hemi thorax, a diagnostic sign in chest x-ray, establishes the diagnosis of DR in asymptomatic trauma patients [3,4]. In the present report, we present a challenging case of a combined abdominal and head trauma patient. Repeated episodes of vomiting dominated on clinical presentation that on the absence of other clues shifted differential diagnosis towards a traumatic brain injury. However, a DR was finally diagnosed that justified the clinical symptoms.

* Correspondence: simeonid@hotmail.com
Department of General Surgery, University Hospital of Larissa, Mezourlo, 41110, Larissa, Greece

Case presentation

A 32-year-old, unrestrained male driver was involved in head-on motor vehicle accident at high speed. He was initially evaluated at the pre-hospital setting and was reported to be hemodynamically stable. On arrival, his score on the Glasgow Coma Scale was 15, blood pressure 110/75 mm Hg, pulse rate 100/min, and respiratory rate 17/min. The patent had a deep scalp laceration, signs of recent nasal bleeding and facial bruising suggestive of a high-energy head injury while he was also complaining of a mild mid-epigastrium pain.

On exam, the patient was alert and oriented. The chest wall was not tender to palpation. Auscultation of the chest wall did not reveal any pathology. The abdomen was non-distended, soft with mild tenderness however to palpation of the upper abdomen (mid-epigastrium). Motor and sensory function of all extremities was intact. The urine was grossly clear. Initial radiographic studies included a supine chest film that besides a widened mediastinum was generally inconclusive. Ultrasonography in the trauma unit did not show any abnormal fluid collection. The initial hematocrit value was 39.5% and blood gas pH was 7.37 with a base deficit of 3.8. Meanwhile the patient started complaining of nausea and several blood-spotted vomiting episodes were noted. An investigation in the direction of a traumatic brain injury was conducted with a standard protocol head Computed Tomography (CT) scan. No evidences of midline shift were observed. The presence of a possible intracranial hematoma or a cranial bone fracture was ruled out. Notable oedema of the facial soft tissues, without however underlining fractures, was an additional finding. Approximately, six hours after the initial imaging evaluation, the persistence of patient's symptoms i. e. vomiting as well as the migration of pain into the lower thorax dictated an additional workup. A second chest x-ray was obtained. Figure 1. An elevated left hemi-diaphragm with the stomach in the left chest was observed. Abdominal CT scan confirmed the presence of a left-sided diaphragmatic tear with herniation of abdominal context within the left hemi-thorax. Figure 2.

The patient underwent emergency laparotomy via a midline incision where a near total herniation of the stomach into the left hemithorax was observed. No resection was necessary as there were no ischemic changes or signs of perforation of the involved organ. The stomach was then successfully reduced into the abdomen revealing the hernia opening about 5 cm in length. Figure 3. A primary repair with interrupted non-absorbable sutures was carried out without the use of a prosthetic mesh. Figure 4. The relatively small size of the hernia opening was the main argument for this approach. A chest tube was not necessary as pleura was not violated and a pneumothorax was not present. Operating time was 45 minutes. The patient had an uneventful postoperative period and was discharged on the fifth postoperative day.

Discussion

DR after blunt abdominal injury is a rare trauma condition. Correct diagnosis is often difficult and is usually established late raising significantly the associated mortality and morbidity. Single or serial plain chest radiographs with a high index of suspicion are diagnostic in many cases of DR [1,4,5]. However, missed cases result in herniation of the abdominal organs into the chest which finally enlarges the diaphragm defect. Chronic intermittent abdominal or chest pain, constipation, strangulation and perforation of the involved abdominal viscera are symptoms and consequences associated with the progressive herniation of the abdominal organs into the chest. As lung on the affected side is compressed, shortness of breath, dyspnea, and respiratory infections appear [3].

Tears of the diaphragm usually originate at the musculotendinous junction, mostly in the posterolateral aspect

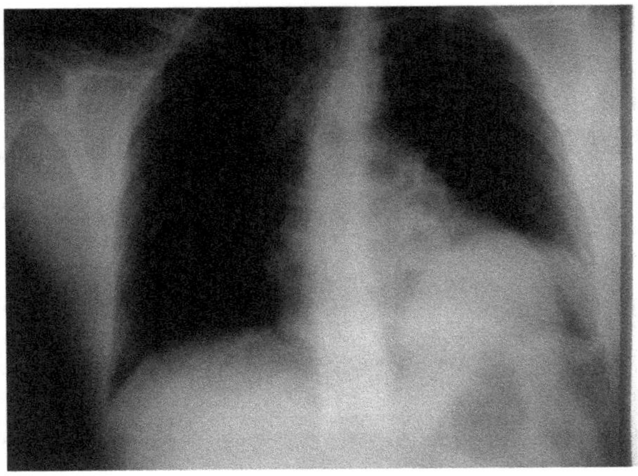

Figure 1 Plain chest x-ray with the stomach in the left hemi-diaphragm.

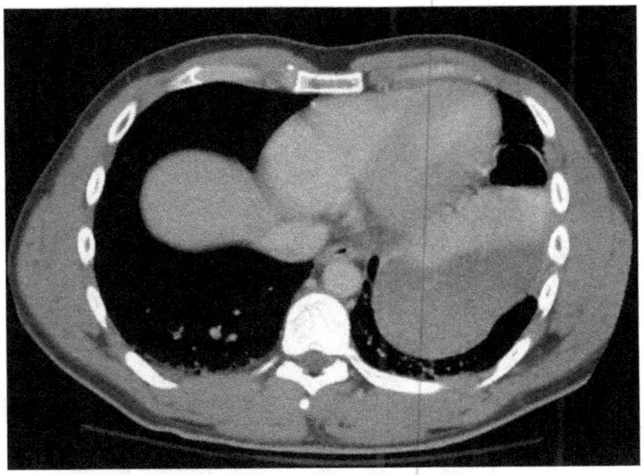

Figure 2 Computed tomography scan image showing the herniation of the stomach into the chest.

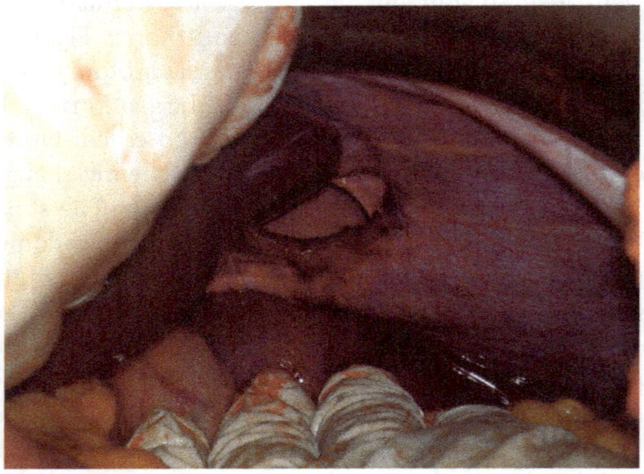

Figure 3 An intraoperative photo showing the diaphragmatic defect after the reduction of the hernia contents .

of the hemidiaphragms. The majority of these tears are on the left side. Either the relative weakness of the left hemidiaphragm or the protective effect of the liver on the right side represents possible explanations. Irrespective of the cause, right-sided rupture is associated with increased severity of injury and, therefore, increased mortality and morbidity rates [6]. Approximately 80-90% of diaphragm injuries are related to automobile accidents. Falls or crush injuries to the diaphragm are rarer injury mechanisms. Lateral-impact automobile accident is three times more likely to cause a DR than any other impact type [7,8].

The usual scenario is the combination of DR with other types of injuries. Thoracic aortic tears, rib fractures, splenic injuries, pelvic fractures and hepatic injuries are the commonest associations [9]. Although this appears more as an observation with limited responsiveness in clinical practice, it could collectively identify patients at risk for blunt diaphragmatic rupture when certain injury patterns show up. A more expeditious and thorough work up in the right direction, i.e. diaphragmatic trauma is the minimum benefit for the multiple trauma patient [9]. On the other hand, head injuries, regardless of the severity, are not usually associated with concurrent blunt DR. Wide variations in the incidence of this injury combination are the rule in the literature. Table 1. Single institutions experience with remarkable variations in diagnostic and treatment tactics expressed via relatively small case series represent the vast majority of the reported cases. However, despite the relatively limited correlation between these two conditions - DR and head injury - complications due to a concurrent head injury accounted for the majority of deaths in a series of sixty patients with blunt abdominal trauma and DR [10].

As soon as the diagnosis of a DR is established a surgical repair is warrant to prevent possible complications. A midline laparotomy is the advocated approach for repair of acute diaphragmatic trauma as it offers the possibility of diagnosing and repairing other associated intra-abdominal injuries. However thoracoscopy or laparoscopy in hemodynamically stable patients represents valid alternatives for the diagnosis and repair of a missed diaphragmatic injury especially in cases of penetrating left thoraco-abdominal trauma. Generally, repair with non-absorbable simple sutures is adequate in most cases [16]. The use of mesh should be reserved for chronic and large defects [16,17].

In our case, the combined abdominal and head injury confused the diagnostic field. Concomitant maxillofacial injuries as well as the deep scalp laceration in a patient with repeated episodes of vomiting rendered traumatic brain injury as the most likely diagnosis. However, the imaging investigation ruled out a central nervous system lesion as the cause of the patient's symptoms i.e. vomiting. The consistency of symptoms as well as the alterations of pain characteristics during the initial phase of patient's observation was the main arguments for the

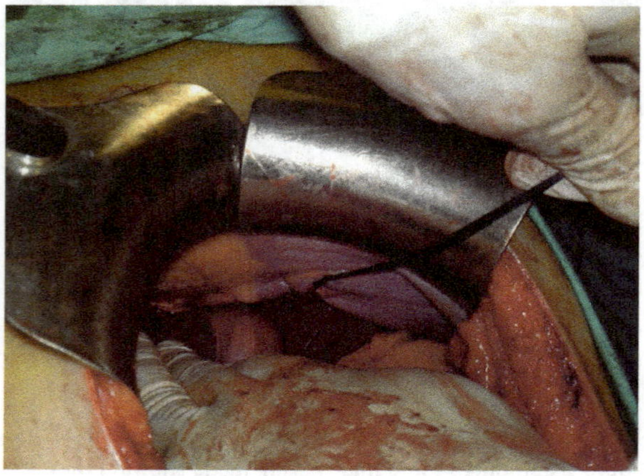

Figure 4 An intraoperative photo showing the final repair result.

Table 1 Representative case series with combined diaphragmatic rupture (DR) and head injury

	Total number of patient with DR	Combined DR and head injury patients	% Co - existence
Simpson et al. 2000 [11]	16	4	**25,0%**
Chen et al. 1991 [12]	62	3	**4,8%**
Pfannschmidt et al. 1994 [13]	58	22	**37,9%**
Balci et al. 2004 [14]	137	33	**24,0%**
Ilgenfritz et al. 1992 [15]	52	21	**40,3%**

additional imaging workup [18]. The pathognomonic sign in the chest x-ray with the stomach or the nasogastric tube in the hemithorax was not present in the chest radiography conducted at the trauma resuscitation unit. However, a nasogastric tube placement was contraindicated in our patient due to maxillofacial injuries and additionally a high quality chest x-ray could not be obtained until a work-up that could reliably rule out a cervical spine injury conducted.

Within the framework of a more meticulous investigation in order to delineate occult pathology to justify the clinical symptoms, a second chest x-ray under more appropriate conditions at the radiology department was obtained. The presence of the stomach within the left hemithorax was observed. Abdominal CT scan confirmed the herniation of the stomach into the chest and additionally ruled out any associated intraabdominal injuries. An urgent laparotomy at the base of DR was conducted. Regarding the repair technique we used intermittent non absorbable suture material in order to approximate the edges of the diaphragmatic defect. We assumed that the use of a prosthetic mesh in the given case with the relatively small diaphragmatic defect would increase the risk of infection and the procedure cost without corresponding benefits in the long term.

Conclusions

Increased level of suspicion is essential in order to diagnose timely blunt DR in multiple trauma patients. Early diagnosis can lead to the proper surgical management and reduce the incidence of hernia related complications.

Consent

Written informed consent was obtained from the patient for publication of this Case report and any accompanying images. A copy of the written consent is available for review by the Editor-in-Chief of this journal.

Competing interests

The authors declare that they have no competing interests.

Authors' contribution

SD, CG, KG and MI acquired the data and drafted the article. SD, SM and TK analysed and interpreted the data. SD and TK critically revised the article. SM, CG, SD and KG performed the surgical operation. All authors read and approved the final manuscript.

References

1. Matsevych OY: **Blunt diaphragmatic rupture: four years' experience.** *Hernia* 2008, **12**(1):73–78.
2. Shah R, Sabanathan S, Mearns AJ, Choudhury AK: **Traumatic rupture of diaphragm.** *Ann Thorac Surg* 1995, **60**(5):1444–1449.
3. Turhan K, Makay O, Cakan A, Samancilar O, Firat O, Icoz G: **Traumatic diaphragmatic rupture: look to see.** *Eur J Cardiothorac Surg* 2008, **33**:1082–1085.
4. Nau T, Seitz H, Mousavi M, Vecsei V: **The diagnostic dilemma of traumatic rupture of the diaphragm.** *Surg Endosc* 2001, **15**(9):992–996.
5. Guth AA, Pachter HL, Kim U: **Pitfalls in the diagnosis of blunt diaphragmatic injury.** *Am J Surg* 1995, **170**(1):5–9.
6. Boulanger BR, Milzman DP, Rosati C, Rodriguez A: **A comparison of right and left blunt traumatic diaphragmatic rupture.** *J Trauma* 1993, **35**(2):255–260.
7. Lee WC, Chen RJ, Fang JF, Wang CC, Chen HY, Chen SC, *et al*: **Rupture of the diaphragm after blunt trauma.** *Eur J Surg* 1994, **160**(9):479–483.
8. Sharma OP: **Traumatic diaphragmatic rupture: not an uncommon entity-personal experience with collective review of the 1980's.** *J Trauma* 1989, **29**(5):678–682.
9. Reiff DA, McGwin G Jr, Metzger J, Windham ST, Doss M, Rue LW 3rd: **Identifying injuries and motor vehicle collision characteristics that together are suggestive ofdiaphragmatic rupture.** *J Trauma* 2002, **53**(6):1139–1145.
10. Chughtai T, Ali S, Sharkey P, Lins M, Rizoli S: **Update on managing diaphragmatic rupture in blunt trauma: a review of 208 consecutive cases.** *Can J Surg* 2009, **52**(3):177–181.
11. Simpson J, Lobo DN, Shah AB, Rowlands BJ: **Traumatic diaphragmatic rupture: associated injuries and outcome.** *Ann R Coll Surg Engl* 2000, **82**(2):97–100.
12. Chen JC, Wilson SE: **Diaphragmatic injuries: recognition and management in sixty-two patients.** *Am Surg* 1991, **57**(12):810–815.
13. Pfannschmidt J, Seiler H, Böttcher H, Karadiakos N, Heisterkamp B: **Diaphragmatic ruptures: diagnosis–therapy-results, experiences with 64 patients.** *Aktuelle Traumatol* 1994, **24**(2):48–51.
14. Balci AE, Kazez A, Eren S, Ayan E, Ozalp K, Eren MN: **Blunt thoracic trauma in children: review of 137 cases.** *Eur J Cardiothorac Surg* 2004, **26**(2):387–392.
15. Ilgenfritz FM, Stewart DE: **Blunt trauma of the diaphragm: a 15-county, private hospital experience.** *Am Surg* 1992, **58**(6):334–338.
16. Hanna WC, Ferri LE: **Acute traumatic diaphragmatic injury.** *Thorac Surg Clin* 2009, **19**(4):485–489.
17. Kuhn R, Schubert D, Wolff St, Marusch F, Lippert H, Pross M: **Repair of diaphragmatic rupture by laparoscopic implantation of a polytetrafluoroethylene patch.** *Surg Endosc* 2002, **16**(10):1495.
18. Patselas TN, Gallagher EG: **The diagnostic dilemma of diaphragm injury.** *Am Surg* 2002, **68**(7):633–639.

7

WSES position paper on vascular emergency surgery

Bruno Monteiro T. Pereira[1], Osvaldo Chiara[2*], Fabio Ramponi[3], Dieter G. Weber[4], Stefania Cimbanassi[2], Belinda De Simone[5], Korana Musicki[3], Guilherme Vieira Meirelles[1], Fausto Catena[5], Luca Ansaloni[6], Federico Coccolini[6], Massimo Sartelli[7], Salomone Di Saverio[8], Cino Bendinelli[4*] and Gustavo Pereira Fraga[1*]

Abstract

Trauma, both blunt and penetrating, is extremely common worldwide, as trauma to major vessels. The management of these patients requires specialized surgical skills and techniques of the trauma surgeon. Furthermore few other surgical emergencies require immediate diagnosis and treatment like a ruptured abdominal aortic aneurysm (rAAA). Mortality of patients with a rAAA reaches 85 %, with more than half dying before reaching the hospital. These are acute events demanding immediate intervention to save life and limb and precluding any attempt at transfer or referral. It is the purpose of this position paper to discuss neck, chest, extremities and abdominal trauma, bringing to light recent evidence based data as well as expert opinions; besides, in this paper we present a review of the recent literature on rAAA and we discuss the rationale for transfer to referral center, the role of preoperative imaging and the pros and cons of Endoluminal repair of rAAA (REVAR) versus Open Repair (OR).

Keywords: Trauma, Vascular injuries, Vascular control, Ruptured abdominal aorta aneurism, Vascular Trauma: Neck, Chest and Extremities

Introduction

Trauma, both blunt and penetrating, is extremely common worldwide. As a result, trauma to major vessels is a not uncommon clinical occurrence. These are acute events demanding immediate intervention to save life and limb and precluding any attempt at transfer or referral. Therefore, the particular specialized surgical skills, techniques and materials for the care of these patients need to be at the disposal of the trauma surgeon. It is the purpose of this position paper to discuss neck, chest and extremities trauma, bringing to light recent evidence based data as well as expert opinions. Also, this will focus on the treatment of injured arteries, although attention will be given to those venous injuries, which require surgical repair rather than simple ligation.

* Correspondence: ochiara@yahoo.com; cino.bendinelli@hnehealth.nsw.gov.au; fragagp2008@gmail.com
[2]Trauma Team, Ospedale Niguarda Milano, Milan, Italy
[4]Department of Traumatology, John Hunter Hospital, Newcastle, NSW, Australia
[1]Division of Trauma Surgery, Department of Surgery, School of Medical Sciences, University of Campinas (Unicamp), Campinas, SP, Brazil

The literature is filled of epidemiological researches demonstrating the features of vascular trauma in a variety of countries [1–9]. There is wide variation in the incidence, cause and mechanism of injury depending on geographic conditions. In Australia vascular injuries represent 1–2 % of total trauma patients [5–9], however it account for 20 % of all trauma related death [5]. Deaths from vascular injury diverge considerably with anatomic location and mechanism of injury. Thoracic vascular injuries routinely have death rates between 30–50 %; vascular injuries to extremities are significantly lower in the range of 5 %, in a civilian reality. In an unparalleled large study from Vietnam, Rich and colleagues [10] reported a total death of only 1.7 % for all vascular injuries. It may be that life-threatening vascular injuries were preselected by their failure to survive transport. In the current warfare conditions of the American intervention in Iraq and Afghanistan,Fox and his group reported that vascular trauma represents 7 % of total battle injuries, 88 % of these were extremity injuries [11]. The amputation rate was only 8 % after vascular repair. In North India [3], with a low risk of personal violence, blunt injuries, mostly motor vehicle accidents, account for 84 %

of vascular injuries. Whereas in Medellin, Colombia [6] 93 % of vascular injuries are penetrating and in Georgia, USA they represent 85 % of the total [2]. Surprisingly, in the western European experience [8], up to 40 % of vascular injuries are iatrogenic, as a result of vascular and other surgical interventions. Jaha et al, recently reported a survival rate of plus 95 % for multiple mechanisms of vascular injuries in Kosovo, most of those were penetrating peripheral vascular trauma (78.3 %) [12]. Kuwait [1] strikes a middle ground with 41 % penetrating, 23 % a result of road traffic accidents (RTA). In Malaysia [4], over 50 % of vascular injuries occur as a result of RTAs differently from a British Trauma Center experience [13]. As far as anatomic site of injury is concerned, variability is less. In Australia [5–9] injuries are split almost equally between thorax, abdomen and upper and lower extremities, with cervical injuries being less common. In Latin America [7], extremity injuries are twice as common as thoracic and abdominal, although these later result in a higher mortality [14, 15]. As far as extremities are concerned upper and lower injuries occur with similar frequency and the brachial, femoral and popliteal arteries are the most commonly injured vessels [16].

General principles for vascular injuries

Before specifically talk about neck, chest and extremities vascular injuries some basic principles must be reviewed.

Traumatic vascular lesions in general have a similar pattern of injury. They are either penetrating or blunt. Still, can be subdivided into high/ low velocity penetrating injury (i.e.: war caliber rifle injury, hand gun injury, shotgun injury, stab wound); blunt vascular injuries caused by joint displacements, bone fractures, contusions; blast injuries provoked by mines, improvised explosion devices, bombs, shrapnel, etc.

In one way or another, the pattern of injury is straight related to the kinetic energy and stretching force, ending up in general, in a similar injury-type such as contusion, total/partial transection and arterio-venous fistulae. Actual management though, may vary depending on the mechanism of injury.

The watershed here is to determine whether or not the presenting patient has palpable pulses. Clinical examination is paramount in these vascular trauma situations and the presence of distal palpable pulse (when possible to measure), even if diminished, already suggests that proximal artery injury is limited. Serial clinical examinations are mandatory. Use of a hand held bedside Doppler is extremely helpful. Table 1 presents hard/soft signs for arterial injuries, which are important to determine medical treatment.

Key management principles on vascular injuries

The care of a trauma victim begins with initial assessment and resuscitation according to the ABC Principles. These do not vary for those trauma patients with vascular injury.

Standard exposures for major arteries and veins are well defined and should be adopted in regular trauma cases. Specific surgical techniques must be mastered if successful vascular repair is to be achieved. These include: proximal and distal exposure for control with vascular clamps and loops; dissection and isolation of injured vessels including veins; heparinization (local and/or systemic); use of vascular sutures; magnification loops; assessment of injury: debridement, contusion, intimal flap and distal dissection and thombosis; selective use of temporary shunting (Argyle); anatomic repairs: with vein patch, end/end anastomosis without tension and reversed autologous vein graft for larger defects; technical details of spatulated ends, running versus interrupted sutures; distal thrombectomy; completion arteriography; fasciotomy and soft tissue coverage. Proper handling of the autogenous vein graft is important.

Attention is needed for peripheral vascular trauma in general when compartment syndrome is a complication risk factor. Suspect of compartment syndrome if prolonged period of shock, arterial occlusion, combined arteriovenous injury, need for arterial or venous ligation, crush injuries, massive tissue damage and swelling. In such cases, fasciotomy is mandatory [20, 21].

Table 1 Hard signs and soft signs of arterial injury [17–19]

Hard signs of arterial injury	Soft signs of arterial injury
(Requires immediate surgery)	(Consider further examination)
External arterial bleeding	History of arterial bleeding at the scene
Rapidly expanding hematoma	Proximity of penetrating/blunt trauma to major artery
Palpable thrill	Diminished unilateral distal pulse
Audible bruit	Small nonpulsatile hematoma
Obvious arterial occlusion (6 p 's: pulseless, pallor, paresthesia, paralysis, poikilothermia)	Neurologic deficit
	Abnormal Ankle-Brachial pressure index (<0.9)
	Abnormal flow-velocity waveform on Doppler ultrasound

Key principles: author's recommendations

- Gain proximal and distal vascular control before attempting to explore a hematoma.
- Avoid large vessels dissections when not necessary, but value good injury exposure.
- Get aware about patient's total trauma burden and physiology.
- Decide for vascular damage control early in time (Argyle shunt).
- Balloon catheters (i.e.: Fogarty) proximal and distal to artery repair, before shunt insertion.
- Regional Heparin (50 units/ml) for arterial injuries (proximal and distal to repair). Analyze if systemic heparinization is possible.
- Completion arteriography, if patient is stable.
- Venous repair is not a must.
- Perform fasciotomy when indicated.

Neck vascular trauma

Blunt neck vascular injuries

Blunt neck trauma (BNT) is known to be rare occurring about 5 % of time of all neck traumas. There are various sources of blunt neck trauma and each is associated with a specific pattern of injury.

Vascular injury occurs in 1–3 % of all BNT and is associated with 20–30 % mortality. It mostly occurs with motor vehicle collisions. Rapid deceleration causes hyperflexion, hyperextension, and rotation of the neck. As a result, the vascular structures are stretched over the cervical spine leading to shearing forces on the vessels and subsequent intimal tears in the vessel wall. Hard signs and soft signs of injury must be detected. Often blunt vascular injury initially manifests in the form of acute ischemic stroke and can be delayed in onset [22]. Classic presentation includes a neurologically intact patient who develops hemiparesis after a high-speed motor vehicle crash. Evaluation by four-vessel angiography remains the gold standard given its sensitivity of 99 % but it is invasive and has a significant complication rate. CT Angiogram (CTA) has excellent accuracy in detecting clinically significant injuries [23, 24]. These modalities can be used as adjuncts to evaluation but are not first-line. Duplex Ultrasound has sensitivity of 90–95 % but it is operator dependent. In general, surgical repair is preferred over ligation and primary repair is preferred over grafting [25].

Penetrating neck vascular injuries

Penetrating neck wounds are often dramatic and require immediate action. When the penetrating mechanism transects the platysma, it is not unclear whether patients without obvious vascular or visceral cervical injuries should not undergo routine exploration: selective exploration is the standard of care [23]. Penetrating injuries to the neck have been divided into three zones: zone 1, from the sternal notch to cricoid cartilage; zone 2, from the cricoid cartilage to the angle of the mandible; zone 3, from the angle of the mandible to the skull base.

Suspected vascular injury in zones 1 and 3 in the presence of hard signs of intra-cranial dysfunction mandates arteriography prior to exploration. Zone 2 injuries are recommended to undergo prompt exploration. Study of the neurologic outcomes in neck injuries shows that the risk of cerebral infarction is unpredictable but that repair of injured vessels gives a more favorable outcome than ligation [27].

Penetrating injuries to the neck also can vary on its mechanism. Glass-Coated kite lines – Fig. 1 [26], Stab wounds, GSW, etc. Gunshot wounds are challenging injuries to repair, are usually related to severe vascular injuries, pharynx, airways, GI, thorax. Help of an interventional radiologist for an endovascular approach is frequently required. Injuries to the vertebral artery can be tricky and very difficult to approach, especially in its zone III topography just before becoming the named basilar artery. Endovascular obliteration of the vertebral artery (VA) as well as its ligation may be preferred and a plausible solution in an *extremis* situation, although exposure of the VA isn't easy and you may not have fast access to the angiographic suite for an endovascular procedure. In such cases, pushing a piece of bone wax into the bleeding hole usually works fine and stops the brisk bleeding coming from the VA. Internal Jugular Vein may also be ligated as a damage control measure.

For the carotid artery (CA) injuries we suggest you to go simple with no cool repairs or exotic maneuvers. Occasions affording simple repairs or end-to-end anastomosis are rare. To our experience they are usually present in low energy clean lacerations such as stab wounds caused by a dagger for instance. Our

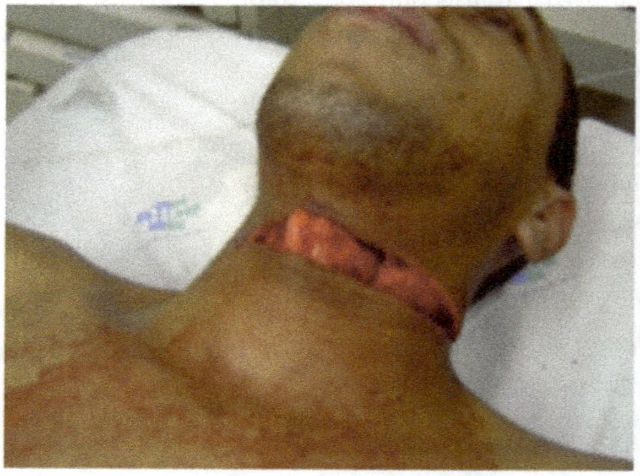

Fig. 1 Glass-coated kite line zone II neck injury

recommendation to these low complex injuries is primary repair, the use of a synthetic graft or patch to reconstruct the carotid depending on how large is the defect, when patient's physiology allows you to proceed with this. When patient is about to breach the physiologic envelope or when there is multiple life threatening injuries associated, ligation of the CA is a valid option. When considering ligation you may be deciding for saving the patient's life with the risk of a neurologic deficit, such as a stroke. When breaking through a zone III CA ligation is your only realistic option [28–30].

Authors recommendations

- Evaluate the neck fully. A C-Spine collar might obscure wounds. Take off the dressings.
- Value the mechanism of injury in blunt neck injuries.
- Be aware of insidious vascular injuries in BNT.
- Clinical signs can be similar to a stroke in BNT.
- Evaluate the location of the wounds to get a sense of the neck zone.
- If the wound does not penetrate the platysma, then it is likely that no further evaluation is required and the patient can be discharged home. If platysmal penetration is not certain, then a CT scan can be performed to rule out penetration.
- A CXR should be obtained in all circumstances (assuming the platysma has been penetrated).
- External hemorrhage should be managed by direct pressure. *Do not* probe/explore the wound. Insertion of an NG tube should be withheld until the patient is in the operating room.
- Patients should be evaluated specifically with a history and physical evaluating for changes in phonation, odynophagia, cranial nerve abnormalities, paresthesia or weakness in the extremities. *Horner's syndrome* (miosis, ptosis, anhydrosis) is often missed as are physical evidence of injuries to the hypoglossal or spinal accessory nerve. If intact, document the normal exam.
- Exploration requires evaluation of the carotid sheath and its structures, the esophagus, and the larynx/trachea. The trajectory of the impaling instrument/missile should be followed. Areas might be omitted from exploration if they are not in the trajectory.

Chest vascular trauma

Blunt thoracic vascular injuries

Blunt thoracic aortic injury is the most severe thoracic vascular injury. This is a specific clinical syndrome related to high impact deceleration injuries and high injury severity scores. Although treatable, it causes significant mortality related partially to delayed diagnosis [25]. About 50 % of victims die on impact, in the rest the bleeding is temporarily contained by the aortic adventitia and pleura and these patients are potentially salvageable. The injury typically occurs at the site of the ligamentum arteriosum, just distal to the take off of the left subclavian artery. Shear forces and stretching of the aorta are likely mechanisms of injury. The classic sign of widened mediastinum is unreliable and investigation should be carried out in cases where there is a high index of suspicion [31]. No controversy remains regarding arch arteriography or CT scanning: Moore et al. demonstrated CT had essentially 100 % negative predictive value [31]. It appears that the use of heparin-bonded shunts allows improved results with a lower incidence of paraplegia. Endovascular techniques are playing an expanding role in the treatment of this problem [32]. Massive hemothorax requiring thoracotomy is defined as plus to 1–1.5 L at the time of insertion of chest drains or 200–300 ml/hr for the subsequent 4 h. Some of these cases will involve injury to the pulmonary vessels [33, 34]. Operative repair of aortic arch is through a median sternotomy and may require use of total cardiopulmonary bypass and insertion of a graft.

The overall incidence of blunt aortic injury has remained the same over the past 12 years despite advances in vehicle restraint systems [33].

Similar mechanisms are implicated in the injury of the non-aortic great vessels as well. Regardless of the mechanism or mechanisms, the result is vessel wall disruption, occlusion, or avulsion. Shearing can result in all of these and compression more often results in occlusion. A small intimal disruption can lead to thrombus formation and subsequent vascular occlusion [34]. Innominate artery and left carotid injuries usually occur proximally at the vessel origin. In contrast, blunt subclavian injuries tend to be more distal [11, 35].

Comparing those patients with penetrating injury, blunt thoracic great vessel injuries are less incident. In general, penetrating injuries result in higher mortality, more combined arterial and venous injures, and lower morbidity than those presenting with blunt trauma. Mortality for blunt injury has been reported between zero and 24 %.

Penetrating thoracic vascular injuries

In thoracic penetrating injuries, the trajectory of the projectile or of the blunt object is the key to determine the anatomic structures involved. In general, missile trajectories that pass through the midline are at more risk for significant vascular injuries [36, 37].

Penetrating injuries involving the ascending arch of the aorta are uncommon. Survival rates approach 50 % for patients having stable vital signs on arrival at a trauma center. Although primary repair of anterior lacerations can be accomplished without adjuncts, cardiopulmonary bypass may be required if there is an additional posterior injury.

For an injury to the transverse aortic arch, extension of the median sternotomy to the neck allows complete exposure of the arch and brachiocephalic branches. If necessary, exposure can be enhanced further by division of the innominate vein. Simple lacerations may be repaired by lateral aortorrhaphy. With difficult lesions such as posterior lacerations or those with concomitant pulmonary artery injuries, cardiopulmonary bypass can be employed [38].

Patients with thoracic vascular injuries are either exsanguinating or have a potential bleeding contained injury. In one way or another one should be followed up in a TICU or SICU.

Bellow you find author's recommendations for both blunt and penetrating mechanism of injury.

Authors recommendations by vessel injury

Innominate Artery& Descending Thoracic Aorta

- The proximal innominate artery and aortic arch are best approached by a median sternotomy. Early ligation of the innominate vein as well as associated thymic tissue in the anterior mediastinum will aid in exposing the aortic arch.
- The proximal descending aorta is approached by a postero-lateral thoracothomy.
- Traumatic blunt ruptures of the aorta are typically found just distal to the ligamentum arteriosum.
- For selected patients with only partial tears of the aortic arch, a continuous lateral arteriorrhaphy using 4–0 polypropylene suture is occasionally possible.
- If patients have stable thoracic hematomas and concomitant abdominal injuries for which they are unstable, laparotomy should be the initial procedure.
- For patients with rapidly expanding mediastinal hematoma, however, repair of thoracic injuries should be the primary therapeutic goal.
- Injury to the descending thoracic aorta is approached by way of a postero-lateral thoracotomy through the fourth intercostal space.
- The current standard technique of repair involves vascular clamping and direct reconstruction. Three commonly employed adjuncts to this approach include pharmacologic agents; temporary, passive bypass shunts; and pump–assisted left heart bypass.
- Vascular clamps are applied to the aortic arch, distal aorta, and left subclavian artery. Close communication between the anesthesiologist and surgeon should occur to maintain stability of hemodynamic parameters. The hematoma is entered, and care is taken to avoid indiscriminate ligation of intercostal vessels; only those required for adequate repair of the aorta should be ligated. The proximal and distal ends of the aorta are completely transected and dissected away from the esophagus. The injury then is repaired by either end–to–end anastomosis or graft interposition.
- The authors have advocated simple clamp-and-repair for injuries to the descending thoracic aorta (without the use of systemic anticoagulation or shunts), a technique that continues to be used with excellent results.
- Regardless of the technique used, paraplegia occurs in approximately 8 % of patients undergoing to descending thoracic aorta repair. Unless operative time is <30 min, partial left heart bypass is superior to clamp-and -sew in preventing paraplegia.

Subclavian vessels

- For subclavian injuries, a cervical extension of a median sternotomy is employed for exposure of right–sided subclavian injuries. For left subclavian artery injures, proximal control is obtained through an anterolateral thoracotomy (third intercostal space), while a separate supraclavicular incision provides distal control.
- In subclavian vascular trauma, a high associated rate of brachial plexus injury is seen.
- Documentation of preoperative neurologic status is important, in all thoracic and neck vascular injuries.
- Repair of subclavian arteries can usually be accomplished with either lateral arteriorrhaphy or graft interposition. Any difficulty in exposure can be managed with division or resection of the clavicle exposing the more distal subclavian.
- Subclavian reconstruction commonly requires the use of a graft (Dacron or PTFE). In the patient, in extremis flow can be reestablished with the use of a shunt, or the artery can be ligated as a life–saving measure.
- Operative exposure of the subclavian veins is equivalent of that described for subclavian artery injuries: median sternotomy with cervical extension for right-sided injuries and left anterolateral thoracotomy with a separate supraclavicular incision for left-sided injuries.
- Repair should be performed by either lateral venorraphy or ligation.

Pulmonary artery & veins

- The intrapericardial pulmonary arteries should be approached via median sternotomy.

- Exposure of the intrapericardial right pulmonary artery is achieved by dissecting between the superior vena cava and the ascending aorta.
- Mortality rates for injury to the central pulmonary arteries or veins are high (>70 %).
- When there is a major hilar injury, rapid pneumonectomy may be a lifesaving maneuver.
- Injuries to the pulmonary veins are difficult to manage through an anterior incision.
- With major bleeding, temporary occlusion of the entire hilum may be necessary.
- If a pulmonary vein must be ligated, the appropriate lobe will need to be resected.

Extremities vascular trauma

Upper extremity

Injuries to the upper extremity vessels are common, usually penetrating and may be associated with significant nerve and orthopedic injury. Blunt injury is usually a result of supracondylar fracture of the humerus or dislocation of the elbow. The amputation rate for ligation of the common brachial vessel varies from 18 to 55 %. With isolated injury to the infra-brachial vessels the amputation rate is lower and ligation of either the radial or ulnar arteries alone is usually well tolerated. A higher level of technical skill is required in dealing with smaller vessels and use of magnification loops is recommended. Spasm of the vessels is frequent and may require topical lidocaine or intra-arterial papaverine. Generally, prosthetic materials are not recommended. Passing of Fogarty catheters proximally and distally is important to remove eventual thrombus. Completion angiograms are important to detect abnormalities, which might result in post-operative thrombosis of the repair. Soft tissue coverage of the repair uses adjacent muscle. Fasciotomy needs to be done if ischemic time is prolonged and orthopaedic stabilization should occur after vascular repair [16–18].

Author recommendations

- Gain rapid access to axillary vessels through the pectoralis major muscle, extending the incision from the mid-clavicle to the deltopectoral groove.
- Damage control options for axillary artery are not many: shunt insertion, fasciotomy and/or less commonly ligation.
- Gain rapid access to the brachial vessels through a incision along the groove between the biceps and triceps muscle.
- Take the median nerve as your anatomic landmark.
- Damage control options for brachial artery are ligation (well tolerated) and fasciotomy.
- Definitive care is usually using a saphena vein interposition graft harvested just above the ankle.

Lower extremity

As for upper extremities, penetrating injuries are more often common in the lower extremities. Pre-operative angiography may not be useful in severe trauma when taken the patient to the operating room for exploration is the best option. Surgically the use of shunts may be helpful as a damage control option, however local heparinization, passing fogarty catheters and completion angiograms can also be obtained. In general, simple vessel injuries are repaired, complex injuries ligated. If grafting is required contralateral reversed saphenous vein is recommended. Fasciotomies should be indicated based on clinical grounds and performed in all cases of prolonged ischemia time, in severe limb injuries or when there are tense compartments, combined arterial and venous lesions, in the presence of motor or sensory defect or in limbs of questionable viability. In war related injuries to the extremity fasciotomies are prophylactically recommended [11]. Primary amputation should be carried out, if the superficial posterior and one other compartment shows non-viability or in cases of devastating injuries to the limb. The amputation rate varies from 16 to 20 % and may be larger in war scenario. Attention should be given to soft tissue injuries associated to vascular lesions. Infectious complications and soft tissue injury contribute to late amputation after severe lower extremity trauma [8, 10–13, 39, 40]. Prepping the contralateral leg for possible harvesting of the long saphenous vein should be remembered.

Femoral vessels

Seventy percent of all peripheral vascular injuries in urban trauma centers are due to femoral injuries. The superficial femoral artery is most incident [41]. The most common complication is compartment syndrome (±19 %) and deep venous thrombosis (±13 %). In an American Civilian Trauma Center the fasciotomy rate for femoral vessels varies in around 14 %. Amputation rate in these centers are low [41].

Authors recommendations

- If there is urgent indication go into the abdomen and control the external iliac artery in the pelvis.
- Vertical groin incision is the simplest way to gain proximal control of the femoral artery.
- Blunt dissection is recommended in devastating vascular trauma.
- The source of persistent back bleeding is frequently the deep femoral artery. This must be identified and controlled.
- Temporary shunt and ligation are plausible damage control options for femoral vessels (Shunting is a much better option for arterial injuries). Don't hesitate in ligate the femoral vein if needed.

- Temporary shunt for common and superficial femoral arteries is an excellent damage control solution. Authors strongly recommend a pre-emptive fasciotomy in such cases.
- Interposition PTFE grafts are well tolerated.
- Always cover your arterial vascular suture with viable well-vascularized soft tissue.
- Decide (with the orthopedic surgeons) to achieve bone alignment prior to arterial repair.

Popliteal vessels Blunt injuries are more often present and carry almost 3 times the risk of amputation in comparison to penetrating injuries. Popliteal vessels are challenging to approach and treat. It is the least accessible vessel in the lower extremity and the collateral flow around the knee is not sufficient to sustain viability of the lower leg if flow of the popliteal artery is interrupted. Popliteal artery traumatic injuries carry the highest limb loss rate of all extremity vascular injuries. Injuries requiring resection of more than 2 cm are not amenable to primary anastomosis. Popliteal vein injuries, which usually occur together with arterial injuries, should be repaired if possible, but never delay the surgery time in physiologically crashed patients. In the case of combined injuries intra-arterial shunts may play a particular role. Prophylactic fasciotomy is recommended in delayed injuries or those with complex soft tissue damage. In the usual case of major soft tissue trauma the decision is often one of primary amputation versus repair. The absolute indications for primary amputation in these cases are: more than 6 h of ischemic time and disruption of the posterior tibial nerve. The relative indications are: severe foot wounds, multiple trauma, injuries requiring extensive soft tissue coverage and tibial reconstruction [42, 43].

Authors recommendations

- Always begin a popliteal repair with a fasciotomy.
- Proximal and distal control are mandatory (as are for all other vascular traumatic injuries).
- Think about systemic heparin whether there are no potential bleeding injuries.
- The posterior edge of the femur is the key anatomical landmark for managing popliteal injuries.
- Careful with the popliteal vein and saphenous nerve is advised when dissecting the popliteal artery.
- Go simple: bypass and exclude the injured popliteal artery.
- Saphenous vein interposition grafts are recommended.

Abdominal vascular injury

Abdominal vascular injury (AVI) is defined as a trauma of the intra- and retro-peritoneal principal arteries and veins, accounting for the 27–33 % of all vascular trauma, and for the 25 % of all the abdominal injuries. The 90–95 % of AVI occurs after penetrating trauma, with incidences of 10 % after stab wounds and 25 % after gunshot wounds, respectively [44]. Particularly, combined injuries involving arteries and veins are common after penetrating trauma and frequent for the iliac and superior mesenteric vessels because of their anatomical proximity [45].

Pathophysiology

Penetrating trauma produces AVI by different mechanisms. Through-and-through perforation or lateral defects in the wall will lead to contained haematomas, which are either pulsatile and expanding (arterial) or non-pulsatile (venous). Only a small number of patients have free haemorrhage into the peritoneal cavity. Complete transections are rarely seen, probably because uncontrolled bleeding from a large-size vessel leads to exsanguination in the pre-hospital setting. On occasion, the trajectory of a missile may be in proximity of a visceral vessel and causes a thrombosis due to the disruption of the intima from the blast effect. The rarest injury related to penetrating trauma is an artero-venous fistula, usually in the upper abdomen or in the iliac area.

Blunt trauma may induce AVI by deceleration forces, direct anterior crushing (lap-type seatbelt) or posterior blow (direct compression) of the structures. Two different types of injury may be caused by deceleration forces. The first one is the avulsion of small branches from the major vessels (i.e intestinal branches from superior mesenteric artery). The second is the partial intimal tear with a secondary thrombosis of the lumen, or full-thickness tear with a secondary pseudoaneurysm. A direct anterior crush and posterior blow may lead to vascular damage by an intimal tear or flap with secondary thrombosis (i.e "seat-belt aorta")[46], and disruption of a vessel (i.e superior mesenteric artery or vein at the base of mesentery). A complete wall disruption leads to a massive intraperitoneal haemorrhage, while partial disruption produces a false aneurysm [47].

Areas of AVI

Although any vessel in the abdomen can be injured, the term *abdominal vascular injury* usually refers to injury of major vessels located in specific "geographic" zones, as listed below:

1. Zone 1: Midline retroperitoneum.

    - Supramesocolic area: suprarenal abdominal aorta, celiac axis, proximal superior mesenteric artery, proximal renal artery, superior mesenteric vein (either supramesocolic or retromesocolic);

- Inframesocolic area: infrarenal abdominal aorta, infrahepatic inferior vena cava;

2. Zone 2: Upper lateral retroperitoneum (renal artery, renal vein)
3. Zone 3: Pelvic retroperitoneum (iliac artery, iliac vein)
4. Portal-retrohepatic area: (portal vein, hepatic artery, retrohepatic vena cava).

As a general rule, all haematomas in zone 1 (either supramesocolic or inframesocolic) from either penetrating or blunt trauma have to be explored. In addition, haematomas from penetrating wounds in zone 2 and 3, and in the porta hepatis need to be opened. In contrast, haematomas from blunt trauma that are located in zones 2 e 3 or in the retrohepatic area are explored only if they are pulsatile, expanding rapidly, or have already ruptured. The classification system is applied to extra- parenchymal vascular injuries, according to the Organ Injury Score (OIS) Table 2 [48]. It is important to be aware that potential visceral injuries (i.e, duodenum, colon, stomach, small bowel, etc.) may be associated to any AVI.

Diagnosis

Upon physical examination, the findings in patients with AVI, after either blunt or penetrating injury mechanisms, depend on whether a *contained haematoma* or *uncontrolled haemorrhage* is present. Patients with a contained haematoma, particularly those with venous injuries, may be hypotensive, but will respond rapidly to infusions. In this case contrast CT scan is the diagnostic tool of choice. Other patients with uncontrolled haemorrhage are hypotensive and non-responsive to fluid infusion, with a tight abdomen, due to intra-peritoneal active bleeding from the damaged vessel. Abdominal distension in association with signs of acute anemia and/or haemorrhagic shock is a strong indicator of a major AVI. Another important physical finding is the loss of the pulse in the femoral artery in one of the lower extremity when the ipsilateral common or external iliac artery has been transected or is thrombosed. Rarely, the patient may be hypotensive, with a copious emesis of dark blood. In this case, a caval-duodenal fistula is suspected. The presence of a wide pulse pressure, abdominal bruit and haematuria suggest an acute aorto-caval fistula. In patients arriving with a blunt or penetrating abdominal trauma with profound hypotension or peritonitis and positive ultrasound (FAST-Focused Abdominal Sonography for Trauma), a time limit of less than 5 min in the emergency room before surgery is mandatory and CT scan is not recommended.

Operative strategy

In the operating theatre, the patient lays in the supine position, with both arms fully abducted. The operative field extends from chin to above the knees and between the posterior axillary lines, in order to provide free access to the abdomen, chest wall and both groins. If the patient arrives profoundly hypotensive or experiences cardiopulmonary arrest in the operating room, an immediate anterolateral thoracotomy with aortic cross-clamping is performed prior to entering the abdomen. Differently, if the patient arrives with some degree of haemodynamic stability, but deteriorates during laparotomy, the abdominal aorta can be controlled digitally at the hiatus through the lesser sac or by cross-clamping. A wide vertical midline incision is carried from the xyphoid to the pubis. All clots are removed and a rapid inspection is performed to visualize a contained haematoma or an ongoing haemorrhage. Active bleeding from a solid organ is controlled by packing, while formal proximal and distal vascular control is essential for an active haemorrhage from major intraabdominal vessels. Once haemorrhage has been controlled, any eventual gastrointestinal spillage is addressed, to avoid further contamination during vascular repair. Conversely, if a contained haematoma is present, occasionally the surgeon has time to control the gastrointestinal contamination first, and subsequently to open the retroperitoneum exposing the underlying vascular injury.

Management of injuries in zone 1: supramesocolic region

Exposure and vascular control

The approach to an injured vessel in the supramesocolic area is different in the presence of a confined haematoma or an active bleeding:

Table 2 Classification system of abdominal vascular system [17–19]

OIS grade	Description of injuries
I	Non-named superior mesenteric artery and vein, and their branches, phrenic artery/vein, lumbar artery/vein, gonadal artery/vein, ovarian artery/vein
II	Right, left, common hepatic artery, splenic artery/vein, right or left gastric arteries, gastroduodenal artery, inferior mesenteric artery/vein, primary branches of mesenteric artery/vein
III	Superior mesenteric vein trunk, renal artery/vein, iliac artery/vein, hypogastric artery/vein, vena cava, infrarenal
IV	Superior mesenteric artery trunk, celiac axis proper, vena cava suprarenal and infrahepatic, aorta, infrarenal.
V	Portal vein, extra-parenchymal hepatic vein, vena cava retrohepatic or suprahepatic, aorta suprarenal, subdiaphragmatic

(a) in the case of a confined haematoma, the vascular control is achieved by a left-sided medial visceral rotation, including the colon, kidney, spleen, tail of the pancreas and the fundus of the stomach. One alternative is to leave the left kidney in its fossa, thereby eliminating the potential damage resulting from rotation of this organ. The transection of the left crus of the diaphragm at 2 o' clock position allows the exposure of the distal thoracic aorta and a vascular clamp is applied to obtain supraceliac aortic proximal control.

(b) in the presence of an active haemorrhage a manual compression may be performed. Alternatively, the lesser omentum is entered manually, the stomach and esophagus are retracted to the left, and the fibers of the aortic hiatus divided manually to obtain a quicker proximal control. Distal control of the aorta in this location is challenging because of the presence of celiac axis and superior mesenteric artery. If the ligation and division of the celiac axis are required, the surgeon must be aware of the potential gallbladder necrosis, as likely consequence. Cholecystectomy is warranted, although it may be performed during re-exploration, if damage control techniques are required. Another possible approach is an extended Kocher manoeuvre, by moving the duodenum and head of the pancreas to the left, in order to expose the suprarenal abdominal aorta.

Vascular repair

Suprarenal aorta (SA)

Small perforating wounds at the SA are repaired by 3–0 or 4–0 polypropylene lateral sutures. If two small perforations are adjacent to one another, they should be connected and the defect closed transversally. If the closure of the perforations results in a significant narrowing of the lumen, or in the presence of a large defect, a patch aortoplasty with polytetrafluoroethylene (PTFE) is required. Occasionally, patients with extensive injuries require insertion of a synthetic vascular conduit or vascular graft, after resection of the involved area [49]. It is important to remember that suprarenal cross-clamping in presence of a haemorrhagic shock induces a severe lower extremities ischemia, with a subsequent reperfusion injury, once the haemodynamic stability has been restored. Compartment pressure of the legs needs to be measured before moving the patient from the operating room, and if this is higher than 30–35 mmHg, two-incision with four-compartment fasciotomies are recommended.

Celiac axis (CA)

Injuries of the branches of the CA are difficult to repair because of the dense neural and lymphatic surrounding tissue, and the small size of these vessels in a patient in shock with secondary vasoconstriction. If the left gastric artery and splenic artery are injured, these vessels should be ligated. Splenectomy must be performed if the splenic artery has been ligated. The larger diameter of the hepatic artery sometimes allows a lateral arteriorraphy, end-to-end anastomosis or the insertion of a graft. However, the surgeon has the option to ligate the vessel proximal to the origin of the gastroduodenal artery, since the collateral flows from the midgut through this artery will maintain the viability of the liver.

Superior mesenteric artery (SMA)

The SMA is anatomically divided into four zones (Fullen zones) (Figs. 2 and 3), and the management of any injury of this vessel depends on the level of injury itself. If the injury is located behind or beneath the pancreas (Fullen zone 1 and zone 2, respectively), the transection of the pancreas, or a left-side medial visceral rotation, or elevation of transverse mesocolon, allow a direct clamping of the proximal SMA. Under all of these conditions, the artery may be ligated, and theoretically, the flow from both the foregut and the hindgut maintains the viability of the midgut (through the middle colic artery). In patients in shock and vasoconstricted collateral flow may be ineffective and the insertion of a temporary intraluminal shunt into the debrided ends of SMA is a better choice, with definitive repair during a second-look procedure. Injuries to the distal SMA (Fullen zone 3, beyond the middle colic branch, and zone 4, at the level of the enteric branches) should be repaired to avoid intestinal ischemia. If this cannot be accomplished, ligation of the artery requires an extensive resection of the ileum and right colon.

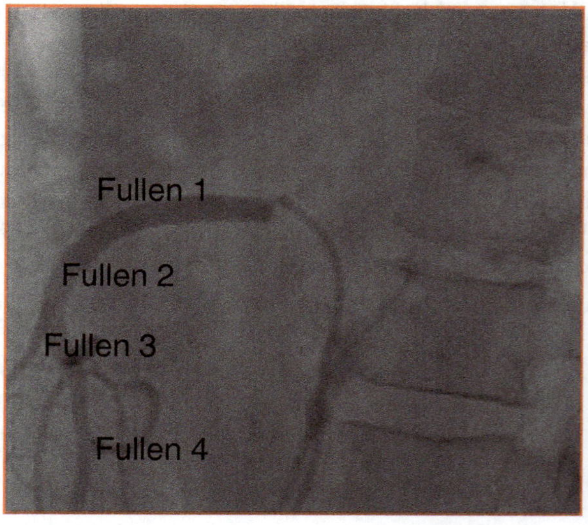

Fig. 2 Zones of superior mesenteric artery: angiographic view was excluded

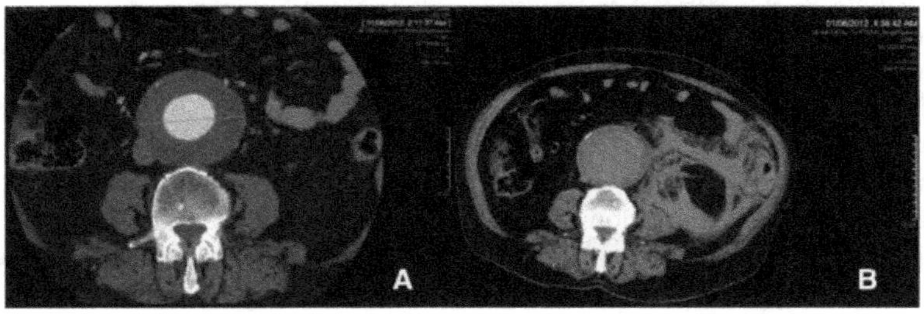

Fig. 3 **a** Abdominal CT with IV contrast of a patient with symptomatic AAA. **b** Non-contrast abdominal CT of the same patient after collapse about 2 h later. The AAA ruptured as is evident from the retroperitoneal hematoma

Superior mesenteric vein (SMV)

A part of the SMV is retro-pancreatic and difficult to expose, and has abundant collaterals. It may be approached through a Kocher and Cattell Braasch maneuver and repaired with a continuous row of 5–0 polypropylene sutures. If multiple vascular and visceral injuries are present, in a young patient, ligation of the SMV can be performed. A vigorous fluid resuscitation is needed, as a splancnic hypervolemia leads to peripheral hypovolemia for at least 3 days after ligation.

Management of injuries in zone 1: inframesocolic region

Exposure and vascular control

To expose an inframesocolic injury of the aorta or caval vein (IVC) the transverse mesocolon is pulled upward, small bowel eviscerated toward the right side, and the midline incised from the left renal vein to the origin of iliac vessels. In case of a large retroperitoneal haematoma, it should be remembered that the hole in the aorta is usually under the highest point of the haematoma (Mount Everest Phenomenon). A rapid finger splitting brings the surgeon to the injured area. Distal vascular control is achieved by dividing the retroperitoneum downward until aortic bifurcation. An injury involving IVC has to be suspected if the haematoma is more extensive to the right side. In this case, IVC control is obtained by a right-sided medial visceral rotation (Kocher and Cattell Braasch). The two areas in which the proximal and distal control of IVC are difficult to obtain are at the confluence of common iliac veins and at the junction of the renal veins. In the first setting it is possible to divide the right common iliac artery allowing the exposure of the iliac vein bifurcation. The artery will be reconstituted by an end-to-end anastomosis. In the second case, the medial rotation of the right kidney permits the application of a clamp. Another technique, which is useful for controlling bleeding from IVC in all locations, is the trans-femoral insertion of a Foley catheter, for tamponade.

Vascular repair

Infrarenal aorta

Injuries of the infrarenal aorta are repaired primarily with 3–0 or 4–0 polypropylene sutures, patch aortoplasty, end-to-end anastomosis, or graft. In the young patient, when a graft is used or an extensive repair has been performed, it is better to cover the suture line by a vascularized pedicle of omentum, in order to prevent an aorto-duodenal fistula.

Infrahepatic IVC

Anterior injuries of the IVC are best repaired transversally with a running suture of 4–0 or 5–0 polypropylene. If a through-and-through perforation is present, the posterior defect is repaired first, from inside the vessel, with the first knot tied outside the lumen. If a long longitudinal suture is performed, the caval vein will appear as an hourglass, and the narrowing will lead to a postoperative occlusion of the vessel. If the patient is unstable, a modification of the repair should not be attempted. In complex injuries of the young patient, the IVC may be ligated [50]. In the postoperative course, the compartment pressure of the legs needs to be measured, and four-compartments fasciotomies must be done if the pressure exceeds 30–35 mmHg. An adequate circulating volume has to be maintained, and elastic compression applied to both lower extremities. Ligation of the suprarenal vena cava is performed only if the patient has an extensive injury at this location and appears to be in profound shock at the end of the operation.

Management of injuries in zone 2

Exposure and vascular control

Patients found to have a perirenal haematoma following a penetrating trauma should undergo the haematoma exploration. If the haematoma is not rapidly expanding, proximal vascular control is obtained, before entering the haematoma, by looping the ipsilateral renal vessels. Proximal renal arteries (RA) are better approached through the base of the mesocolon, beneath the left renal vein. Conversely, if there is an active bleeding, the exposure of the proximal part of the left RA is accomplished by a left-sided medial visceral rotation and of the right RA by a Kocher maneuver. The retroperitoneum is opened lateral to the injured organ, the kidney is manually lifted upward and a vascular clamp is applied proximal to the hilum. If a non-expanding haematoma is detected after blunt trauma, surgical exploration should not be attempted and post-operative angiography with interventional radiology repair should be planned.

Vascular repair

Renal arteries (RA)

Small perforations from penetrating injury can be repaired by lateral sutures or resection with an end-to-end anastomosis. In the presence of large defects, graft interposition should be considered only if there is a reasonable possibility to save the kidney. After a blunt trauma, a patient with an injury to one kidney should be considered for revascularization only in the presence of stable haemodynamics and short time of ischemia (less than 5 h).

Renal veins (RV)

A lateral venorrhaphy is the preferred technique for repair. If right RV has to be ligated, a nephrectomy should be performed at the same time or at the reoperation if damage control has been necessary. Left proximal RV can be ligated as long as the gonadal veins and the left adrenal vein are intact.

Management of injuries in zone 3

Exposure and vascular control

The proximal vascular control of the iliac vessels is obtained by eviscerating the small bowel to the right and opening the retroperitoneum over the aortic bifurcation. Distal vascular control is achieved at the point the vessels come out of the pelvis proximal to the inguinal ligament [51]. When bilateral injuries are present, the only way to achieve bleeding control is the total pelvic vascular exclusion, with a proximal cross-clamping of the aorta or vena cava, above their bifurcation, and a distal cross-clamping of the external iliac arteries or veins on both sides.

Vascular repair

Iliac arteries (IA)

Injuries of the common IA should be sutured or temporarily shunted if possible. Ligation of these vessels in the hypotensive patient leads to limb ischemia. In a stable or stabilized patient, depending on the type of injury, it is possible to perform a lateral arteriorraphy, an end-to-end anastomosis and an insertion of saphenous vein or PTFE graft. External IA may be ligated if omolateral internal IA is intact.

Iliac veins (IV)

Injuries of the IV are best repaired with a 4–0 or 5–0 polypropylene lateral suture or with ligation. If a significant narrowing of the lumen has occurred after the repair, postoperative anticoagulation therapy should be started to avoid thrombosis and pulmonary embolism.

Management of injuries in the porta hepatis

Exposure and vascular control

It is important to be aware that vascular injuries at this location are frequently associated with an injury of the common bile duct. Because of this anatomic proximity, no suture should be placed until the vascular injury is precisely defined. If haematoma or haemorrhage are present the Pringle's maneuver (compression of the hepatoduodenal ligament between non crushing clamps, fingers or loops) should be used. The injuries of the portal vein are best exposed with a wide Cattel-Braasch maneuver. Exposure of the posterior position of the vessel requires an extensive Kocher maneuver in association with a mobilization of the common bile duct toward the left and the cystic duct superiorly. The approach to retropancreatic portion of the vessel requires pancreatic transection followed by distal pancreatectomy once the repair is made.

Hepatic artery (HA)

Lateral repair or shunt of HA are difficult because of its small caliber, but desirable. In fact, the portal vein alone is not always sufficient for liver viability [52]. Ligation of the gastro-hepatic artery, proximal to the origin of gastroduodenal artery is usually well tolerated. Ligation of the right HA requires a cholecystectomy.

Portal vein (PV)

Direct lateral venorraphy with a 4–0 or 5–0 polypropylene suture is the technique of choice. It is better to avoid any attempt to perform a porto-systemic shunt, because of the possible onset of encephalopathy at a later stage. Ligation of PV has a very high mortality. Massive fluid sequestration induces transient splancnic hypervolemia that requires a large amount of fluid restoration to avoid peripheral hypoperfusion.

Recommendations

All trauma surgeons must be skilled in the techniques of emergency abdominal vascular control and repair. The reduced functional reserve of the unstable patient with AVI and the presence of multiple injuries require a damage control approach with staged surgical strategy. Moreover, an abdominal vascular ligation or repair in more stable patients needs to be re-explored for the assessment of visceral viability. Finally, AVI are unusual after blunt trauma, which in Europe account for 95 %

of trauma admissions. Further, training for the treatment of these injuries is generally low. For all these considerations, a patient with an AVI represents one of the most challenging scenarios for a trauma team and mortality remains elevated.

Non traumatic emergency vascular surgery

Ruptured aneurysms of the abdominal aorta: current management and results

Few other surgical emergencies require immediate diagnosis and treatment like a ruptured abdominal aortic aneurysm (rAAA). Mortality of patients with a rAAA reaches 85 %, with more than half dying before reaching the hospital. Open repair (OR) of rAAA is associated with perioperative mortality of 40–70 %. Patient age, haemodinamic instability and pre-existing comordibitidies are significantly associated with perioperative deaths. Endoluminal repair of rAAA (REVAR) has emerged as an alternative to OR. Since the first experience with this technique in the early 1990s, a substantial decrease in perioperative and long term mortality has been demonstrated after REVAR when compared with OR. In addition to the advances of REVAR, modern resuscitation techniques including hemostatic resuscitation and permissive hypotension, and the availability of endoluminal aortic occlusive balloons for supraceliac aortic control in the emergency room, has assisted salvaging patients that historically died before reaching surgery. REVAR mandates pre-operative imaging, a dedicated team, an angio suite and ready access to suitable stents.

In this paper we present a review of the recent literature on rAAA. We discuss the rationale for transfer to referral center, the role of preoperative imaging and the pros and cons of REVAR versus OR.

Where should ruptured abdominal aortic aneurysms be repaired?

A positive correlation between sub-specialization, high volume and improved outcome has been demonstrated in multiple surgical procedures, including open and endovascular operations. Thus, a dilemma occurs: should an open repair be attempted immediately, by a team and center with limited experience, or should the patient be transferred to the referral centre for sub-specialized care with obvious delay to treatment and risk of decompensation during transfer? Relatively sparse data is available on the true effects of transfer of patients with an unsecured rAAA. A recent case-series in Canada suggests that while the transfer caused treatment delays (from approximately 3 to 6 h), it did not significantly impact mortality (50 vs 54 %) [53]. However, the retrospective design of this study may have biased by selection of likely survivors for transfer, and palliation of the sicker patients. Unfortunately, for vascular emergencies, the last decade has seen an unchecked drive towards elective subspecialization with a surge of endovascular procedures and a rapid reduction of open vascular procedures. In this environment, the General and Acute Care Surgeons have lost almost all training in vascular surgery. The large variations in local practices and expertise, retrieval teams, and geography preclude a universal recommendation on a transfer policy.

We suggest preemptive, careful design of pathway and protocols for patients with a rAAA which should be tailored to individual hospitals and area health. In any case, preoperative resuscitation should follow the concept of "permissive hypotension" with the aim of maintaining consciousness and prevent ST changes, and a systolic blood pressure between 70 and 80 mmHg [54, 55]. This can be achieved by limiting infusion of fluids and blood products and/or pharmacologically reducing the blood pressure [56].

Role of preoperative imaging

While open repair of a rAAA can be "attempted" with minimal imaging by most surgeons familiar with abdominal surgery, REVAR introduced the need of pre-operative CT scan. To allow immediate and accurate imaging reconstruction, CT should be performed with intravenous contrast, by a trained radiographer, with the correct bolus timing, no oral contrast and possibly the availability of thin axial slices. A good quality CT scan is of paramount importance to properly assess feasibility of endoluminal repair and graft sizing (Fig. 3, Fig. 4, Fig. 5). The main concern of running a potentially unstable patient through a scanner is the possible delay from ED admission to surgery. According to Lloydet al.,in not operated patients with rAAA the mean time from onset of symptoms and ED admission to death was 16 and 11 h respectively; only 13 % of patients died within 2 h of admission. In case of transfer, the CT scans can be reviewed online and EVAR suitability and measurements can be completed before the patient arrives to the hospital. The lack of protocols for efficient transfer and management of patients with rAAA, rather than the time spent in radiology, seems to cause most delays to surgery [57–59].

Patients with a systolic blood pressure above 80mmHG should be preoperatively investigated with CT with IV contrast. Patients with a systolic less then 80 mmHg should be immediately transferred to theatre with an aortic occlusive balloon (endoclamp) ready to be inflated in the supracoeliac aorta. REVAR assessment can then be done with a digital subtraction angiogram on the operative table.

Open repair

The open approach to the rAAA has been standard for several decades. During this time, relatively little has changed regarding the surgical procedure: first, rapid

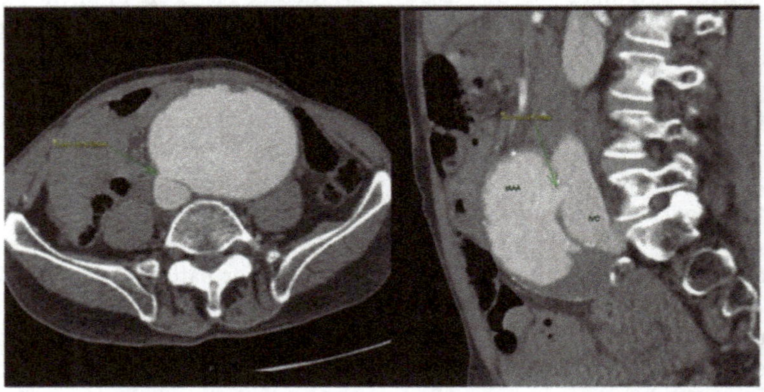

Fig. 4 Abdominal CT with IV contrast demonstrating a large infrarenal AAA ruptured in the inferior vena cava in axial and sagittal view

proximal control of the aneurysm is achieved immediately on induction of anesthesia; second, distal control; and finally, after a small period of time is afforded to the anesthetic team to further resuscitate the patient, the aneurysm is opened and a graft used to bypass the diseased aorta [60, 61].

Preoperative CT imaging is not strictly necessary, but still very useful as it can guide in location to achieve proximal control and possible anatomical variation (such as a retroaortic renal vein or a horseshoe kidney) or presence of additional aneurysms.

The rAAA is classically approached through a midline laparotomy, facilitating a transperitoneal repair. This approach provides good exposure of the abdominal aorta and common iliac arteries. The peritoneal exploration also allows inspection of the abdominal viscera for secondary pathology. However a retroperitoneal approach may be preferable in cases such as known supraceliac

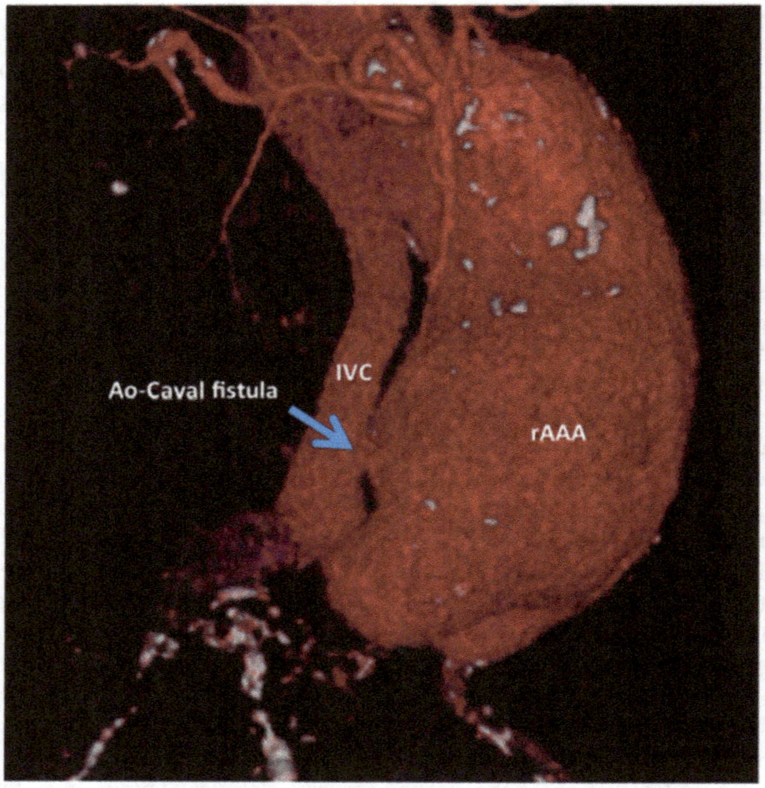

Fig. 5 3D reconstruction of large infrarenal AAA ruptured into the inferior vena cava

extension of the aneurysm, a battle-scarred abdomen, or in patients with atypical anatomy such as a horseshoe kidney. While there are no randomized data to guide the type of incision for a rAAA, in cases of elective repair, randomized trials have produced conflicting results regarding possible reductions in postoperative ileus and shorter hospital stays associated with a retroperitoneal approach [62, 63].

After entering the peritoneal cavity, routine supraceliac control has traditionally been the first maneuver. However, when the aneurysm is limited to the infrarenal aorta, aortic control may be achieved below the renals in a similar time frame and is a feasible alternative: the assistant temporarily compresses the supraceliac aorta against the vertebral body at the diaphragm's aortic hiatus, while the surgeon uses fingertip exploration of the periaortic hematoma to guide an infrarenal clamp. Care is required to avoid venous injuries to the left renal, gonadal and inferior mesenteric veins during infrarenal clamping, as injuries to these veins are associated with a significantly worse prognosis [60]. For supraceliac control, however, the left lobe of the liver is first mobilized and retracted to the right. The nasogastric tube then facilitates identification of the esophagus, which together with the stomach is retracted towards the left. This allows access to the aorta at its diaphragmatic hiatus, through the lesser sac. Caution is required to avoid the not infrequent presence of an aberrant left hepatic artery travelling through the lesser omentum. The aorta can then be clamped as it emerges between the crura of the diaphragm.

When the rAAA is approached from a retroperitoneal dissection, the incision is usually placed through a 10th intercostal space, though in the cases of very proximal aneurysmal disease, a formal throacoabdominal incision, with a transpleural aortic cross-clamp, may be required. Retrospective series report reduced gastrointestinal and respiratory morbidity, reduced hospital stays and possible reduced mortality, favoring a retroperitoneal approach [64, 65]. During this approach, a left medial visceral rotation facilitates the aortic exposure.

Distal control is usually easier to achieve; the level of control, and the site for the distal anastomoses, will be guided by associated vascular pathology in the iliac and femoral vessels. If a bifurcated graft is used to bypass iliac disease, attempts should be made to perfuse at least one internal iliac artery to avoid ischaemic complications of the pelvis and lower abdominal viscera.

Endoluminal balloons provide an alternative to the traditional atraumatic clamps, limited by the need for a careful dissection to avoid injury to adjacent structures. First described with Foley catheters deployed through the aneurysm and inflated in the proximal aorta, endoluminal balloons have become increasingly available and are associated with reduced intraoperative mortality [66]. Furthermore, aortic occlusion catheter kits are commercially available to facilitate blind insertion and aortic control in the emergency department [67]. However, blind application of this device is not recommended in rAAAs.

After proximal and distal control, the largely decompressed aneurysm may be opened to allow the graft repair. Red cell scavenging forms a standard part of arAAA repair. Its use has been clearly linked to improved survival and reduced post-operative complications [68, 69]. It does not replace the need to careful assessment and targeted replacement of blood components, but it does provide a feasible, cost-effective, method to replace red cell loss from the vascular space.

Once the aortic reconstruction is completed before the proximal clamp is released to establish distal flow, the distal vessels are generously back bled, to prevent embolization of soft clot that may have formed. This is particularly important if the patient is neither systemically nor peripherally heparinized. As indicated by a recent review, the pro-coagulant, inflammatory stimulus from the trauma associated with a rAAA and its surgery, likely favors routine heparin administration. However, unfortunately a limited number of studies are available to guide the decision regarding the use of heparin in rAAA. As such, there remains no clear consensus or practice guideline to delineate the standard practice [70, 71].

At the completion of the vascular repair, approximately one quarter of patients will have abdominal contents too swollen to allow a non-tensioned abdominal closure, and around half of patients will exhibit an intra-abdominal pressure > 20 mmHg. Historically, these patients had their abdomens closed under tension with deleterious consequences. The resultant abdominal compartment syndrome (ACS) is responsible of multiorgan failure and increased mortality. A proactive approach to allow early diagnosis and intervention is required. Temporary abdominal closure devices with negative pressure dressing have redefined the standard of care of these patients [72, 73].

Endoluminal repair: protocols and technique

Endovascular aneurysm repair (EVAR) is the endoluminal exclusion of an aneurysm sac from the circulation by the use of an endograft; initially described by Parodi et al. in 1991 [73], this technique has evolved and has been proven safe and effective when compared to traditional OR in the elective settings [75, 76]. In 1994 the first successful endoluminal repair of a rAAA was performed in New York [77]. Today REVAR represents the most important innovation in rAAA management over the last 50 years [78, 79]. The protocol introduced by the Albany group [80] is efficient and applicable in most tertiary centers (Fig. 6); it requires multidisciplinary teamwork and appropriate team training. Once the ED physician has a suspect of rAAA (clinical or supported with ultrasound) the vascular team and theatre staff needs to be immediately notified. A dedicated theatre fully equipped for open and endovascular surgery is mandatory; a hybrid suite is ideal, but a standard theatre with a mobile C-arm intensifier is enough. Stable patients (SBP ≥ 70–80 mmHg) will have an expeditious CT scan; unstable patients will be directly transferred to theatre for endovascular-first approach and conversion to open if necessary. Patients are usually excluded from REVAR if (i) the aortic neck length ≤ 10 mm, (ii) the aortic neck diameter ≥ 32 mm, (iii) neck angulation ≥ 75° and (iv) bilateral iliac diameter ≤ 5 mm. Using those anatomical criteria almost 80 % of patients are feasible for REVAR [80]; Mayer et al. have recently reported 100 % feasibility of REVAR over a period of 32 consecutive months, with an exclusion rate of only 4 % [81]. STAT VASCULAR is the program implemented by Hodgonsat the University of Southern Illinois (Fig. 7) [82]. It emphasizes the importance of CT angiography for all patients suspected of having an acute aortic event either abdominal or thoracic; positive CT finding activates STAT VASCULAR and the on-call vascular team. REVAR can be safely and more effectively performed under local anesthesia supplemented by analgo-sedation [83]. Femoral access is achieved either with a cut-down or percutaneously. The percutaneous approach requires familiarity with preclose techniques with ProGlide or ProStar closure devices [84]. Once vascular access is established an initial glidewire is exchanged for a stiff one over a 5Fr catheter and a 12–14Fr 45 cm long sheath is placed at the level of the renal arteries to support an aortic occlusion balloon (femoral approachis preferred over brachial) [80, 85].

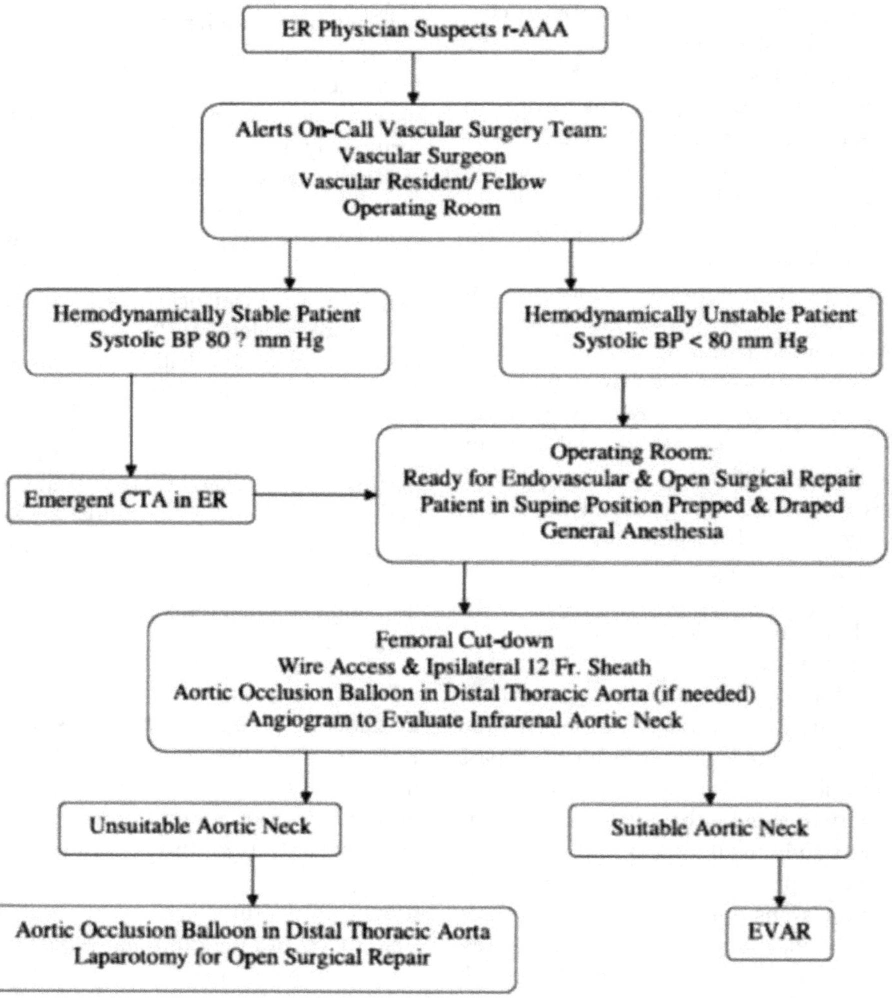

Fig. 6 Flowchart of the rAAA protocol introduced by the Albany Group [80]

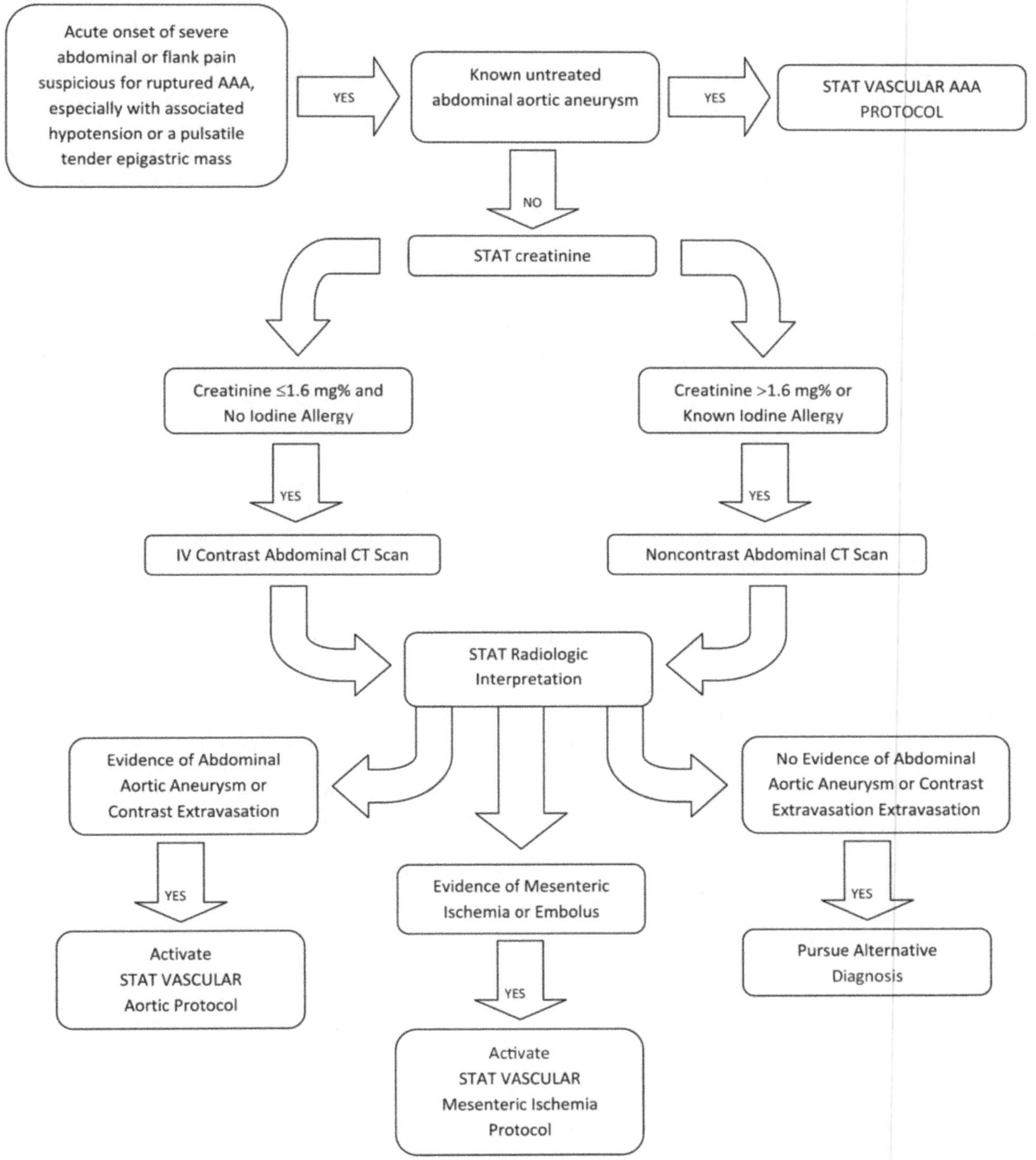

Fig. 7 Flowchart of the STAT VASCULAR program from the University of Illinois [82]

In hemodynamically stable patients the balloon can be removed after the initial angiogram and the main body of the endograft will be delivered through the ipsilateral groin. In patients in hemorrhagic shock, when the balloon needs to remain inflated to maintain brain and heart perfusion, the endograft is delivered through the contralateral groin and quickly deployed after the balloon is deflated and retrieved proximally.

Different endografts are available for treatment of rAAA in both bifurcated and aorto-uniiliac (AUI) configuration and the device choice depends on the patient's anatomy and the surgeon preference. Table 3 summarizes the characteristics of the most commonly used devices. The use of AUI devices should be limited to when (i) rapid cannulation of the contralateral gate is not possible or when (ii) the contralateral iliac is difficult to access because of occlusive disease. It is important to have a wide range of sizes and configurations available off the shelf in order to accommodate different anatomies. Adjunctive procedures (extension cuffs, giant Palmaz stents and embolization) might become necessary to seal on the table a proximal type for type IIendoleak, especially if causing ongoing hemorrhage [84, 86]. Finally extending the indications for REVAR to "all comers" might require visceral debranching (open or endoluminally with Chimney grafts) if the native neck is too short [87, 88].

The obvious advantage of avoiding a laparotomy carries the intrinsic risks of increased incidence of ACS. Metha reports an incidence of ACS of 18 %, occurring mainly in patients with pre-operative hemodynamic instability [89]. They suggest to routinely withhold systemic heparin in REVAR and to closely monitor the bladder pressure during and after the case. Increased bladder pressure alone or signs of end-organ dysfunction associated with abdominal distention, regardless of the bladder pressure, warrants decompressive laparotomy. Mayeret al. suggested an intravescical pressure > 20 mmHg or an abdominal perfusion pressure < 50–60 mmHg as indication for open abdominal treatment [90, 91]. Finally, on-table conversion to open surgical repair might be needed; the use of the occlusive aortic balloon as endoclamp can be very valuable to maintain haemodinamic stability. This needs to be supported to avoid its prolapse into the AAA with consequent loss of aortic occlusion.

Open or endovascular repair for rAAA?

Patients presenting with a ruptured aorta represent a medical and surgical challenge for everyone involved in their care. Rapid diagnosis of this catastrophic condition triggers an immediate and coordinated series of actions involving different health care providers. Despite the advances in medical care and surgical technique, the perioperative mortality rate of OR has seen only a modest improvement in the last 50 years [92, 93]. Among many theories, the "two-hit" hypothesis has been suggested to explain high mortality secondary to multi-organ failure [94]; this is summarized by the combination of two consecutive ischemic events (hemorrhagic shock and aortic clamping) followed by reperfusion injury. This sequence seems to be responsible of cardiac contractile dysfunction and massive neutrophils activation with resultant generalized peroxidation injury.

In the last twenty years multiple centers around the world have reported a dramatic reduction in perioperative mortality following REVAR [54, 74, 79, 95–100]; those excellent outcomes have been challenged as being the result of patient selection or publication biases [78, 100–103]. A meta-analysis of 18 observational studies (>10 cases) of patients undergoing REVAR; the pooled mortality among 436 pts who underwent REVAR was 21 % (95 % CI 13 to 29) but with substantial heterogeneity among different studies; however, 90 % of the heterogeneity between studies was not explained by chance alone. Surgical volume explained substantial heterogeneity [78]. A prospective study from 49 centers from all over the world showed an overall mortality at 30-days of 21.2 % but those results had an intrinsic selection bias due to the limited use of REVAR in "stable" patients in most of the centers. Thirteen centers performed "REVAR whenever possible" including haemodinamically unstable patients, and 30-days mortality was 19.7 % for REVAR compared with 36.3 % for OR ($p < .0001$) [79].

So the question is: which patient with a rAAA would benefit the most of an endograft? Do we have the data to justify the "EVAR-first" approach on everyone? Mayer et al. have reported a progressive increase in the use of REVAR over the years, reaching the up to a "100 % EVAR" approach. Adjusted 30-days mortality in the "EVAR/OPEN period" was 15.7 % for EVAR and 37.4 % for OR ($p = 0.004$). When all rAAA were treated endoluminally, 30-days mortality climbed to 24.3 % of "*all comers*" [81, 90]. Extending the indications for REVAR to "*all comers*" had multiple consequences: "exclusion from treatment" rate fell from 10 to 4 %, at the expenses of a higher REVAR mortality and more complex procedures. In addition, in order to accommodate also unsuitable anatomies, adjunctive procedures were used in 24 % of the cases, adding a considerable degree of complexity to an already challenging procedure. A Kaplan-Meier analysis based on more than 40.000 patients from the US Medicare dataset showed a survival benefit for REVAR over OR for the first 90 days; after propensity score matching the benefit persisted over 4 years [98]. Similar findings on long-term survival were also reported by Mehta et al.(37 vs 26 % REVAR and OR; $p < .005$) [95]. In this series almost a fourth of patients treated with an endograft, required re-intervention for endoleaks or graft migration, highlighting the importance of close follow-up.

A recent review based on US Medicare data beneficiaries used propensity score matching to show a survival benefit for REVAR (33.8 vs 47.7 %) which persisted at 4 years. At 36 months, EVAR patients had higher rates of AAA-related re-interventions than OR patients whereas OR patients had more laparotomy-related complications [103]. Based on a cohort of 1447 patients with rAAA, unstable patients showed less favorable outcomes: the 30-day mortality for unstable patients was

Table 3 Characteristics of the most commonly used endografts for rAAA

	Cook Zenith®		Medtronic®	Gore®
	LP AAA	Flex AAA, Spiral-Z Iliac	Endurant II	Excluder AAA
	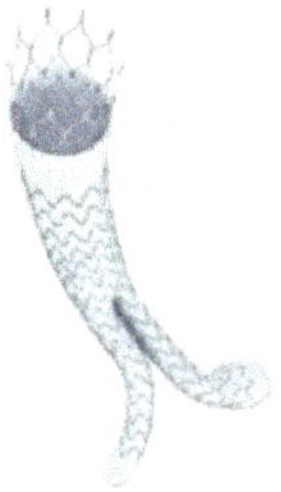	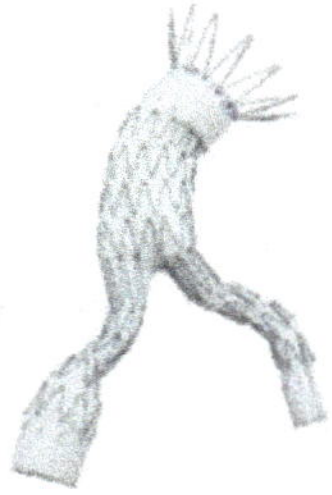	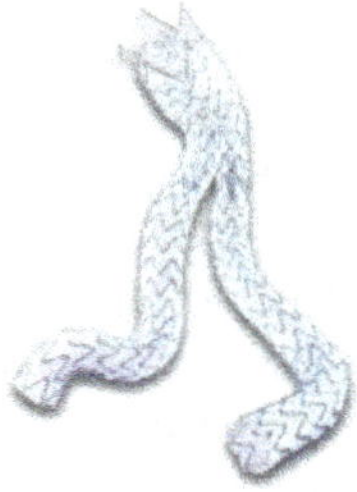	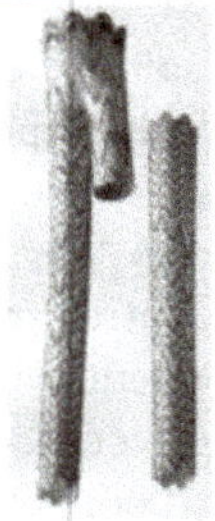
Indications for use				
Infrarenal neck fixation				
Diameter	18–28 mm	18–32 mm	19–32 mm	19–32 mm
Length	≥15 mm	≥15 mm	≥10 mm or ≥15 mm	≥15 mm
Angle (to suprarenal)	<45 deg	<45 deg	≤45 deg or ≤60 deg	≤60 deg
Angle (to aneurysm)	<60 deg	<60 deg	≤60 deg or ≤75 deg	≤60 deg
Iliac (ipsi/contra) fixation				
Diameter	8–20 mm	7.5–20 mm	8–25 mm	8–25 mm
Length	>10 mm	>10 mm	≥15 mm	≥10 mm
Iliofemoral access				
Sheath inner diameter	16Fr (5.3 mm)	18–22Fr (6.0–7.3 mm)	–	18–20Fr (6.1–6.8 mm)
Sheath out diameter	18Fr (6.0 mm)	21–26Fr (7.1–8.5 mm)	18–20Fr (6.0–6.7 mm)	20–27Fr (6.8–7.5 mm)
Graft specifications				
Materials				
Stents	Nitinol (self-expanding)	Stainless steel and nitinol	Nitinol	Nitinol
Grafts	Polyester (& PTFE)	Polyester	Polyester	ePTFE (& FEP)
Modular system, bifurcated main body device				
Fixation/sealing	Suprarenal bare stent, barbs, radial force	Suprarenal bare stent, barbs, radial force	Suprarenal bare stent, barbs, radial force	Graft sealing cuff, barbs, radial force
Diameter (~15 % oversize)	22–32 mm	22–36 mm	23–36 mm	23–35 mm
Length (body-ipsilateral)	94–152 mm	112–170 mm	124–166 mm	120–180 mm
Length - body-contralateral	70–128 mm	82–140 mm	70–80 mm	70–90 mm
Modular system, iliac extension device				
Diameter (~15 % oversize)	10–24 mm	9–24 mm	10–28 mm	12–27 mm
Length (limb)	36–120 mm	39–122 mm	82–199 mm	70–140 mm
Aortouniiliac device				
Fixation/sealing	–	Suprarenal bare stent, barbs, radial force	Suprarenal bare stent, barbs, radial force	Graft sealing cuff, barbs, radial force
Diameter (~15 % oversize)	–	22–36 mm	23–36 mm	23–31 mm
Length (body-ipsilateral)	–	130–161 mm	102 mm	120–180 mm
Ancillary components				
Main body extension	45–58 mm length	39–73 mm length	49–70 mm length	33–45 mm length
Converters	66 mm length	80–82 mm length	–	–
Iliac plugs	–	14–24 mm diameter	–	–

52.8 % for OR and 35.6 % for REVAR ($P < .001$),while for stable patients mortality was 26.3 % for OR and 16.4 % for REVAR ($P = .001$). Also, in this study REVAR was associated with a diminished 30-day mortality and morbidity [104]. Despite the excellent immediate and mid-term REVAR results reported by observational and population-based studies, the level of evidence to support "EVAR-first" for rAAA is still debatable [105] and all three randomized control trials conducted so far failed to prove a survival benefit with REVAR [106–110]. The first study was a single center trial conducted in the UK and published in 2006; it failed to prove a survival benefit for REVAR over OR, but results were considered inaccurate because the trial was interrupted when only a third of the predetermined number of patients was recruited.

The AJAX study [108] is a three-centers trial conducted in the Netherlands where 116 patients with rAAA anatomically suitable for "both" EVAR or OR were randomized to either treatment. This trial did not show a significant difference in combined death and severe complications between the two modalities; 30-days mortality was 21 % post REVAR compared to 25 % with OR (ARR = 4.4 %; 95 % confidence interval:−11 to +20 %). The authors explain the unusually low surgical mortality with the introduction of round-the-clock acute aneurysm service, centralization of aneurysm care and routine preoperative CTA. This study has indeed some significant statistical and technical limitations. Only 22 % (116/520) of rAAA diagnosed in the seven years study period met anatomical criteria for randomization: this limited the yearly caseload per trial center and affected the power of the study with regard to the primary endpoints.

IMPROVE [107] is a multicenter "pragmatic" trial a total of 613 patients with rAAA randomized to REVAR or OR. REVAR was not associated with significant reduction in either 30 day mortality or cost ("endovascular strategy" 35.4 % *vs* OR 37.4 %; odds ratio 0.92; 95 % confidence interval 0.66 to 1.28; $P = 0.62$). Only potential advantages of REVAR were: (i) lower 30 day mortality in the female population ($P = 0.02$) and (ii) earlier recovery with direct discharge to home (189/201 (94 %) *vs*141/183 (77 %); $P < 0.001$ %). Despite the considerable size and the "real world" design of this study, the results from the IMPROVE trial have to be considered carefully. Among the 316 patients randomized to *"endovascular strategy"*(mortality 35.4 %; 112/316) only less than half were considered endoluminal candidate based on CTA and actually underwent REVAR (30 day mortality 25 %; 38/150). The rest were either considered anatomically unsuitable for REVAR and underwent OR (mortality 38 %; 43/112), died during conversion from REVAR to OR (100 %; 4/4), died without treatment (mortality 94 %; 16/17) or didn't have a confirmed rAAA (mortality 33 %; 11/33); this clearly influenced the overall 30 day mortality of 35.4 % of the *"endovascular"* arm of the study. Finally strategy decision and technical expertise, with only a minimum of 5audited REVAR on the logbook, is questionable.

We conclude with a recommendation to transfer patients with clinical suspect of rAAA to centers that can offer *both treatments* with audited results.

Competing interests

The authors declare that they have no competing interests.

Authors' contributions

Dr. BMTP, Dr. OC and Dr. FR contributed equally the same to this study and all three certify that each had a "first author" role equally. Dr. BMTP has written the section "vascular trauma: neck, chest and extremities", Dr. OC has written the section "abdominal vascular injury" and Dr. FR has written the section "ruptured aneurysms of the abdominal aorta: current management and results". All authors reviewed and approved the final manuscript.

Author details

[1]Division of Trauma Surgery, Department of Surgery, School of Medical Sciences, University of Campinas (Unicamp), Campinas, SP, Brazil. [2]Trauma Team, Ospedale Niguarda Milano, Milan, Italy. [3]Department of Cardiothoracic Surgery, John Hunter Hospital, Newcastle, NSW, Australia. [4]Department of Traumatology, John Hunter Hospital, Newcastle, NSW, Australia. [5]Department of Emergency and Trauma Surgery of the University Hospital of Parma, Parma, Italy. [6]Department of general and emergency surgery, Papa Giovanni XIII Hospital, Bergamo, Italy. [7]Department of surgery, Macerata Hospital, Macerata, Italy. [8]Department of surgery, Maggiore Hospital of Bologna, Bologna, Italy.

References

1. Asfar S, Al Ali J, Safar H, Al Bader M, Farid E, Ali A, et al. 155 vascular injuries: a retrospective study in Kuwait, 1992–2000. Eur J Surg. 2002;168(11):626–30.
2. Razmadze A. Vascular injuries of the limbs: a fifteen-year Georgian experience. Eur J Vasc Endovasc Surg. 1999;18(3):235–9.
3. Menakuru SR, Behera A, Jindal R, Kaman L, Doley R, Venkatesan R. Extremity vascular trauma in civilian population: a seven-year review from North India. Injury. 2005;36(3):400–6.
4. Lakhwani MN, Gooi BH, Barras CD. Vascular trauma in Penang and Kuala Lumpur Hospitals. Med J Malays. 2002;57(4):426–32.
5. Sugrue M, Caldwell EM, Damours SK, Crozier JA, Deane SA. Vascular injury in Australia. Surg Clin N Am. 2002;82(1):211–9.
6. Morales-Uribe CH, Sanabria-Quiroga AE, Sierra-Jones JM. Vascular trauma in Colombia: experience of a level I trauma center in Medellin. Surg Clin N Am. 2002;82(1):195–210.
7. Sonneborn R, Andrade R, Bello F, Morales-Uribe CH, Razuk A, Soria A, et al. Vascular trauma in Latin America: a regional survey. Surg Clin N Am. 2002;82(1):189–94.
8. Fingerhut A, Leppaniemi AK, Androulakis GA, Archodovassilis F, Bouillon B, Cavina E, et al. The European experience with vascular injuries. Surg Clin N Am. 2002;82(1):175–88.
9. Gupta R, Rao S, Sieunarine K. An epidemiological view of vascular trauma in Western Australia: a 5-year study. ANZ J Surg. 2001;71(8):461–6.
10. Rich NM. Complications of Vascular Injury Management. Surg Clin N Am. 2002;82(1):143–74.
11. Fox CJ, Gillespie DL, O'Donnell SD, Rasmussen TE, Goff JM, Johnson CA, et al. Contemporary management of wartime vascular trauma. J Vasc Surg. 2005;41(4):638–44.
12. Jaha L, Andreevska T, Rudari H, Ademi B, Ismaili-Jaha V. A decade of civilian vascular trauma in Kosovo. World J Emerg Surg. 2012;7(1):24.
13. Perkins ZB, De'Ath HD, Aylwin C, Brohi K, Walsh M, Tai NR. Epidemiology and outcome of vascular trauma at a British Major Trauma Centre. Eur J Vasc Endovasc Surg. 2012;44(2):203–9.
14. Gonçalves R, SaadJúnior R. Surgical accesses to the major mediastinalvessels in thoracic trauma. Rev Col Bras Cir. 2012;39(1):64–73. Review.

15. Pereira BM, Nogueira VB, Calderan TR, Villaca MP, Petrucci O, Fraga GP. Penetrating cardiac trauma: 20-y experience from a university teaching hospital. J Surg Res. 2013;183:792.
16. Prichayudh S, Verananvattna A, Sriussadaporn S, Sriussadaporn S, Kritayakirana K, Pak-art R, et al. Management of upper extremity vascular injury: outcome related to the Mangled Extremity Severity Score. World J Surg. 2009;33(4):857–63.
17. Feliciano DV, Shackford SR. Vascular injury: 50th anniversary year review article of The Journal of Trauma. J Trauma. 2010;68(4):1009–13.
18. Rozycki GS, Tremblay LN, Feliciano DV, McClelland WB. Blunt vascular trauma in the extremity: diagnosis, management, and outcome. J Trauma. 2003;55(5):814–24.
19. Feliciano DV, Moore FA, Moore EE, West MA, Davis JW, Cocanour CS, et al. Evaluation and management of peripheral vascular injury. Part 1. Western Trauma Association/critical decisions in trauma. J Trauma. 2011;70(6):1551–6.
20. Rasmussen TE, Woodson J, Rich NM, Mattox KL. Vascular trauma at a crossroads. J Trauma. 2011;70(5):1291–3.
21. Hirshberg A, Mattox KL. Top Knife. The art & craft of trauma surgery. TFM, Castle Hill Barns, Harley, UK, 2005:(1).
22. Thakore N, Abbas S, Vanniasingham P. Delayed rupture of common carotid artery following rugby tackle injury: a case report. World J Emerg Surg. 2008;3:14.
23. Sperry JL, Moore EE, Coimbra R, Croce M, Davis JW, Karmy-Jones R, et al. Western Trauma Association critical decisions in trauma: penetrating neck trauma. J Trauma Acute Care Surg. 2013;75(6):936–40.
24. Ofer A, Nitecki SS, Braun J, Daitzchman M, Goldsher D, Hoffman A, et al. CT angiography of the carotid arteries in trauma to the neck. Eur J Vasc Endovasc Surg. 2001;21(5):401–7.
25. Dua A, Desai SS, Kuy S, Patel B, Dua A, Desai PJ, et al. Predicting outcomes using the national trauma data bank: optimum management of traumatic blunt carotid and blunt thoracic injury. Perspect Vasc Surg Endovasc Ther. 2012;24(3):123–7.
26. Ventura J, Hirano ES, Fraga GP. Glass-coated kites and cervical injuries. Clinics. 2011;66(5):923–5.
27. duToit DF, van Schalkwyk GD, Wadee SA, Warren BL. Neurologic outcome after penetrating extracranial arterial trauma. J Vasc Surg. 2003;38(2):257–62.
28. Lleva P, Ahluwalia BS, Marks S, Sahni R, Tenner M, Risucci DA, et al. Traumatic and spontaneous carotid and vertebral artery dissection in a level 1 trauma center. J Clin Neurosci. 2012;19(8):1112–4.
29. Maillard AA, Urso RG, Jarolimek AM. Trauma to the intracranial internal carotid artery. J Trauma. 2010;68(3):545–7.
30. Shiroff AM, Gale SC, Martin ND, Marchalik D, Petrov D, Ahmed HM, et al. Penetrating neck trauma: a review of management strategies and discussion of the 'No Zone' approach. Am Surg. 2013;79(1):23–9.
31. Dyer DS, Moore EE, Ilke DN, McIntyre RC, Bernstein SM, Durham JD, et al. Thoracic aortic injury: how predictive is mechanism and is chest computed tomography a reliable screening tool? A prospective study of 1,561 patients. J Trauma. 2000;48(4):673–82. discussion 682–3.
32. O'Connor JV, Byrne C, Scalea TM, Griffith BP, Neschis DG. Vascular injuries after blunt chest trauma: diagnosis and management. Scand J Trauma Resusc Emerg Med. 2009;17:42.
33. Schulman CI, Carvajal D, Lopez PP, Soffer D, Habib F, Augenstein J. Incidence and crash mechanisms of aortic injury during the past decade. J Trauma. 2007;62:664–7.
34. Horton TG, Cohn SM, Heid MP, Augenstein JS, Bowen JC, McKenney MG, et al. Identification of trauma patients at risk of thoracic aortic tear by mechanism of injury. J Trauma. 2000;48:1008–13.
35. Symbas JD, Halkos ME, Symbas PN. Rupture of the innominate artery from blunt trauma: current options for management. J Card Surg. 2005;20:455–9.
36. Okoye OT, Talving P, Teixeira PG, Chervonski M, Smith JA, Inaba K, et al. Transmediastinal gunshot wounds in a mature trauma centre: Changing perspectives. Injury. 2013;44:1198.
37. Ruano RM, Pereira BM, Biazzoto G, Bortoto JB, Fraga GP. Management of Severe Thoracic Impalement Trauma Against Two-Wheeled Horse Carriage: A Case Report and Literature Review. Indian J Surg. 2014;76(4):297–302.
38. DuBose JJ, Savage SA, Fabian TC, Menaker J, Scalea T, Holcomb JB, et al. The American Association for the Surgery of Trauma PROspective Observational Vascular Injury Treatment (PROOVIT) registry: multicenter data on modern vascular injury diagnosis, management, and outcomes. J Trauma Acute Care Surg. 2015;78(2):215–22. discussion 222–3.
39. Penn-Barwell JG. Outcomes in lower limb amputation following trauma: a systematic review and meta-analysis. Injury. 2011;42(12):1474–9.
40. Huh J, Stinner DJ, Burns TC, Hsu JR. Infectious complications and soft tissue injury contribute to late amputation after severe lower extremity trauma. J Trauma. 2011;71(1 Suppl):S47–51.
41. Peña D, Pereira BM, Prichayudh S, Tsunoyama T, Ruiz F, Capin A, et al. Femoral Vessel Injuries: Analysis of the NTDB. J Am Coll Surg. 2009;209(3):s140.
42. Frykberg ER. Popliteal vascular injuries. Surg Clin North Am. 2002;82(1):67–89.
43. Simmons JD, Gunter 3rd JW, Schmieg Jr RE, Manley JD, Rushton Jr FW, Porter JM, et al. Popliteal artery injuries in an urban trauma center with a rural catchment area: do delays in definitive treatment affect amputation? Am Surg. 2011;77(11):1521–5.
44. Chapellier X, Sockeel P, Baranger B. Management of penetrating abdominal vessel injuries. J Visc Surg. 2010;147:e1–12.
45. Johnson GE, Sandstrom CK, Kogut MJ, Ingraham CR, Stratil PG, Valji K, et al. Frequency of external iliac artery branch injury in blunt trauma: improved detection with selective external iliac angiography. J Vasc Interv Radiol. 2013;24:363–9.
46. Shalhub S, Starnes BW, Tran NT, Hatsukami TS, Lundgren RS, Davis CW, et al. Blunt abdominal aortic injury. J Vasc Surg. 2012;55:1277–86.
47. Aladham F, Sundaram B, Williams DM, Quint LE. Traumatic aortic injury: computerized tomographic findings at presentation and after conservative therapy. J Comput Assist Tomogr. 2010;34:388–9.
48. Moore EE, Cogbill TH, Jurkovich GJ, McAninch JW, Champion HR, Gennarelli TA, et al. Organ injury scaling III: Chest wall, abdominal vascular, ureter, bladder, and urethra. J Trauma. 1992;30:337–40.
49. Deree J, Shenvi E, Fortlage D, Potenza B, Hoyt DB, Coimbra R. Patient factors and operating room resuscitation predict mortality in traumatic abdominal aortic injury; a 20-years analysis. J Vasc Surg. 2007;45:493–7.
50. Sullivan PS, Dente CJ, Patel S, Carmichael M, Srinivasan JK, Wyrzykowski AD, et al. Outcome of ligation of inferior vena cava in the modern era. Am J Surg. 2010;199:500–6.
51. Requarth JA, Miller PR. Aberrant obturator artery is a common arterial variant that may be a source of unidentified hemorrhage in pelvic fracture patients. J Trauma. 2011;70:366–72.
52. Mohan B, Bodhay HS, Aslam N, Kaur H, Chhabra S, Sood N, et al. hepatic vascular injury: clinical profile, endovascular management and outcomes. Ind Heart J. 2012;65:59–65.
53. HamesH FTL, HarrisJR LDK, DeRose G, Harris KA. The effect of patient transfer on outcomes after rupture of an abdominal aortic aneurysm. Can J Surg. 2007;50:43–7.
54. IMPROVE trial investigators, Powell JT, Hinchliffe RJ, Thompson MM, Sweeting MJ, Ashleigh R, et al. Observations from the IMPROVE trial concerning the clinical care of patients with ruptured abdominal aortic aneurysm. Br J Surg. 2014;101:216–24.
55. Veith FJ, Ohki T. Endovascular approaches to ruptured infrarenalaorto-iliac aneurysms. J Cardiovasc Surg. 2002;43:369–78.
56. van der Vliet JA, van Aalst DL, Schultze Kool LJ, Wever JJ, Blankensteijn JD. Hypotensive hemostasis (permissive hypotension) for ruptured abdominal aortic aneurysm: are we really in control? Vascular. 2007;15:197–200.
57. Lloyd GM, Bown MJ, Norwood MG, Deb R, Fishwick G, Bell PR, et al. Feasibility of preoperative computer tomography in patients with ruptured abdominal aortic aneurysm: a time-to-death study in patients without operation. J Vasc Surg. 2004;39:788–91.
58. Mehta M, Taggert J, Darling 3rd RC, Chang BB, Kreienberg PB, Paty PS, et al. Establishing a protocol for endovascular treatment of ruptured abdominal aortic aneurysms: outcomes of a prospective analysis. J Vasc Surg. 2006;44:1–8.
59. Moore R, Nutley M, Cina CS, Motamedi M, Faris P, Abuznadah W. Improved survival after introduction of an emergency endovascular therapy protocol for ruptured abdominal aortic aneurysms. J Vasc Surg. 2007;45:443–50.
60. Lindsay TF. Abdominal aortic aneurysms: ruptured. Chapter 133. In Cronenwett: Rutherford's Vascular Surgery, 8th Ed. Philadelphia: Saunders, Elsevier. 2005.
61. O'Hara PJ, Hertzer NR. Infrarenal abdominal aortic aneurysm: open repair. Chapter 30. In Hallett: Comprehensive Vascular and Endovascular Surgery, 2nd Ed. Philadelphia: Mosby, Elsevier. 2009.
62. Sicard GA, Reilly JM, Rubin BG, Thompson RW, Allen BT, Flye MW, et al. Transabdominalversus retroperitoneal incision for abdominal aortic surgery: report of a prospective randomized trial. J Vasc Surg. 1995;21:174–81.
63. Cambria RP, Brewster DC, Abbott WM, Freehan M, Megerman J, LaMuraglia G, et al. Transperitoneal versus retroperitoneal approach for aortic reconstruction: a randomized prospective study. J Vasc Surg. 1990;11:314–8.

64. Darling III RC, Shah DM, Chang BB, Paty PS, Leather RP. Current status of the use of retroperitoneal approach for reconstructions of the aorta and its branches. Ann Surg. 1996;224:501–8.
65. Chang BB, Paty PK, Shah DM, Leather RP. Selective use of retroperitoneal aortic exposure in the emergency treatment of ruptured and symptomatic abdominal aortic aneurysms. Ann Surg. 1988;156:108–10.
66. Raux M, Marzelle J, Kobeiter H, Dhonneur G, Allaire E, Cochennec F, et al. Endovascular balloon occlusion is associated with reduced intraoperative mortality of unstable patients with ruptured abdominal aortic aneurysm but fails to improve other outcomes. J Vasc Surg. 2014;61:304–8.
67. Martinelli T, Thorny F, Declety P, Sengel C, Broux C, Tonetti J, et al. Intra-aortic balloon occlusion to salvage patients with life-threatening hemorrhagic shocks from pelvic fractures. J Trauma. 2010;68:942–8.
68. Marty-Ane CH, Alric P, Picot MC, Picard E, Colson P, Mary H. Ruptured abdominal aortic aneurysm: influence of intraoperative management on surgical outcome. J Vasc Surg. 1995;22:780–6.
69. Serracino-Inglott F, Awad S, Barclay A, Nasim A. The use of a cell saver during repair of ruptured abdominal aortic aneurysms increases early survival. Ann R Coll Surg Engl. 2005;87:475.
70. Graham AP, Fitgerald O'Connor E, Hinchliffe RJ, Loftus IM, Thompson MM, Black SA. The use of heparin in patients with ruptured abdominal aortic aneurysms. Vascular. 2012;20:61–4.
71. Wiersema AM, Jongkind V, Bruijninckx CM, Reijnen MM, Vos JA, van Delden OM, et al. Prophylactic perioperative anti-thrombotics in open and endovascular abdominal aortic aneurysm surgery: a systematic review. Eur J Vasc Endovasc Surg. 2012;44:359–67.
72. Rasmussen TE, Hallett Jr JW, Noel AA, Jenkins G, Bower TC, Cherry Jr KJ, et al. Early abdominal closure with mesh reduces multiple organ failure after ruptured abdominal aortic aneurysm repair: guidelines from a 10 year case-control study. J Vasc Surg. 2002;35:246–53.
73. Björck M. Management of the tense abdomen or difficult abdominal closure after operation for ruptured abdominal aortic aneurysms. SeminVasc Surg. 2012;25:35–8.
74. Parodi JC, Palmaz JC, Barone HD. Transfemoral intraluminal graft implantation for abdominal aortic aneurysms. Ann Vasc Surg. 1991;5:491–9.
75. Prinssen M, Buskens E, de Jong SE, Buth J, Mackaay AJ, van Sambeek MR, et al. A randomized trial comparing conventional and endovascular repair of abdominal aortic aneurysms. N Engl J Med. 2004;351:1607–18.
76. Greenhalgh RM, Brown LC, Kwong GP, Powell JT, Thompson SG, EVAR trial participants. Comparison of endovascular aneurysm repair with open repair in patients with abdominal aortic aneurysm (EVAR trial 1), 30-day operative mortality results: randomized controlled trial. Lancet. 2004;364:843–8.
77. Marin ML, Veith FJ, Cynamon J, Sanchez LA, Lyon RT, Levine BA, et al. Initial experience with transluminally placed endovascular grafts for the treatment of complex vascular lesions. Ann Surg. 1995;222:449–65.
78. Mastracci TM, Garrido-Olivares L, Cinà CS, Clase CM. Endovascular repair of ruptured abdominal aortic aneurysms: a systematic review and meta-analysis. J Vasc Surg. 2008;47:214–21.
79. Veith FJ, Lachat M, Mayer D, Malina M, Holst J, Mehta M, et al. Collected world and single center experience with endovascular treatment of ruptured abdominal aortic aneurysm. Ann Surg. 2009;250:818–24.
80. Metha M. Endovascular aneurysm repair for ruptured abdominal aortic aneurysm: the Albany Vascular Group approach. J Vasc Surg. 2010;52:1706–12.
81. Mayer D, Aeschbacher S, Pfammatter T, Veith FJ, Norgren L, Magnuson A, et al. Complete replacement of open repair for ruptured abdominal aortic aneurysms by endovascular aneurysm repair: a two-center 14-year experience. Ann Surg. 2012;256:688–95.
82. Hodgson KJ. EVAR for ruptured aneurysms: are the data complete? SeminVasc Surg. 2012;25:217–26.
83. Lachat ML, Pfammatter T, Witzke HJ, Bettex D, Künzli A, Wolfensberger U, et al. Endovascular repair with bifurcated stent-grafts under local anaesthesia to improve outcome of ruptured aortoiliac aneurysms. Eur J VascEndovasc Surg. 2002;23:528–36.
84. Lee WA, Brown MP, Nelson PR, Huber TS. Total percutaneous access for endovascular aortic aneurysm repair ("Preclose" technique). J Vasc Surg. 2007;45:1095–101.
85. Malina M, Veith F, Ivancev K, Sonesson B. Balloon occlusion of the aorta during endovascular repair of ruptured abdominal aortic aneurysm. J Endovasc Ther. 2005;12:556–9.
86. White GH, Yu W, May J, Chaufour X, Stephen MS. Endoleak as a complication of endoluminal grafting of abdominal aortic aneurysms: classification, incidence, diagnosis, and management. J Endovasc Surg. 1997;4:152–68.
87. Rancic Z, Mayer D, Pfammatter T, Frauenfelder T, Falk V, Ueda H, et al. A new sutureless telescoping anastomotic technique for major aortic branch revascularization with minimal dissection and ischemia. Ann Surg. 2010;252:884–9.
88. Pecoraro F, Pfammatter T, Mayer D, Frauenfelder T, Papadimitriou D, Hechelhammer L, et al. Multiple periscope and chimney grafts to treat ruptured thoracoabdominal and pararenal aortic aneurysms. J Endovasc Ther. 2011;18:642–9.
89. Mehta M, Darling 3rd RC, Roddy SP, Fecteau S, Ozsvath KJ, Kreienberg PB, et al. Factors associated with abdominal compartment syndrome complicating endovascular repair of ruptured abdominal aortic aneurysms. J Vasc Surg. 2005;42:1047–51.
90. Mayer D, Pfammatter T, Rancic Z, Hechelhammer L, Wilhelm M, Veith FJ, et al. 10 years of emergency endovascular aneurysm repair for ruptured abdominal aortoiliac aneurysms: lessons learned. Ann Surg. 2009;249:510–5.
91. Mayer D, Rancic Z, Meier C, Pfammatter T, Veith FJ, Lachat M. Open abdomen treatment following endovascular repair of ruptured abdominal aortic aneurysms. J Vasc Surg. 2009;50:1–7.
92. Bown MJ, Sutton AJ, Bell PR, Sayers RD. A meta-analysis of 50 years of ruptured abdominal aortic aneurysm repair. Br J Surg. 2002;89:714–30.
93. Visser P, Akkersdijk GJ, Blankensteijn JD. In-hospital operative mortality of ruptured abdominal aortic aneurysm: a population-based analysis of 5593 patients in The Netherlands over a 10-year period. Eur J Vasc Endovasc Surg. 2005;30:359–64.
94. Lindsay TF, Luo XP, Lehotay DC, Rubin BB, Anderson M, Walker PM, et al. Ruptured abdominal aortic aneurysm, a "two-hit" ischemia/reperfusion injury: evidence from an analysis of oxidative products. J Vasc Surg. 1999;30:219–28.
95. Mehta M, Byrne J, Darling 3rd RC, Paty PS, Roddy SP, Kreienberg PB, et al. Endovascular repair of ruptured infrarenal abdominal aortic aneurysm is associated with lower 30-day mortality and better 5-year survival rates than open surgical repair. J Vasc Surg. 2013;57:368–75.
96. Starnes BW, Quiroga E, Hutter C, Tran NT, Hatsukami T, Meissner M, et al. Management of ruptured abdominal aortic aneurysm in the endovascular era. J Vasc Surg. 2010;51:9–17.
97. Brossier J, Coscas R, Capdevila C, Kitzis M, Coggia M, Goeau-Brissonniere O. Anatomic feasibility of endovascular treatment of abdominal aortic aneurysms in emergency in the era of the chimney technique: impact on an emergency endovascular kit. Ann Vasc Surg. 2013;27:844–50.
98. Egorova N, Giacovelli J, Greco G, Gelijns A, Kent CK, McKinsey JF. National outcomes for the treatment of ruptured abdominal aortic aneurysm: comparison of open versus endovascular repairs. J Vasc Surg. 2008;48:1092–100.
99. Coppi G, Silingardi R, Gennai S, Saitta G, Ciardullo AV. A single-center experience in open and endovascular treatment of hemodynamically unstable and stable patients with ruptured abdominal aortic aneurysms. J Vasc Surg. 2006;44:1140–7.
100. Karkos CD, Sutton AJ, Bown MJ, Sayers RD. A meta-analysis and metaregression analysis of factors influencing mortality after endovascular repair of rupturedabdominal aortic aneurysms. Eur J Vasc Endovasc Surg. 2011;42:775–86.
101. Lee RW, Rhodes JM, Singh MJ, Davies MG, Wolford HY, Diachun C, et al. Is there a selection bias in applying endovascular aneurysm repair for rupture? Ann Vasc Surg. 2008;22:215–20.
102. Badger S, Bedenis R, Blair PH, Ellis P, Kee F, Harkin DW. Endovascular treatment for ruptured abdominal aortic aneurysm. Cochrane Database Syst Rev. 2014;7:1–37.
103. Edwards ST, Schermerhorn ML, O'Malley AJ, Bensley RP, Hurks R, Cotterill P, et al. Comparative effectiveness of endovascular versus open repair of ruptured abdominal aortic aneurysm in the Medicare population. J Vasc Surg. 2014;59:575–82.
104. Gupta PK, Ramanan B, Engelbert TL, Tefera G, Hoch JR, Kent KC. A comparison of open surgery versus endovascular repair of unstable ruptured abdominal aortic aneurysms. J Vasc Surg. 2014;60:1439–45.
105. Veith FJ, Powell JT, Hinchliffe RJ. Is a randomized trial necessary to determine whether endovascular repair is the preferred management strategy in patients with ruptured abdominal aortic aneurysms? J Vasc Surg. 2010;52:1087–93.
106. Hinchliffe RJ, Bruijstens L, MacSweeney ST, Braithwaite BD. A randomised trial of endovascular and open surgery for ruptured abdominal aortic

aneurysm - results of a pilot study and lessons learned for future studies. Eur J Vasc Endovasc Surg. 2006;32:506–13.
107. IMPROVE Trial Investigators, Powell JT, Sweeting MJ, Thompson MM, Ashleigh R, Bell R, et al. Endovascular or open repair strategy for ruptured abdominal aortic aneurysm: 30 day outcomes from IMPROVE randomized trial. BMJ. 2014;348:7661.
108. Reimerink JJ, Hoornweg LL, Vahl AC, Wisselink W, van den Broek TA, Legemate DA, et al. Endovascular repair versus open repair of ruptured abdominal aortic aneurysms: a multicenter randomized controlled trial. Ann Surg. 2013;258:248–56.
109. Hoornweg LL, Storm-Versloot MN, Ubbink DT, Koelemay MJ, Legemate DA, Balm R. Meta-analysis on mortality of ruptured abdominal aortic aneurysms. Eur J Vasc Endovasc Surg. 2008;35:558–70.
110. Mureebe L, Egorova N, Giacovelli JK, Gelijns A, Kent KC, McKinsey JF. National trends in the repair of ruptured abdominal aortic aneurysms. J Vasc Surg. 2008;48:1101–7.

8

Allocating operating room resources to an acute care surgery service does not affect wait-times for elective cancer surgeries

Ram Venkatesh Anantha[1], Dave Paskar[1], Kelly Vogt[2], Silvie Crawford[3], Neil Parry[1,4,5] and Ken Leslie[1,6*]

Abstract

Introduction: Acute care surgical services provide timely comprehensive emergency general surgical care while optimizing the use of limited resources. At our institution, 50% of the daily dedicated operating room (OR) time allocated to the Acute Care Emergency Surgery Service (ACCESS) came from previous elective general surgery OR time. We assessed the impact of this change in resource allocation on wait-times for elective general surgery cancer cases.

Methods: We retrospectively reviewed adult patients who underwent elective cancer surgeries in the pre-ACCESS (September 2009 to June 2010) and post-ACCESS (September 2010 to June 2011) eras. Wait-times, calculated as the time between booking and actual dates of surgery, were compared within assigned priority classifications. Categorical and continuous variables were compared using chi-square and Mann–Whitney U tests respectively.

Results: A total of 732 cases (367 pre-ACCESS and 365 post-ACCESS) were identified, with no difference in median wait-times (25 versus 23 days) between the eras. However, significantly fewer cases exceeded wait-time targets in the post-ACCESS era ($p < 0.0001$). There was a significant change ($p = 0.027$) in the composition of cancer cases, with fewer breast cancer operations (22% versus 28%), and more colorectal (41% versus 32%) and hepatobiliary cancer cases (5% versus 2%) in the post-ACCESS era.

Conclusion: These results suggest that shifting OR resources towards emergency surgery does not affect the timeliness of surgical cancer care. This study may encourage more centres to adopt acute care surgical services alongside their elective or subspecialty practices.

Keywords: Acute care surgery, Cancer wait-times, Resource allocation, Health outcomes research

Introduction

Acute care surgery (ACS) is a distinct surgical care model that provides dedicated comprehensive care for general surgical emergencies such as acute appendicitis, cholecystitis, bowel obstruction, perineal sepsis, and perforated viscus [1-3]. This model has proven to be an innovative and cost-effective strategy of delivering emergency surgical care to patients [1,3], resulting in significantly shorter wait-times for urgent and emergent operations [4-7], more efficient disposition from the emergency room [4-7], and considerably reduced hospital costs [5,8,9] in many centres. Surgeons also benefit from this model as it offers more predictable scheduling, reduced nocturnal workload, and enables them to focus on elective patient care or academic endeavours when they are not on call for ACS [1].

The local delivery and structure of ACS services can vary significantly from hospital to hospital, particularly in terms of the availability of dedicated ACS operating room (OR) time. Because of the financial constraints associated with a publicly-funded healthcare system, Canadian hospitals have typically funded dedicated ACS OR time by reallocating existing OR resources,

* Correspondence: ken.leslie@lhsc.on.ca
[1]Division of General Surgery, Department of Surgery, Schulich School of Medicine and Dentistry, Western University, London, ON, Canada
[6]Victoria Hospital, London Health Sciences Centre, Room E2-217, 800 Commissioners Road East, London, ON N6A 5W9, Canada

rather than providing additional funding *de novo*. At the London Health Sciences Centre (LHSC) - Victoria Hospital, the Acute Care and Emergency Surgery Service (ACCESS) was established in July 2010 when the growing need for organized emergency general surgery coverage was recognized by the Division of General Surgery, the Emergency Department, and hospital leadership. In this model, a single staff surgeon suspends their elective practice while covering ACCESS for one week at a time (Monday to Monday), and their previously-allocated elective OR time for the week (15 hours) is subsumed into the daily dedicated ACCESS OR time. An additional 15 hours of OR time per week was funded by the South West Local Health Integration Network (the health authority responsible for administering public healthcare services within Southwestern Ontario) specifically for the ACCESS initiative, for a total of 30 hours per week dedicated to the service. The team is also assigned a full complement of housestaff.

In 2004, Ontario's Ministry of Health and Long-Term Care (MOHLTC) implemented a Wait Time Strategy [10-13] to improve access to healthcare services for adult patients in five "key" populations, one of which was those requiring cancer surgery. Target wait-times were developed by Cancer Care Ontario (CCO) and the Surgical Access to Care and Wait Times Subcommittee [10,14], and provincial funding for centres providing surgical care for cancer patients was based on adherence to these suggested guidelines [10,13]. Since all the surgeons at LHSC who participate in ACCESS also perform cancer operations as part of their subspecialty practices, we sought to determine if the weekly suspension of one surgeon's elective practice and diversion of their elective OR time for the week had a negative impact on wait-times for cancer surgeries.

Methods

All clinical activity reviewed occurred at Victoria Hospital (VH), LHSC in London, Canada, which serves as a regional tertiary-care hospital and Level I trauma centre for Southwestern Ontario. The Division of General Surgery at VH is a diverse group of sub-specialists, including colorectal, hepatobiliary, endocrine, surgical oncology, trauma, and minimally invasive surgeons. All eight general surgeons at Victoria Hospital were involved with ACCESS during the study period, and performed oncological surgeries as part of their subspecialty practices, including thyroid, breast, colorectal, hepatobiliary (HPB), foregut (gastric and duodenal), endocrine, and melanoma surgery. Other surgical specialties, including plastic, orthopaedic, urologic, gynecologic, and head and neck surgery, also routinely perform cancer operations at VH.

Ethics approval for this single-centre retrospective cohort study was provided by the Western University Research and Ethics Board (REB Number 102988). The LHSC-VH operative database was queried for all elective cancer operations performed by all surgical specialties between September 1, 2009 and June 30, 2010 (pre-ACCESS) and between September 1, 2010 and June 30, 2011 (post-ACCESS). Cancer surgeries were defined as oncological operations booked electively. As part of the provincial Wait-Time Strategy initiative, all cancer operations were assigned a certain priority status by the surgeon at the time of booking based on the perceived urgency of the intervention (Table 1). Recommended wait-times for surgery are determined by the assigned priority and range from immediate (for patients with life-threatening malignancies; "P1" status) to 84 days (for patients with indolent tumours; "P4" status). Wait-times are defined as the length of time between the decision-to-treat date (defined as the date on which the surgeon and patient made the decision to pursue surgery) and the date that the operation was actually performed.

All adults (age 18 and older) undergoing elective cancer surgery with curative intent and whose decision-to-treat and operation dates fell within the defined study periods

Table 1 Recommended target wait times (days) for cancer operations based on assigned priority category, as established by the Cancer Care Ontario sub-committee on cancer wait times

Priority category	Clinical conditions	Consult to decision-to-treat*	Ready-to-treat to operation
P1	Patients requiring surgery to remove known or suspected cancers that have immediately life-threatening conditions (e.g., airway obstruction, hemorrhage, neurological compromise)	Immediate	Immediate
P2	Patients diagnosed with very aggressive tumours, such as central nervous system (CNS) cancer	14	14
P3	All patients with known or suspected invasive cancer that does not meet the criteria of urgency category II or IV	14	28
P4	Patients diagnosed with indolent tumours	14	84

*From the date of the patient's first visit to the operating surgeon for this specific problem until the decision-to-treat date. The decision-to-treat date is the date on which sufficient pre-treatment testing is complete, the physician can reasonably assume that the patient will be treated, and the patient has agreed to the treatment. By this date, sufficient assessment will have been completed in order to reasonably assume that the procedure will go ahead, and an operating room booking is requested.

were included. We excluded patients whose cases were booked in emergency or ACCESS OR time, and patients who were assigned a P1 priority status, since they required an imminent operation and thus were typically operated on non-electively. We also excluded patients who underwent surgery to remove benign or pre-malignant tumours, to correct or repair defects from previous cancer operations (reconstructive surgery), or to provide palliation.

Analyses were carried out on the basis of surgeries performed by general surgeons, as well as the overall patient population. Continuous variables were compared using the Mann–Whitney U-test. Categorical variables were compared using chi-square or Fisher's exact tests where indicated. P-values less than 0.05 were considered statistically significant. Statistical analysis was performed using Graphpad Prism Version 5 (Graphpad, La Jolla, California).

Results

We identified a total of 732 patients who underwent cancer surgery by the general surgeons at VH across the two study periods (Table 2). There were 365 elective cancer surgeries performed in the post-ACCESS, compared to 367 cases performed in the pre-ACCESS period. Overall, there was no difference in the median wait-times (25 versus 23 days) between the eras for elective general surgery cancer operations ($p = 0.82$).

The distribution of general surgery cancer cases by priority level was significantly different ($p < 0.0001$) between the eras: in the post-ACCESS period, P2 and P3 cases declined by 95% and 40%, respectively, while P4 cases rose by 185%. There was no significant change in wait-times for elective general surgery cancer cases pre- and post-ACCESS, according to priority status. However, the proportion of cases that exceeded assigned wait-time targets in the post-ACCESS era declined by 100% and 55% for P2 and P3 cases, respectively ($p < 0.0001$), while the proportion of P4 cases that exceeded wait-time targets did not change (Table 2). There was also a significant change in the type of cancer operated by general surgeons post-ACCESS: breast cancer, skin carcinoma, and skin melanoma cases declined by 24%,

Table 2 Distribution of elective cancer operations performed by general surgeons at Victoria Hospital, before (pre-ACCESS) and after (post-ACCESS) the implementation of ACCESS

Variable	Pre-ACCESS	Post-ACCESS	Change, n (%)	P value
Number of cases, n	367	365	−2 (−1)	-
Number of cases by priority, n (%)				<0.0001
P2	21 (6)	1 (0.3)	−20 (−95)	
P3	277 (75)	167 (46)	−110 (−40)	
P4	69 (19)	197 (54)	+128 (+185)	
Number of cases exceeding wait-time targets, n (%)				<0.0001
P2	13 (62)	0 (0)	−13 (−100)	
P3	92 (33)	41 (25)	−51 (−55)	
P4	2 (3)	2 (1)	0 (0)	
Median wait-times by priority, days (range)				0.94
P2	15 (2–29)	9 (N/A)	−6 (−40)	
P3	21 (0–90)	15 (0–90)	−6 (−29)	
P4	33 (6–92)	22 (0–90)	−11 (−33)	
Type of cancer, n (%)				0.027
Breast	104 (28)	79 (22)	−25 (−24)	
Colorectal	119 (32)	151 (41)	+32 (+27)	
Hepatopancreatobiliary	8 (2)	18 (5)	+10 (+125)	
Gastric	10 (3)	5 (1)	−5 (−50)	
Endocrine	100 (27)	94 (26)	−6 (−6)	
Lymph	1 (0)	0 (0)	−1 (−100)	
Soft-tissue sarcoma	6 (2)	8 (2)	+2 (+33)	
Skin carcinoma[1]	4 (1)	2 (1)	−2 (−50)	
Skin melanoma	15 (4)	7 (2)	−8 (−53)	

[1]Includes basal and squamous cell carcinoma.

50%, and 53%, respectively, whereas colorectal and hepatobiliary cases increased by 27% and 125%, respectively ($p = 0.027$).

There were 3309 cancer surgeries performed by non-general surgeon specialists at VH during the study periods (Table 3). There was a 4% reduction in the total number of cancer surgeries performed in the post-ACCESS era. The distribution of cancer cases by priority level was also significantly different post-ACCESS ($p < 0.0001$): P2 and P3 cases declined by 49% and 25%, respectively, while P4 cases rose by 62%. Furthermore, the number of cases that exceeded wait-time targets based on their designated priority levels declined by 100% and 55% for P2 and P3 cases, respectively, post-ACCESS ($p < 0.0001$). There was no significant change in the length of wait-times for elective cancer cases pre- and post-ACCESS. Additionally, the proportions by type of cancer treated at VH was significantly different post-ACCESS ($p < 0.0001$): esophageal, prostate, and gynaecological cancer cases declined by 19%, 20%, and 19%, respectively, while head and neck cancer, and lung cancer cases increased by 79% and 15%, respectively.

Discussion

As ACS continues to flourish around the world, an increasing number of studies have emphasized the benefits of this care model for patients with general surgical emergencies [2,5,8,15-18]. Surgical departments, however, have historically been expensive to run because of the costly equipment, support staff, as well as the specialized nursing and medical staff required [19]. The operating room, therefore, is viewed as a necessary but expensive liability in the financially-constrained Canadian healthcare system. Consequently, funding for the implementation of surgical programs such as ACS services often requires the reallocation of pre-existing operating room resources.

Prior to the implementation of ACCESS at our institution, there was no structured system for performing

Table 3 Distribution of elective cancer operations performed by subspecialty surgical oncologists (non-general surgeons) at Victoria Hospital, before and after the implementation of ACCESS (pre- and post-ACCESS, respectively)

Variable	Pre-ACCESS, n (%)	Post-ACCESS, n (%)	Change, n (%)	P value
Number of cases, n	1685	1624	−61 (−4)	-
Number of cases by priority level, n (%)				<0.0001
P2	187 (11)	95 (6)	−92 (−49)	
P3	1027 (61)	768 (47)	−259 (−25)	
P4	471 (28)	761 (47)	+290 (+62)	
No. of cases exceeding wait-time targets by priority, n (%)				0.39
P2	120 (64)	61 (64)	−59 (−49)	
P3	485 (47)	297 (39)	−188 (−39)	
P4	122 (26)	118 (16)	−4 (−3)	
Median wait-times by priority, days (range)				0.52
P2	19 (1–215)	17 (1–55)	−2 (−10)	
P3	27 (0–274)	23 (0–108)	−4 (−14)	
P4	66 (0–246)	41 (0–207)	−25 (−37)	
Type of cancer, n (%)				< 0.0001
Gastric	21 (1)	10 (0.6)	−11 (−52)	
Endocrine	238 (14)	172 (11)	−66 (−28)	
Genitourinary (excluding prostate)	228 (14)	230 (14)	+2 (+1)	
Gynecological	350 (21)	284 (17)	−66 (−19)	
Head and neck (excluding thyroid)	154 (9)	276 (17)	+122 (+79)	
Lung	168 (10)	194 (12)	+26 (+15)	
Lymph	2 (0.1)	3 (0.2)	+1 (+50)	
Peripheral nervous system	1 (0.1)	3 (0.2)	+2 (+200)	
Prostate	132 (8)	105 (6)	−27 (−20)	
Skin carcinoma[1]	8 (0.5)	7 (0.4)	−1 (−13)	
Skin melanoma	49 (3)	30 (2)	−19 (−39)	

[1]Includes basal and squamous cell carcinoma.

emergency general surgery cases during the daytime. Emergency patients would usually have their operation in the evening or night, after the completion of the daytime elective caseload, or they would have their operation during the daytime at the expense of cancelling one or more elective cases. Alternatively, patients would stay in the hospital—sometimes for days— before a surgeon was able to perform an operation during his elective schedule. The goal of ACCESS, therefore, was to provide more timely access to the OR for emergency general surgery, while decreasing the amount of expensive "after-hours" surgeries, all the while without increasing the overall general surgery operating volume.

The general surgeons at our institution agreed to participate in ACCESS for several reasons: they would be provided with 28 hours of operating time per week, almost two times more than their weekly allotted elective OR time; they would operate less at night because most emergency cases could be performed during the subsequent day; they would have significant control over their billing during ACCESS since they were paid by fee-for-service; and, most importantly, they would be able to focus on their elective practice and academic pursuits when they were not covering ACCESS. With respect to the latter, all emergency general surgery patients were admitted to ACCESS, even if they were operated by an on-call surgeon in the evening or night-time, thereby reducing the inpatient load for all non-ACCESS surgeons.

Since more than 50% of the dedicated OR time for ACCESS came from previous elective OR time, one of the concerns stemming from this reallocation was that there may be an impact on the timeliness of care for patients awaiting elective surgery, particularly for the treatment of cancer. Surgery is a key component of curative treatment for many cancers. Delays in cancer treatment can increase the risk of metastases, potentially precluding the opportunity for cure, as well as the risk of oncologic emergencies such as luminal obstruction [20,21]. Additionally, longer waits for cancer treatment can lead to significant psychological stress and anxiety in patients [20-24]. While surgical wait-times could be reduced by the provision of additional OR resources, the challenge faced by healthcare professionals and hospital administrators is to balance the medical and psychosocial costs of waiting against other demands on healthcare resources.

Initiatives such as the Ontario Wait Time Strategy have been implemented to ensure that wait times remain appropriate [10,12,14,25,26]. A fundamental component of this strategy was the development of the Wait Time Information System (WTIS) to collect wait-time data from hospitals throughout the province [26]. To complement the WTIS, the MOHLTC and CCO developed wait time targets for cancer surgery, based on evidence-based medicine and expert consensus [10,11]. CCO determined that most patients with suspected or confirmed invasive cancer could be assigned to a single priority category (P3). However, three additional categories (P1 for emergent cases, P2 for very aggressive tumours, and P4 for indolent tumours) were created to reflect the heterogeneity of tumour biology. Finally, using a "pay for performance" approach, hospital funding for surgical cancer care was tied to the achievement of wait-time milestones [11,13].

At VH, the impetus to reallocate general surgery operating resources to ACS was done as we felt this would help improve overall patient care. Another goal was to reduce the long stays in the emergency department for general surgery patients requiring emergency operations, without adversely affecting wait-times for elective cases. Along with the implementation of ACCESS at VH, the performance of cancer operations not requiring inpatient admission (such as breast cancer and melanoma) was shifted to a nearby ambulatory-care centre. During the study period, CCO also mandated a shift in the treatment of select malignancies (particularly hepatobiliary and colorectal cancer) away from community hospitals to high-volume tertiary-care centres such as VH. Consequently, there was a significant change observed in the composition of cancer surgeries performed at VH after the implementation of ACCESS, with fewer breast and melanoma surgeries, and increased proportions of colorectal and hepatobiliary cases.

Interestingly, we observed a significant change in the distribution of cancer cases by priority post-ACCESS, for all surgeons (including general surgeons) at Victoria Hospital: the proportion of P2 and P3 cases declined, while the proportion of P4 cases increased significantly. Since the general surgeons participating in ACCESS also perform cancer surgeries during their elective practices, they may have been performing P2 and P3 cancer cases on standby during ACCESS time (when there was a paucity of emergency general surgery cases), thereby contributing to the decline in P2 and P3 cases electively. If this was the case, surgeons may have had more time during their elective OR time to operate on patients with P4 cancers. This possible change may also partially explain the significant reduction in the number of general surgery cancer cases that exceeded the wait-time targets. Alternatively, surgeons at VH may have become more conservative in assigning priority levels for cancer patients in order to avoid missing wait-time targets and the associated penalties. This explanation may be more likely given the down-grading present across all surgical specialties at VH, although a case–control analysis of cancer patients may determine if this has been occurring since the implementation of the Wait Time Strategy. One of the limitations of this study was our inability to accurately determine the number of cancer surgeries performed during ACCESS time because standby cancer operations were usually reported as emergency cases rather than elective surgeries. With the recent integration of operative databases for emergency and elective cases at our institution, however, future prospective analyses may provide this important information.

Overall, there was no significant change in cancer surgery wait times pre- versus post-ACCESS. Therefore, the implementation of ACCESS, and the resultant reallocation of OR time from elective to emergency case loads, did not negatively impact wait times for elective cancer surgery. Additionally, wait-times remained unchanged despite the significant increase in the performance of hepatobiliary and colorectal surgeries post-ACCESS, which are typically longer and more complex than the breast cancer and melanoma cases that were moved offsite. Finally, while general surgery OR resources were redistributed to accommodate ACCESS at a single institution (VH), other hospitals within the city and region may have also adjusted their practices, contributing to keeping wait-times on target.

To our knowledge, this is the first study to examine the impact of implementing an ACS service on wait-times for elective surgeries. Miller *et al.* [27] and Barnes *et al.* [15] observed a 23% and 44% increase in operative productivity in terms of elective caseloads, respectively, but an overall decline in general surgery operative volumes because of a reduction in emergent cases [15]. However, neither study considered wait-times for elective cases. While many studies examining the impact of ACS services originate from the United States, American ACS services often differ significantly from Canadian models. In Canada, general surgeons participating in ACS services often also perform cancer operations as part of their elective practices, whereas many American acute care surgeons are trauma specialists who do not routinely perform oncological operations.

One of the limitations of this study is that the effect of ACCESS on wait-times for non-cancer elective operations, such as elective bowel resections for non-malignant pathology or hernia repair, was not explored. Because of the lack of organized databases to measure wait-times for elective non-cancer operations, it was difficult to ascertain the impact of ACCESS on wait-times for these cases. However, surgeons are given the discretion to book elective cases during ACCESS OR time if there are no emergency cases on the board. Most have reported excellent patient satisfaction with the development of "standby lists", whereby patients who are booked for elective non-cancer surgeries are called into the hospital on the day of their operation. Additionally, as discussed earlier, the recent integration of elective and emergency operating databases, which also include non-cancer operations, may allow for future prospective studies to address this important issue.

In conclusion, the reallocation of operating room resources from elective surgical practice towards an ACS service did not appear to affect the timeliness of care provided to patients waiting for elective cancer surgeries, and thus such concerns should not serve as a barrier for centres considering implementing an ACS service.

Competing interest
The authors do not have any actual or potential conflicts of interest to declare.

Authors' contributions
RVA, NP, and KL conceived and designed the study. RVA and KV collected the data and performed the statistical analysis. RVA drafted the manuscript. DP helped to draft the manuscript. RVA, DP, KV, SC, NP, and KL provided critical revisions of the manuscript for important intellectual content. All authors read and approved the final manuscript.

Author details
[1]Division of General Surgery, Department of Surgery, Schulich School of Medicine and Dentistry, Western University, London, ON, Canada. [2]Division of Trauma and Acute Care Surgery, Department of Surgery, Los Angeles County and University of Southern California Medical Center, Los Angeles, CA, USA. [3]Executive Leadership (Patient Centred Care), London Health Sciences Centre, London, ON, Canada. [4]Trauma Program, London Health Sciences Centre, London, ON, Canada. [5]Division of Critical Care, Department of Medicine, Schulich School of Medicine and Dentistry, Western University, London, ON, Canada. [6]Victoria Hospital, London Health Sciences Centre, Room E2-217, 800 Commissioners Road East, London, ON N6A 5W9, Canada.

References

1. Ball CG: **Acute care surgery: a new strategy for the general surgery patients left behind.** *Can J Surg* 2010, **53:**84–85.
2. Davis KA: **Acute care surgery in evolution.** *Crit Care Med* 2010, **38:**S405–S410.
3. Hameed SM, Brenneman FD, Ball CG, Pagliarello J, Razek T, Parry N, Widder S, Minor S, Buczkowski A, Macpherson C, Johner A, Jenkin D, Wood L, McLoughlin K, Anderson I, Davey D, Zabolotny B, Saadia R, Bracken J, Nathens A, Ahmed N, Panton O, Warnock GL: **General surgery 2.0: the emergence of acute care surgery in Canada.** *Can J Surg* 2010, **53:**79–83.
4. Britt RC, Weireter LJ, Britt LD: **Initial implementation of an acute care surgery model: implications for timeliness of care.** *J Am Coll Surg* 2009, **209:**421–424.
5. Cubas RF, Gomez NR, Rodriguez S, Wanis M, Sivanandam A, Garberoglio CA: **Outcomes in the management of appendicitis and cholecystitis in the setting of a new acute care surgery service model: impact on timing and cost.** *J Am Coll Surg* 2012, **215:**715–721.
6. Gandy RC, Truskett PG, Wong SW, Smith S, Bennett MH, Parasyn AD: **Outcomes of appendicectomy in an acute care surgery model.** *Med J Aust* 2010, **193:**281–284.
7. Geere SL, Aseervatham R, Grieve D: **Outcomes of appendicectomy in an acute care surgery model.** *Med J Aust* 2011, **194:**373–374.
8. Ciesla DJ, Cha JY, Smith JS 3rd, Llerena LE, Smith DJ: **Implementation of an acute care surgery service at an academic trauma center.** *Am J Surg* 2011, **202:**779–785. discussion 785–776.
9. Procter L, Bernard AC, Korosec RL, Chipko PL, Kearney PA Jr, Zwischenberger JB: **An acute care surgery service generates a positive contribution margin in an appropriately staffed hospital.** *J Am Coll Surg* 2013, **216:**298–301.
10. **Ontario Wait Times.** http://waittimes.hco-on.ca/en/search/surgery/adult.
11. Carruthers C: **Sustaining the wait time strategy.** *Healthc Pap* 2006, **7:**51–54. discussion 74–57.
12. MacLeod H, Hudson A, Kramer S, Martin M: **The times they are a-changing: what worked and what we learned in deploying Ontario's Wait Time Information System.** *Healthc Q* 2009, **12 Spec No Ontario:**8–15.
13. Trypuc J, Hudson A, MacLeod H: **Evaluating outcomes in Ontario's wait time strategy: part 4.** *Healthc Q* 2007, **10:**58–67. 54.

14. Bruni RA, Laupacis A, Levinson W, Martin DK: **Public involvement in the priority setting activities of a wait time management initiative: a qualitative case study.** *BMC Health Serv Res* 2007, **7**:186.
15. Barnes SL, Cooper CJ, Coughenour JP, MacIntyre AD, Kessel JW: **Impact of acute care surgery to departmental productivity.** *J Trauma* 2011, **71**:1027–1032. discussion 1033–1024.
16. Kreindler SA, Zhang L, Metge CJ, Nason RW, Wright B, Rudnick W, Moffatt ME: **Impact of a regional acute care surgery model on patient access and outcomes.** *Can J Surg* 2013, **56**:318–324.
17. Britt RB: **Impact of acute care surgery on biliary disease.** *J Am Coll Surg* 2010, **210**:595–599.
18. Earley AP: **An acute care surgery model improves outcomes in patients with appendicitis.** *Ann Surg* 2006, **244**:498–503.
19. Macario A, Vitez TS, Dunn B, McDonald T: **Where are the costs in perioperative care? Analysis of hospital costs and charges for inpatient surgical care.** *Anesthesiology* 1995, **83**:1138–1144.
20. Visser MR, van Lanschot JJ, van der Velden J, Kloek JJ, Gouma DJ, Sprangers MA: **Quality of life in newly diagnosed cancer patients waiting for surgery is seriously impaired.** *J Surg Oncol* 2006, **93**:571–577.
21. Oudhoff JP, Timmermans DR, Knol DL, Bijnen AB, van der Wal G: **Waiting for elective general surgery: impact on health related quality of life and psychosocial consequences.** *BMC Public Health* 2007, **7**:164.
22. Ganz PA, Schag CA, Cheng HL: **Assessing the quality of life–a study in newly-diagnosed breast cancer patients.** *J Clin Epidemiol* 1990, **43**:75–86.
23. Dickerson SS, Alqaissi N, Underhill M, Lally RM: **Surviving the wait: defining support while awaiting breast cancer surgery.** *J Adv Nurs* 2011, **67**:1468–1479.
24. Drageset S, Lindstrom TC, Giske T, Underlid K: **Being in suspense: women's experiences awaiting breast cancer surgery.** *J Adv Nurs* 2011, **67**:1941–1951.
25. Bruni RA, Laupacis A, Levinson W, Martin DK: **Public views on a wait time management initiative: a matter of communication.** *BMC Health Serv Res* 2010, **10**:228.
26. Martalog J, Bains S: **Turning data into meaningful information.** *Healthc Q* 2009, **12 Spec No Ontario**:76–77.
27. Miller PR, Wildman EA, Chang MC, Meredith JW: **Acute care surgery: impact on practice and economics of elective surgeons.** *J Am Coll Surg* 2012, **214**:531–535. discussion 536–538.

9

Intra-abdominal hypertension; prevalence, incidence and outcomes in a low resource setting

Job Kuteesa[1,4*], Olivia Kituuka[1], Dan Namuguzi[1], Cynthia Ndikuno[2], Samuel Kirunda[1], David Mukunya[3] and Moses Galukande[1]

Abstract

Background: Intra-abdominal hypertension (IAH) is defined as a sustained elevation in intra-abdominal pressure (IAP) greater than or equal to 12 mmHg. IAH has been shown to cause organ derangements and dysfunction in the body. Objective screening of IAH is neither done early enough nor at all thus leading to significant morbidity and mortality among surgical patients. The epidemiology and outcome of IAH among surgical patients has not been documented in Uganda. The aim of this study was to determine the prevalence, incidence and outcome of intra-abdominal hypertension among patients undergoing emergency laparotomy.

Methodology: Prospective observational study, conducted from January to April 2015 among patients undergoing emergency laparotomy. Inclusion criteria was; age >7 yrs, scheduled for emergency laparotomy, able to lie supine. Exclusion Criteria: pregnant, failed urethral catheterization, known cardiac, renal and respiratory disorders. Consecutive sampling was used. IAP, blood pressure, heart rate, respiratory rate, Sp02, Serum creatinine, Serum urea, and Urine output were measured preoperatively and postoperatively at 0, 6, 24 and 48 h. IAH was defined as IAP > 12 mmHg on three consecutive readings 3 min apart.

Results: In total 192 patients were enrolled. Mean age ± SD was 14.25 (±3.16) yrs in the paediatrics and 34.4(±13.72) yrs in the adults with male preponderance 65 and 80.7 % respectively. The prevalence of IAH was 25 % paediatrics and 17.4 % adults and the cumulative incidence after surgery was 20 % paediatrics and 21 % adults. In paediatrics, IAH was associated with mortality at 0 h postoperatively, RRR = 1:24, 95 % CI (1.371–560.178), *p*-value 0.048. In adults, the statistically significant outcomes associated with IAH were respiratory system dysfunction RRR1:2.783, *p*-value 0.023, 95 % CI (1.148–6.744) preoperatively and mortality RRR 1:2.933, *p*-value 0.034, 95 % CI (1.017–8.464) at 6 h, RRR 1:3.769, *p*-value 0.033, 95 % CI (1.113–12.760) at 24 h postoperatively.

Conclusion: The prevalence and incidence of IAH in the paediatrics and adults group in our study population were high. IAH was associated with mortality in both adult and paediatrics groups and respiratory system dysfunction in adult group. This calls for objective monitoring of intraabdominal pressure in patients undergoing emergency laparotomy with the aim of reducing associated mortality.

Keywords: Intra-abdominal pressure, Intra-abdominal hypertension, Emergency laparotomy, Mortality

* Correspondence: kuteesajob@gmail.com
[1]Department of Surgery, College of Health Sciences, Makerere University, Mulago Hill road, P.O Box 7072, Kampala, Uganda, East Africa
[4]Department of Surgery, School of Medicine, College of Health Sciences, Makerere University, P.O Box 7072 Kampala, Uganda
Full list of author information is available at the end of the article

Background

Intra-abdominal hypertension is a sustained or repeated elevation in Intra-Abdominal pressure (IAP) greater than or equal to 12 mmHg [1]. IAP is the steady-state pressure concealed within the abdominal cavity [1]. It's usually increased in abdominal surgical emergencies. This increased IAP leads to significant organ dysfunction; respiratory, cardiac, renal, gastrointestinal which inevitably leads to increase morbidity and mortality [2–5].

The elevated Intra abdominal pressure leads to a splinting effect on the diaphragm resulting in reduction in lung and chest wall compliance hence the respiratory dysfunction [6, 7]. When the IAP is ≥ 15 mmHg; there is impairment of venous return from the inferior vena cava. At about ≥20 mmHg, there is substantial collapse of abdominal veins (mesenteric, renal and inferior vena-cava, etc.) hence the significant drop in venous return and this will lead to reduced cardiac output [7–9]. The second effect on the heart is the elevated after load due to increased systemic vascular resistance mainly from the high intra-abdominal pressure and increased intrathoracic pressure [8]. The reduced after load in addition to the venous compression will in turn affect the central nervous system, renal and gastrointestinal system through ischaemia [7, 9].

Despite the growing awareness of the IAH and its adverse consequences; this has coincided with a significant increase in the number of publications related to the theme, many clinicians are not able to recognise or diagnose it early [10, 11] and it's currently not a routine practice to measure IAP in Uganda.

Therefore in this study we aimed to determine the prevalence, incidence and outcome of IAH among patients undergoing emergency laparotomy.

Methods

Study design

A prospective observational study.

Study setting

This study was conducted in the surgery department of Mulago National Referral Hospital (MNRH), Kampala district. MNRH is Uganda's national referral hospital. It is also the teaching hospital for the Makerere University College of Health Sciences. It has a total bed capacity of 1500, an inpatient turnover of 120,000 patients and attends to over 480,000 outpatients annually. The study was conducted between January and April 2015. Patients were followed up until discharge or death.

Participants

All patients above 7 yr that were scheduled for emergency laparotomy in the surgery department of MNRH were eligible for the study provided they were not pregnant, urinary catheterization was possible and did not have any of the following; pelvic fractures, haematuria, neurogenic bladder, cardiac, renal or respiratory conditions.

Study procedure, measurements and sample collection procedure

A patient was included in the study only after a decision to operate upon him/her was taken by the attending surgical team. Patient particulars (age, sex, tribe, weight, height, past medical history) were noted along with the diagnosis and indication for surgery. Measurement of IAP was taken three times on each occasion and the average was recorded. The measurements were done in the preoperative period and then postoperatively at 0, 6, 24 and 48 h. Zero hour was taken as time of up to 3 h after surgery. If IAP remained below 12 mmHg, measurements were discontinued after 24 h. Other parameters were measured preoperatively and then after surgery at 0, 6, 24 and 48 h. These included; blood pressure, pulse rate, respiratory rate, oxygen saturation (SpO2), temperature, urine output, Glasgow coma score, duration of surgery, blood urea, serum creatinine. Zero hour was taken as time of up to 3 h after surgery.

Post-operational findings to note include: duration of hospital stay, morbidity (burst abdomen), and mortality. The patients were followed up until discharge for morbidity (burst abdomen, relaparotomy, wound dehiscence and wound sepsis) and mortality.

Details of the measurement of the IAP

The patient was placed in supine position and catheterized with a Foley's catheter. The bladder was drained until no urine was flowing out from the catheter. The Unometer (UnoMeter™ Abdo-Pressure™ manufactured Unomedical, Uno label 005–2) was connected to the Foley's Catheter then 20 mls (10–20 mls in Paediatrics) of sterile saline was infused into the bladder through an opening on the Unometer (as recommended by the manufacturer of the Unometer). The tubing of the collecting bag was clamped. The symphysis pubis was the point of zero reference. The patient was told to expire and hold their breath, in that moment the pressure was measured in millimeters of mercury. The measurement was repeated three times with a gap of about 3 min between the readings.

Study variables

Independent variables

Patient's age (in complete years), gender, weight (in kilograms), height (in meters), diagnosis, duration of surgery (in minutes).

Dependent variables

Renal dysfunction(creatinine, urea and urine output), respiratory dysfunction(Respiratory rate, SpO_2, cardiovascular dysfunction(MAP, Heart rate), central nervous system dysfunction(GCS), intra-abdominal pressure duration of hospital stay, morbidity (burst abdomen, relaparotomy, wound dehiscence and wound sepsis), and mortality.

Interpretation of findings

Grading of intra-abdominal hypertension for adults

1. Grade I: 12–15 mmHg;
2. Grade II: 16–20 mmHg;
3. Grade III: 21–25 mmHg; and
4. Grade IV: >25 mm Hg

Grading of intra-abdominal hypertension for paediatrics

1. Grade I: 10–12 mmHg,
2. Grade II: 13–15 mmHg,
3. Grade III: 16–19 mmHg; and
4. Grade IV: ≥ 20 mmHg

Patients (adults) were considered to have ACS when they had IAH > 25 mmHg with evidence of a newly developed organ dysfunction. In Paediatric group, ACS was sustained IAP of greater than 10 mmHg associated with new organ dysfunction/failure. Intervention was left for the attending surgeon to decide.

Organ system derangement

Cardiovascular system

1. MAP < 60 mmHg
2. Heart rate > 100/min
3. Both of the above

Respiratory system

1. Respiratory rate > 20/min or
2. SpO2 < 90 % or
3. Patient in need of ventilatory support or
4. Any two or all of the above

Renal system

1. Serum creatinine > 106 umol/L or
2. Blood urea > 6.4 umol/L or
3. Urine output < 25 ml/h or
4. Any two or all of the above

Central nervous system

Glasgow Coma Scale: 15–14; Mild, 13–9; Moderate, <8; Severe.

Below 14//15, was be considered as CNS dysfunction

Study size

The sample size for prevalence and incidence was calculated using the modified Keish and Leslie formula using an estimated proportion of 50.5 %, from a multicentre epidemiological study [12], and a precision of 0.05. The estimated sample size for comparing IAH and outcomes was derived from a general formula for calculating the total sample size using the z statistic for comparison of two proportions with an estimated proportion of 80 % from an Indian study [13]. The larger sample size of 141 patients was considered.

Statistical methods

Data entry

Data was double entered into Epi Data version 3.1 with range, consistency and validity checks embedded to ensure accuracy of data. The data was stored on a computer hard drive that is password protected to ensure confidentiality and backed up on separate external hard drives kept in separate locations.

Data analysis

Univariate analysis was performed for baseline factors of the study. For continuous variables such as age; means (standard deviations) and median (interquartile range) if data was skewed, were reported. For categorical variables, proportions and percentages were reported and findings displayed in frequency distribution tables.

Multivariate analysis using the multinomial logistic regression at 95 % confidence interval and *P*-value <0.05 statistical significance, organ dysfunction, morbidity rate, mortality rate were considered as outcomes of IAH. Results were reported in relative risk ratios and *p*-value.

Quality control

The recruited research assistants were trained on the use of the data collection tool, how to do the different measurements and patient approach. The data collection tool was pretested. We cross-checked the data daily to ensure completeness with double data entry. An accurate history and physical examination of the patients was done.

Measurements of the IAP were done three times 3 min apart and the average was recorded and to increase accuracy. Standardized machines were used to measure other parameters such as SpO2, MAP, and PR etc.

Data cleaning and entry was done occasionally. There was periodic data evaluation. All questionnaires were safely stored to enable reference in case of data loss.

Ethical consideration

Informed written consent was obtained from the participants; a translated consent form was availed to non-English speaking respondents. Accent was obtained from the children and written informed consent from the guardian. Confidentiality was observed through strict storage of data and no use of names. Ethical Approval was obtained from; Mulago Hospital ethics committee, Makerere University school of medicine ethics and research committee and the Uganda National council science and technology.

Results

Characteristics of the study participants

A total of 192 patients were enrolled in this study. Of these, in the paediatric group 13 (65.5 %) patients and in adult group 138 (80.7 %) were male. Patients' age ranged from 9–86 years, paediatrics (9–18) years and adults (19–86) years. The paediatric mean age was 14.25 years (SD ± 3.16) and adult age was 34.4 yrs (SD ± 13.72). The paediatric age median was 15 years and adult median 30 years (See Table 1).

Intra-abdominal hypertension

IAH was reported as No IAH for values (<10 mmHg) paediatrics, (<12 mmHg) adult or IAH for values (≥10 mmHg) paediatrics and (≥12 mmHg) adults. Table 2 shows the different percentages of the patients who presented with or developed IAH and those who did not develop IAH both preoperatively and postoperatively.

Prevalence and incidence of IAH

The prevalence of IAH in this study was 25 % paediatrics and 17.4 % adults. Overall incidence of IAH was 20 % paediatrics and 21 % adults. The incidence of IAH at 0, 6, 24 and 48 h is presented in the Table 2.

Outcomes associated with IAH among patients scheduled for emergency laparotomy

Multivariate analysis was carried out using the multinomial logistic regression in order to determine the significant outcome factors for IAH. Tables 3, 4, 5, and 6 below show IAH as a predictor of the outcomes of organ dysfunction (respiratory and renal), morbidity and mortality in paediatrics and adults groups.

In the paediatrics group, Patients with IAH postoperatively at 6 h were more than twenty four times at risk of dying as compared to those without IAH, RRR = 1:24, 95 % CI (1.371–560.178), *p*-value 0.048.

In the adults group, patients with IAH preoperatively were 2.7 times more likely to develop respiratory dysfunction compared to those without IAH, RRR = 1:2.783, 95 % CI (1.148–6.744), and *p*-value 0.023.

Table 1 A table showing descriptive characteristics of the study participants

Characteristic	Paediatric		Adults	
	Frequency (*N* = 20)	Proportion (%)	Frequency (*N* = 172)	Proportion (%)
Age				
Mean (SD)	14.25(±3.16)		34.46(±13.72)	
Median	15.0		30.0	
Gender				
Male	13	65.5	138	80.7
BMI				
Underweight (<18.5)	10	50.0	14	8.1
Normal weight (18.5–24.9)	10	50.0	132	76.7
Overweight (25.0–29.9)	–	0.0	14	8.1
Class I obesity (30.0–34.9)	–	0.0	5	2.9
Class II obesity (35.0–39.9)	–	0.0	2	1.2
Referral				
Yes	12	60.0	93	54.4
Indication for emergency laparotomy				
Intra-abdominal sepsis	14	70.0	113	66.1
Intestinal obstruction	5	25.0	11	6.4
Trauma	1	5.0	43	25.1
Others[1]	0	0.0	4	2.3
Operative findings				
Trauma related	4	20.0	10	5.8
Non trauma relate	15	75.0	144	84.2
Duration of surgery				
<60 min	4	20	48	27.9
60 min–<90 min	9	45.0	50	29.1
90 min–<2 hours	6	30.0	40	23.3
>2 hours	0	0.0	15	8.7
Morbidity				
Present	4	20.0	42	24.4
Mortality				
Death occurred	4	20.0	42	24.4

Paediatric IAH ≥10 mmHg and Adult IAH ≥ 12 mmHg

Table 2 ATable showing prevalence and incidence of IAH before and after emergency laparotomy

Characteristic	Paediatric		Adults	
	Frequency($n = 20$)	Proportion (%)	Frequency ($n = 172$)	Proportion (%)
Preoperative				
No IAH	13	65.0	134	77.9
IAH	5	25.0	30	17.4
Overall Postoperative				
No IAH	15	75.0	110	63.9
IAH	4	20.0	37	21.5
IAH at 0 hours ($n = 153$)				
No	14	70.0	122	70.9
Yes	3	15.0	14	8.1
IAH at 6 hours ($n = 148$)				
No	18	90.0	108	62.8
Yes	0	0.0	22	12.8
IAH at 24 hours ($n = 148$)				
No	15	75.0	117	68.1
Yes	1	5.0	15	8.7
IAH at 48 hours ($n = 83$)				
No	5	10.0	63	36.6
Yes	0	0.0	15	8.7

Patients with IAH postoperatively at 6 h and at 24 h were noted to be more than 2.933 and 3.769 times more likely to die than those without IAH, 95 % CIs (1.017–8.464) (1.113–12.760) and p-values 0.047, 0.033 respectively

There was an increasing likelihood or risk of dying with increasing time (hrs) among patients postoperatively with IAH.

Discussion

This study was conducted to find out the epidemiology of IAH and the association of IAH with organ dysfunction, morbidity (e.g. burst abdomen, re-laparotomy) and mortality among surgical patients undergoing emergency laparotomy. We found the prevalence to be 25 % paediatrics and 17.4 % adults, and incidence to be 20 % paediatrics and 21 % adults. IAH is a significant predictor of mortality and respiratory dysfunction.

Basic Characteristics of the study participants

In both the paediatrics and adults groups, there was a male predominance that is 65 % in paediatrics and 80.7 % in adults; a similarity is seen in a number of studies. A study done in India had 76 % males [13], a study in children 57 % male [14], in USA two studies were done which reflected males 70 % [15] and 72 % [16]. The mean age in the paediatrics group was 14.25 years (SD ± 3.16) and adult age was 34.4 yrs (SD ± 13.72). The median age for paediatric and adults group was 15 and 30 years respectively which is consistent with the Uganda population statistics which show that Uganda has a young population [17]. In this study, intra-abdominal sepsis had 66 % of the study population, which is similar with findings from Khan et al. (2010) where 64 % presented with intra-abdominal sepsis.

Intra-abdominal pressures

The mean IAP before and after emergency laparotomy were 15.4 (SD ± 3.6) mmHg and 14.21 (SD ± 5.0) mmHg, respectively. The mean IAP in the study group of Khan et al. before and after decompressions were 16.6 (SD ± 9.4) mmHg and 10.3 (SD ± 3.1) mmHg, respectively [13]. Meldrum et al. reported higher values of preoperative IAP, 27 (SD ± 2.3) [15]. This can be explained by the observation that in our study, 66 % of the patients had peritonitis secondary to gut perforation leading to elevated IAP which, after decompression and removal of liters of fluids and gas, returned to normal level immediately.

Prevalence of IAH

The prevalence of IAH in our study was 25 % paediatrics and 17.4 % adults. In the adults group, this was slightly lower than Murtaza et al. who showed a prevalence of 28 % [18], however this can be

Table 3 Multivariate analysis showing IAH as a predictor of respiratory dysfunction and renal dysfunction among adult patients scheduled and underwent emergency laparotomy

Variable	RRR	95 % CI	*P*-value
Respiratory dysfunction			
IAH preoperative			
No IAH	1		
IAH	2.783	1.148–6.744	**0.023**
IAH Postoperative			
No IAH	1		
IAH	1.399	0.661–2.962	0.379
IAH Postop 0 hr			
No IAH	1		
IAH	0.873	0.285–2.669	0.811
IAH Postop 6 hrs			
No IAH	1		
IAH	0.952	0.379–2.396	0.917
IAH Postop 24 hrs			
No IAH	1		
IAH	1.989	0.664–5.963	0.219
IAH Postop 48 hrs			
No IAH	1		
IAH	0.606	0.193–1.905	0.391
Renal Dysfunction			
IAH preoperative			
No IAH	1		
IAH	0.538	0.201–1.439	0.217
IAH Postoperative			
No IAH	1		
IAH	0.522	0.218–1.255	0.147
IAH Postop 0 hr			
No IAH	1		
IAH	1.139	0.358–3.621	0.826
IAH Postop 6 hrs			
No IAH	1		
IAH	0.588	0.201–1.722	0.333
IAH Postop 24 hrs			
No IAH	1		
IAH	0.138	0.017–1.084	0.060
IAH Postop 48 hrs			
No IAH	1		
IAH	0.331	0.068–1.606	0.170

Highlighted variables statistically significant findings since p-value < 0.05

Table 4 Multivariate analysis showing IAH as a predictor of respiratory dysfunction and renal dysfunction among Pediatric patients scheduled and underwent Emergency laparotomy

Variable	RRR	95 % CI	*P*-value
Respiratory dysfunction			
IAH preoperative			
No IAH	1		
IAH	3.333	0.319–34.829	0.315
IAH Postoperative			
No IAH	1		
IAH	6.500	0.555–76.175	0.136
IAH Postop 0 hr			
No IAH	1		
IAH	3.000	0.177–50.784	0.447
IAH Postop 6 hrs			
No IAH	1		
IAH	1	–	–
IAH Postop 24 hrs			
No IAH	1		
IAH	$1.900*10^8$	0	0.998
IAH Postop 48 hrs			
No IAH			
IAH			
Renal Dysfunction			
IAH preoperatively			
No IAH	1		
IAH	$6.31*10^8$	0	0.998
IAH Post-operatively			
No IAH	1		
IAH	1.5	0.164–13.749	0.720
IAH 0 hrs Postop			
No IAH	1		
IAH	2.667	0.193–36.756	0.464
IAH 6 hrs Postop			
No IAH	1		
IAH	1		
IAH 24 hrs Postop			
No IAH	1		
IAH	$3.35*10^7$	0	0.994
IAH 48 hrs Postop			
No IAH			
IAH			

Highlighted variables statistically significant at p-value < 0.05

explained by the fact that Murtaza et al. looked at ICU patients who are generally sicker than the general patients we looked at. Again in the paediatrics group, the prevalence was lower compared to Ozden et al. with 49.3 %, this is still explained by the different study populations, and this study was carried out in the emergency ward setting compared to NICU or PICU.

Table 5 Multivariate analysis showing IAH as a predictor of morbidity rate and mortality among adults patients scheduled and underwent Emergency laparotomy

Characteristic	RRR	95 % CI	*P*-value
Morbidity Rate			
IAH preoperatively			
No IAH	1		
IAH	1.955	0.844–4.529	0.118
IAH Postoperatively			
No IAH	1		
IAH	1.078	0.476–2.444	0.857
IAH 0 hrs Postop			
No IAH	1		
IAH	0.398	0.085–1.869	0.243
IAH 6 hrs Postop			
No IAH	1		
IAH	0.668	0.227–1.964	0.464
IAH 24 hrs Postop			
No IAH	1		
IAH	1.125	0.359–3.528	0.840
IAH 48 hrs Postop			
No IAH	1		
IAH	1.433	0.449–4.578	0.543
Mortality Rate			
IAH preoperatively			
No IAH	1		
IAH	2.249	0.918–5.506	0.076
IAH Postoperatively			
No IAH	1		
IAH	1.043	0.399–2.729	0.930
IAH 0 hrs Postop			
No IAH	1		
IAH	1.829	0.523–6.395	0.345
IAH 6 hrs Postop			
No IAH	1		
IAH	2.933	1.017–8.464	**0.047**
IAH 24 hrs Postop			
No IAH	1		
IAH	3.769	1.113–12.760	**0.033**
IAH 48 hrs Postop			
No IAH	1		
IAH	0.338	0.040–2.843	0.318

Highlighted variables statistically significant at *p*-value < 0.05

Table 6 IAH as a predictor of morbidity rate and mortality among Pediatric patients scheduled and underwent Emergency laparotomy

Characteristic	RRR	95 % CI	*P*-value
Morbidity rate			
IAH preoperative			
IAH	1		
No IAH	1.25	0.087–17.975	0.870
IAH Postoperative			
IAH	1		
No IAH	1.333	0.099–17.823	0.828
IAH Postop 0 hr			
IAH	1		
No IAH	$3.67*10^8$	–	0.998
IAH Postop 6 hrs			
IAH	1		
No IAH		–	–
IAH Postop 24 hrs			
IAH	1		
No IAH	$1.900*10^8$		0.998
IAH Postop 48 hrs			
IAH			
No IAH			
Mortality Rate			
IAH preoperative			
No IAH	1		
IAH	$5.39*10^9$	–	0.999
IAH Postoperative			
No IAH	1		
IAH	13	0.771–219.107	0.075
IAH Post op 0 hr			
No IAH	1		
IAH	24	1.028–560.178	**0.048**
IAH Post op 6 hrs			
No IAH			
IAH			
IAH Post op 24 hrs			
No IAH	1		
IAH	$7.51*10^7$	–	0.997
IAH Post op 48 hrs			
No IAH	1		
IAH	0.339	0.041–2.833	0.318

Highlighted variables statistically significant at *p*-value < 0.05

Incidence of IAH

In the adult group, the incidence of IAH in literature varies from 2 to 81 % depending on the values used to defined IAH and patient population [19, 20]. However, only a few studies have reported the incidence in paediatrics, 12.6 % Thabet et al. [21], and 9 % Divarci et al. [14]. The incidence of IAH in our study was 20 % paediatrics and 21 % adults. The incidence in the adult group at the 0, 6, 24 and 48 h postoperatively was 8.1, 12.8, 8.7 and 8.7 % respectively. At 6 h the incidence of IAH increases and then drop at 24 and 48 h, this is similar to Khan et al. reported 0 % at 0 h, 3.55 % at 6 h and 0 % at 24 h [13]. The incidence of 21 % in the adults group is high therefore close attention should be paid to these patients postoperatively to avoid poor outcome. The incidence in paediatrics group at 0, 6, 24 and 48 h was 15, 0, 5 and 0 %.

Outcome factors associated with IAH

In the adults group, the statistically significant outcomes associated with IAH include mortality and respiratory system dysfunction. Preoperative IAH was significantly associated with respiratory system dysfunction while post-operative IAH was significantly associated with mortality. Khan et a[13]l reported similar findings and the preoperative respiratory dysfunction is explained by the splintage of the diaphragm as the IAP progressively raises, however the after surgery respiratory function could have improved due to the decompression from surgery.

The mortality associated with IAH postoperatively at 6 and 24 h shows at need to objectively measure IAP in patients at risk hence early recognition and proceeds with effective intervention.

In the paediatrics group, the significant outcome associated with IAH after multivariate analysis was mortality at 0 h, which could be explained by probable delay in surgical intervention or recognition and appropriate treatment of IAH.

Limitation of the study

The measurements may have varied depending on whether if they were taken at end of inspiration or at the end of expiration which may have led to under estimation of the readings. Sessions were conducted to train the research assistants to correctly measure the IAP.

IAP measurements were between 6 h interval; hence we may have missed episodes of IAH between measurements.

At IAP measured omitted at 48 h if pt has no episode of IAH, pre-op and post-op up to 24 h. This was done for the concern of causing urinary tract infections in the patients, hence the reading 48 h was to be assumed as normal (but this was not analysed) hence our few numbers at 48 h.

Conclusion

The prevalence and incidence of IAH in both paediatrics and adult groups in this study were high. IAH was significantly associated with mortality postoperatively and respiratory dysfunction preoperatively in the adult group but only mortality postoperatively in the paediatrics group. These conclusions add emphasis to the need to objectively monitor IAP in these patients undergoing emergency laparotomy so as to recognise and treatment IAH early.

Recommendations

Objective routine IAP measurements should be considered for all patients undergoing emergency laparotomy. Clinical protocols should be designed to guide the management of patients with IAH in the accidents and emergency surgery wards. Resources should also be channeled towards procurement of equipment required to monitor the IAP in these patients. More studies are needed to demonstrate proper guidelines on monitoring of IAP in patients undergoing emergency laparotomy.

Competing interests

All authors declare no conflict of interest.

Authors' contributions

JK, MG, OK, DN, SK, CN, DM participated in the conception, study design, data analysis and manuscript preparation. JK, CN participated in the data collection. JK,MG,SK,DM participated in the data preparation and analysis and manuscript preparation. All authors read and approved the final manuscript.

Authors' information

JK Registrar surgery (Surgical trainee) MBChB (MakCHS) MCS (ECSA)
MG Associate professor MBChB, M.Med (Surgery) (MakCHS), MScHPE (Maastricht), FCSGen (ECSA).
OK Senior lecturer MBChB, M.Med (Surgery) (MakCHS), FCSGen (ECSA)
DN Senior lecturer MBChB, M.Med (Surgery) (MakCHS), FCSUro (ECSA)
SK Registrar surgery (Surgical trainee) MBChB (MUST)
DM Researcher MBChB (MakCHS), PHD fellow (International health)
CN Nurse BSN (MakCHS).

Acknowledgements

We want to acknowledge Jovito Ojieri, Ibrahim Ssemirimo and Emmanuel Rwamutwe, who helped in data collection. Sister Janat Nawamwena and Sister Brenda Tumuhimbise for the invaluable assistance. Edwin Mwaka, Dr Moses Arinaitwe and Peter Babigumira Ahabwe for help in data management. Dr Edward Mpoza, Dr Mary Nakibirango, Hillary Turyagenda for all support and help. Friends of Kagando, Dr Peter and Liz Lunn, Kagando Hospital for the funding and extraordinary support to acquire the tools needed to carry out this research.

Author details

[1]Department of Surgery, College of Health Sciences, Makerere University, Mulago Hill road, P.O Box 7072, Kampala, Uganda, East Africa. [2]Department of Nursing, College of Health Sciences, Makerere University, Kampala, Uganda. [3]Department of Paediatrics, College of Health Sciences, Makerere University, Kampala, Uganda. [4]Department of Surgery, School of Medicine, College of Health Sciences, Makerere University, P.O Box 7072 Kampala, Uganda.

References

1. Kirkpatrick AW, Roberts DJ, De Waele J, Jaeschke R, Malbrain ML, De Keulenaer B, et al. Intra-abdominal hypertension and the abdominal compartment syndrome: Updated consensus definitions and clinical practice guidelines from the World Society of the Abdominal Compartment Syndrome. Intensive Care Med. 2013;39(7):1190–206.
2. Kirkpatrick AW, Pelosi P, De Waele JJ, Malbrain ML, Ball CG, Meade MO, et al. Clinical review: Intra-abdominal hypertension: Does it influence the physiology of prone ventilation? Crit care. 2010;14(4):232.

3. Correa-Martin L, Castellanos G, Garcia M, Sanchez-Margallo FM. Renal consequences of intraabdominal hypertension in a porcine model. Search for the choice indirect technique for intraabdominal pressure measurement. Actas Urol Esp. 2013;37(5):273–9.
4. Scollay JM, de Beaux I, Parks RW. Prospective study of intra-abdominal pressure following major elective abdominal surgery. World J Surg. 2009; 33(11):2372–7.
5. Sugrue M, Buhkari Y. Intra-abdominal pressure and abdominal compartment syndrome in acute general surgery. World J Surg. 2009;33(6):1123–7.
6. da Silva Almeida JR, Machado FS, Schettino GP, Park M, Azevedo LC. Cardiopulmonary effects of matching positive end-expiratory pressure to abdominal pressure in concomitant abdominal hypertension and acute lung injury. J Trauma. 2010;69(2):375–83.
7. Moore AF, Hargest R, Martin M, Delicata RJ. Intra-abdominal hypertension and the abdominal compartment syndrome. Br J Surg. 2004;91(9):1102–10.
8. Kashtan J, Green JF, Parsons EQ, Holcroft JW. Hemodynamic effect of increased abdominal pressure. J Surg Res. 1981;30(3):249–55.
9. Carr JA. Abdominal compartment syndrome: A decade of progress. J Am Coll Surg. 2013;216(1):135–46.
10. Kimball EJ, Rollins MD, Mone MC, Hansen HJ, Baraghoshi GK, Johnston C, et al. Survey of intensive care physicians on the recognition and management of intra-abdominal hypertension and abdominal compartment syndrome. Crit Care Med. 2006;34(9):2340–8.
11. Ravishankar N, Hunter J. Measurement of intra-abdominal pressure in intensive care units in the United Kingdom: A national postal questionnaire study. Br J Anaesth. 2005;94(6):763–6.
12. Malbrain ML, Chiumello D, Pelosi P, Wilmer A, Brienza N, Malcangi V, et al. Prevalence of intra-abdominal hypertension in critically ill patients: A multicentre epidemiological study. Intensive Care Med. 2004;30(5):822–9.
13. Khan S, Verma AK, Ahmad SM, Ahmad R. Analyzing intra-abdominal pressures and outcomes in patients undergoing emergency laparotomy. J Emerg Trauma Shock. 2010;3(4):318–25.
14. Divarci E, Karapinar B, Yalaz M, Ergun O, Celik A: Incidence and prognosis of intraabdominal hypertension and abdominal compartment syndrome in children. Journal of Pediatric Surgery 2014. doi: 10.1016/j.jpedsurg.2014.03.014.
15. Meldrum DR, Moore FA, Moore EE, Franciose RJ, Sauaia A, Burch JM. Prospective characterization and selective management of the abdominal compartment syndrome. Am J Surg. 1997;174(6):667–72. discussion 672–663.
16. Hong JJ, Cohn SM, Perez JM, Dolich MO, Brown M, McKenney MG. Prospective study of the incidence and outcome of intra-abdominal hypertension and the abdominal compartment syndrome. Br J Surg. 2002; 89(5):591–6.
17. United-Nations-Population-Division. World population prospects: The 2012 revision. New York: Population Division of the Department of Economic and Social Affairs of the United Nations Secretariat; 2013.
18. Murtaza G, Pal KM, Jajja MR, Nawaz Z, Koondhar R, Nasim S. Intra abdominal hypertension; incidence, prevalence and outcomes in a mixed intensive care unit: Prospective cohort study. Int J Surg. 2015;9:67–71.
19. Malbrain ML, Chiumello D, Cesana BM, Reintam Blaser A, Starkopf J, Sugrue M, et al. A systematic review and individual patient data meta-analysis on intra-abdominal hypertension in critically ill patients: The wake-up project. World initiative on Abdominal Hypertension Epidemiology, a Unifying Project (WAKE-Up!). Minerva Anestesiol. 2014;80(3):293–306.
20. Cheatham ML, Malbrain ML, Kirkpatrick A, Sugrue M, Parr M, De Waele J, et al. Results from the International Conference of Experts on Intra-abdominal Hypertension and Abdominal Compartment Syndrome. II. Recommendations. Intensive Care Med. 2007;33:951–62. 2007/03/23 edn.
21. Thabet FC, Bougmiza IM, Chehab MS, Bafaqih HA, AlMohaimeed SA, Malbrain ML: Incidence, Risk Factors, and Prognosis of Intra-Abdominal Hypertension in Critically Ill Children: A Prospective Epidemiological Study. Journal of intensive care medicine 2015.

10

Examining the safety of colon anastomosis on a rat model of ischemia-reperfusion injury

David Czeiger[1], Anton Osyntsov[2], Lidia Osyntsov[3], Chad G Ball[4], Roy Gigi[5] and Gad Shaked[1,2*]

Abstract

Introduction: Intestinal ischemia and reperfusion can impair anastomotic strength.
The purpose of this study was to evaluate the safety of delayed colon anastomosis following remote ischemia-reperfusion (IR) injury.

Methods: Rats divided into two groups underwent bilateral groin incisions, however only the study group had femoral artery clamping to inflict IR injury. Twenty-four hours following this insult, the animals underwent laparotomy, incision of the transverse colon and reanastomosis. End points included anastomotic leakage, strength and histopathological features.

Results: Anastomotic leak among IR animals (22.2%) was not statistically different in comparison to the controls [10.5% ($p = 0.40$)]. Anastomotic mean burst pressures showed no statistically significant difference [150.6 ± 15.57 mmHg in the control group vs. 159.9 ± 9.88 mmHg in the IR group ($p = 0.64$)]. The acute inflammatory process in the IR group was similar to controls ($p = 0.26$), as was the chronic repair process ($p = 0.88$). There was no significant difference between the inflammation:repair ratios amongst the two groups ($p = 0.67$).

Conclusion: Primary colon repair is safe when performed 24 hours following systemic IR injury.

Keywords: Ischemia-reperfusion, Injury, Colon, Intestinal anastomosis, Rat model, Emergency surgery

Introduction

Ischemia-reperfusion (IR) injury represents a fundamental common pathway of tissue damage in a wide variety of disease and surgical processes such as major trauma, acute mesenteric ischemia, septic and hypovolemic shock, abdominal aortic aneurism surgery, and cardiopulmonary bypass [1,2]. Interruption of blood supply results in ischemic injury to all body systems and especially to high metabolically active tissues; the intestine is a prominent example of a sensitive tissue to IR injury which is associated with high morbidity and mortality [1]. Paradoxically, restoration of blood flow to the ischemic tissue augments cell injury by delivering toxic mediators induced in the ischemic tissue into the circulation thus affecting distant organs. This might lead to the development of systemic inflammatory response syndrome, which can progress to multiple organ failure and death [2]. Among the toxic mediators produced in the IR injured tissue are acute-phase proteins, pro-inflammatory cytokines, oxygen free radicals, and components of the complement system [3]. Emergency surgery and trauma situations may require abbreviated procedures during the initial phase of shock and organ ischemia. Definitive procedures including anastomosis to restore bowel continuity are undertaken 24 hours or more afterward. Two common examples of such situations are the strategy of damage control surgery in seriously injured patients, and acute mesenteric ischemia. In damage control laparotomy the goal in the emergency surgery is to stop bleeding and to control spillage from the intestine. In the second operation, which is done after the patient's deranged physiology is corrected, bowel anastomosis may be created. In mesenteric ischemia gangrenous segments of the bowel are resected, while fluid resuscitation continues. Not infrequently, the patient condition does not allow performing primary anastomosis. This may be done during a second look operation 24 hours later. The spectrum of the effects of IR injury on the intestine is broad and ranges from a

* Correspondence: shakedg@bgu.ac.il
[1]Department of General Surgery and Trauma Unit, Soroka University Medical Center and Ben-Gurion University, Beer Sheva, Israel
[2]Department of General Surgery, Soroka University Medical Center and Ben-Gurion University, Beer Sheva 84101, Israel

transient absorptive impair following mucosal damage to frank gangrene of the bowel [4]. Previous reports have shown that ischemia and reperfusion of the intestinal wall can lead to impaired anastomotic strength [5-8]. However, there is not enough evidence in the literature to show the safety of delayed bowel anastomosis following systemic IR injury. We hypothesized that IR injury would adversely affect the safety of colonic anastomoses performed 24 hours following the injury. To evaluate this hypothesis we investigated the effects of IR injury on the healing of colon anastomoses in a rat model.

Materials and methods

The protocol employed in this study was approved by the Committee for the Ethical Care and Use of Laboratory Animals of the Ben-Gurion University of the Negev (approval code IL-41-7-2006). It included a provision that any rat exhibiting evidence of distress (such as restlessness or aggressive behavior) be immediately euthanized. Rats were acclimated to the laboratory for 2 weeks prior to the study and had free access to water and food at all times. A total of 40 male Sprague–Dawley rats (average weight 350 g) were used. The number of animals in each group was considered satisfactory based on a two-sided sample size determination (power analysis), assuming power of 0.80 and significance of 0.05. All rats were anesthetized with inhaled isoflurane 1% at a rate of 3–5 L/min. The study group (n = 20) underwent bilateral groin incision and clamping the femoral arteries for 30 minutes. The control group (n = 20) had a similar sham operation without inducing extremities ischemia. All wounds were then sutured with 4/0 silk. Twenty-four hours following this insult, all animals were anesthetized and underwent a midline laparotomy, full circumference incision of the transverse colon (including resection of 0.5 cm of mesentery on each side of the colon) and reanastomosis (end-to-end) using 4/0 polyglycolic acid sutures. The animals were then followed up and sacrificed one week later. The peritoneal cavity was subsequently explored for the presence of perforation, and local or generalized peritonitis.

Anastomotic healing was assessed by determining anastomotic burst pressures, as well as by formal histopathological examination. The transverse colon was dissected free of adhesions and resected. One end of this segment was ligated, and a catheter connected to a sphygmomanometer was secured to the other end. Air was then pumped into the segment of colon, which was submerged in water. Intraluminal pressure was monitored continuously while the air was injected. The intraluminal pressure at which air leakage from the anastomosis occurred was recorded as the burst pressure. More specifically, this parameter represents the mechanical strength of the anastomosis. The colon specimen was then processed and evaluated for three parameters of acute inflammation: (1) total number of polymorphonuclear cells, (2) total number of red blood cells and (3) the amount of fibrin, as well as for three parameters of chronic wound healing: (1) total number of mononuclear cells, (2) total number of fibroblasts and (3) total amount of collagen. Each parameter was graded from 0 to 4. The colon surgeon and the pathologist were each blinded with regard to the individual group allocation history of the animals. Statistical analysis was performed using GraphPad Prism version 4.00 for Windows, GraphPad Software, San Diego, California, USA. Parametric results are expressed as mean ± SEM and were compared using an unpaired t-test. Two-tailed $p < 0.05$ was considered as having a statistical significance.

Results

Three animals were excluded from the study because they died before the completion of the surgical procedure (1 control and 2 IR). One rat in the IR group also died during the 7-day follow-up period ($p > 0.05$). Autopsy of this animal revealed an anastomotic leak and diffuse peritonitis. Among the animals that completed the follow-up period, anastomotic leak and a severe peritoneal reaction was observed in 3 animals within the IR cohort, and in 2 control animals. The anastomotic leak rate among IR animals (22.2%) was not statistically different in comparison to the controls [10.5% ($p = 0.40$)]. The anastomotic mean burst pressures also showed no statistically significant difference [150.6 ± 15.57 mmHg in the control group vs. 159.9 ± 9.88 mmHg in the IR group ($p = 0.64$)]. The specific distribution of individual burst pressures is displayed in Figure 1. More specifically, the burst pressures among the IR group display significantly less variance than the control group. The F test used to compare variances shows a significant difference ($p = 0.025$). To statistically compare histopathological results, 3 grades were assigned for both the inflammatory process and chronic repair process for each animal. Student's t-test comparing the means of sums and Fisher's exact test comparing inflammation:repair ratios of the two groups revealed no significant statistical differences. The acute inflammatory process in the IR group was similar to controls ($p = 0.26$), as was the chronic repair process ($p = 0.88$). There was also no significant difference between the inflammation:repair ratios in the two groups ($p = 0.67$).

Discussion

The goal of this study was to examine the safety of colon anastomosis performed 24 hours after profound systemic ischemia-reperfusion injury. Our results show that resection and anastomosis of the colon is safe, when performed twenty-four hours following profound, remote IR injury. This is based on similar mortality and anastomotic leak ratios (although a non-significant trend towards a higher incidence of anastomotic leak among the IR animals was

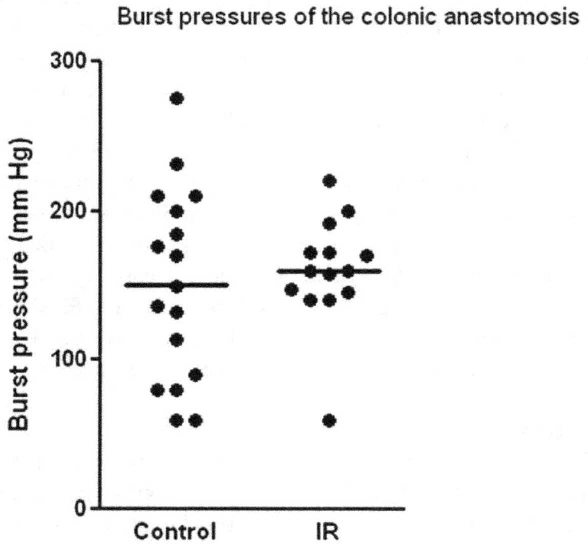

Figure 1 Colon anastomotic strength is reflected by burst pressure expressed by mmHg. Individual values and means are shown for the IR and control groups. The variance of distribution of burst pressures around the mean pressure is significantly smaller in the IR group compared to the control group (p = 0.025).

noted), comparable anastomotic mechanical strengths, and equivalent histological features of the anastomosis between the IR and the control groups.

Today, in 2013, anastomotic leak after colorectal resection still has lethality of 6-22% and morbidity leading to reoperation and permanent stoma in 56% [9]. There is convincing evidence in the literature that primary repair or anastomosis is appropriate for the management of most colonic injuries and for other emergent surgical situations [10-17]. In contrast, there is little methodologically sound evidence outlining the outcome of a colon anastomosis in the setup of severe IR. Damage control surgery (DCS) is probably one of the most common situations where the surgeon faces the dilemma of creating colonic anastomosis in a delayed fashion after IR injury. Clinical retrospective series have revealed contradictory conclusions regarding the safety of this procedure. Miller et al. [18] concluded that delayed anastomoses in patients undergoing DCS is safe, whereas Weinberg and colleagues reported a significant colon related complication rate in patients who were treated by resection and anastomosis [19]. A third group also identified a higher incidence of colonic anastomotic leakage among DCS patients who had resection followed by anastomosis; however they declared that resection and anastomosis is still considered safe [20]. Ott pointed in a recently published manuscript that colon anastomosis is safe unless the abdomen remains open. He also regards the left colon as more vulnerable to leak under these conditions [21]. It is obvious that limitations in these studies include heterogeneous patient populations, variance in patients' clinical condition and surgeons' preference, and even the very definition of DCS by different surgeons.

To overcome these limitations inherent in clinical retrospective studies we created a rat model of IR injury followed by resection and reansatomosis of the transverse colon. IR injury has been intensively investigated since the 1970s. The IR phenomenon represents the common underlying pathophysiological process to a variety of medical conditions and surgical procedures. Tissue ischemia with inadequate oxygen supply followed by successful reperfusion initiates a wide and complex array of inflammatory responses that may both aggravate local injury, as well as induce impairment of remote organ function [22]. Review of the literature reveals experimental studies evaluating the effect of transient preoperative IR on gut anastomotic strength [6,8,23-29]. The results of these studies were equivocal. This may partially be explained by the degree and duration of the inflicted ischemia [26]. Also, the surgical procedure was done on small bowel in some of the studies [30], while in others large bowel anastomoses were tested [31]. Furthermore, in the previous models the ischemia was done by clamping the blood supply of the resected segment of intestine, and/or performed the intestinal anastomosis immediately following the IR injury. Kuzu et al. attempted to demonstrate the systemic nature of IR by occluding the superior mesenteric artery and its collaterals and immediately thereafter they resected and reansatomose the left colon [7]. Posma described the effect of a prolonged interval between IR and anastomotic construction on the anastomosis healing, but used a model of local mesenteric ischemia [26].

We believe that the present model, with severe systemic remote ischemia, performance of a colon anastomosis 24 hours later, and testing the anastomotic strength after one week, more closely resembles the true conditions of some emergent conditions that the surgical approach for them is still uncertain. Several mechanisms have been suggested to explain the blunting of the IR deleterious effect on bowel anastomoses when these are constructed late after the insult. One is subsidence of the harmful effects over the time elapsed from the insult to the creation of the anastomosis. Another explanation is the protective effect of ischemic preconditioning [30,32]. Recently, studies have been published on prevention/alleviation the effect of IR injury by inhibiting compliment system activation [33], by applying antioxidants [34,35], and trace elements [36]. Another trend for attenuating effects of IR injury is ischemic postconditioning [37-39].

In our experiment we amplified the local ischemia at the site of anastomosis by resecting 0.5 cm of mesentery on each side of the divided transverse colon. Even under these stringent conditions we did not observe the expected IR harmful effects. On the other hand, our results showed no benefit to the ischemic group. This should question the protective effect of ischemic preconditioning in this setup.

In summary, this rat model augments the literature which support delayed primary repair after ischemia-reperfusion injury. However, more laboratory and clinical evidence is required before final conclusion can be drawn. More studies are also needed to understand the attenuation of the harmful effects of IR on intestinal anastomosis when performed 24 hours after the injury.

Competing interests

The authors declare that they have no competing interests.

Authors' contributions

DC participated in the design of the study, performed the statistical analysis, and revised the manuscript, AO carried out the operations, LO performed the pathological examinations and the evaluations of the specimens, CB was involved in drafting the manuscript and revising it critically, RG participated in the laboratory work and animal assays, GS initiate the study, created its design and wrote the manuscript. All authors read and approved the final manuscript.

Acknowledgements

This work was not supported by any third party such as pharmaceutical or industrial company, or grants. No author has conflict of interest regarding the publication of this work. The study has not been presented, yet, at a scientific or medical conference.
The manuscript is not under consideration for publication by any other journal.

Author details

[1]Department of General Surgery and Trauma Unit, Soroka University Medical Center and Ben-Gurion University, Beer Sheva, Israel. [2]Department of General Surgery, Soroka University Medical Center and Ben-Gurion University, Beer Sheva 84101, Israel. [3]Pathology Institute, Soroka University Medical Center and Ben- Gurion University, Beer Sheva, Israel. [4]Department of Surgery, University of Calgary, Calgary, Alberta, Canada. [5]Department of Orthopedics, Tel Aviv Sourasky Medical Center, Tel Aviv, Israel.

References

1. Mallick IH, Yang W, Winslet MC, Seifalian AM: **Ischemia-reperfusion injury of the intestine and protective strategies against injury.** *Dig Dis Sci* 2004, **49**(9):1359–1377.
2. Leng YF, Zhang Y, Zhang Y, Xue X, Wang T, Kang YQ: **Ischemic post-conditioning attenuates the intestinal injury induced by limb ischemia/reperfusion in rats.** *Braz J Med Biol Res* 2011, **44**(5):411–417.
3. Grootjans J, Lenaerts K, Derikx JP, Matthijsen RA, de Bruine AP, van Bijnen AA, van Dam RM, Dejong CH, Buurman WA: **Human intestinal ischemia-reperfusion-induced inflammation characterized: experiences from a new translational model.** *Am J Pathol* 2010, **176**(5):2283–2291.
4. Haglund U, Bulkley GB, Granger DN: **On the pathophysiology of intestinal ischemic injury. Clinical review.** *Acta Chir Scand* 1987, **153**(5–6):321–324.
5. Posma LA, Bleichrodt RP, Lomme RM, de Man BM, van Goor H, Hendriks T: **Early anastomotic repair in the rat intestine is affected by transient preoperative mesenteric ischemia.** *J Gastrointest Surg* 2009, **13**(6):1099–1106.
6. Kologlu M, Yorganci K, Renda N, Sayek I: **Effect of local and remote ischemia-reperfusion injury on healing of colonic anastomoses.** *Surgery* 2000, **128**(1):99–104.
7. Kuzu MA, Tanik A, Kale IT, Aslar AK, Koksoy C, Terzi C: **Effect of ischemia/reperfusion as a systemic phenomenon on anastomotic healing in the left colon.** *World J Surg* 2000, **24**(8):990–994.
8. Posma LA, Bleichrodt RP, van Goor H, Hendriks T: **Transient profound mesenteric ischemia strongly affects the strength of intestinal anastomoses in the rat.** *Dis Colon Rectum* 2007, **50**(7):1070–1079.
9. Daams F, Luyer M, Lange JF: **Colorectal anastomotic leakage: aspects of prevention, detection and treatment.** *World J Gastroenterol* 2013, **19**(15):2293–2297.
10. Demetriades D, Murray JA, Chan L, Ordonez C, Bowley D, Nagy KK, Cornwell EE 3rd, Velmahos GC, Munoz N, Hatzitheofilou C, Schwab CW, Rodriguez A, Cornejo C, Davis KA, Namias N, Wisner DH, Ivatury RR, Moore EE, Acosta JA, Maull KI, Thomason MH, Spain DA, Committee on Multicenter Clinical Trials, American Association for the Surgery of Trauma: **Penetrating colon injuries requiring resection: diversion or primary anastomosis? An AAST prospective multicenter study.** *J Trauma* 2001, **50**(5):765–775.
11. Gonzalez RP, Merlotti GJ, Holevar MR: **Colostomy in penetrating colon injury: is it necessary?** *J Trauma* 1996, **41**(2):271–275.
12. Sasaki LS, Allaben RD, Golwala R, Mittal VK: **Primary repair of colon injuries: a prospective randomized study.** *J Trauma* 1995, **39**(5):895–901.
13. Stone HH, Fabian TC: **Management of perforating colon trauma: randomization between primary closure and exteriorization.** *Ann Surg* 1979, **190**(4):430–436.
14. Chappuis CW, Frey DJ, Dietzen CD, Panetta TP, Buechter KJ, Cohn I Jr: **Management of penetrating colon injuries. A prospective randomized trial.** *Ann Surg* 1991, **213**(5):492–497. discussion 497–8.
15. Singer MA, Nelson RL: **Primary repair of penetrating colon injuries: a systematic review.** *Dis Colon Rectum* 2002, **45**(12):1579–1587.
16. Jimenez Fuertes M, Costa Navarro D: **Resection and primary anastomosis without diverting ileostomy for left colon emergencies: is it a safe procedure?** *World J Surg* 2012, **36**(5):1148–1153.
17. Constantinides VA, Tekkis PP, Athanasiou T, Aziz O, Purkayastha S, Remzi FH, Fazio VW, Aydin N, Darzi A, Senapati A: **Primary resection with anastomosis vs. Hartmann's procedure in nonelective surgery for acute colonic diverticulitis: a systematic review.** *Dis Colon Rectum* 2006, **49**(7):966–981.
18. Miller PR, Chang MC, Hoth JJ, Holmes JH 4th, Meredith JW: **Colonic resection in the setting of damage control laparotomy: is delayed anastomosis safe?** *Am Surg* 2007, **73**(6):606–609. discussion 609–10.
19. Weinberg JA, Griffin RL, Vandromme MJ, Melton SM, George RL, Reiff DA, Kerby JD, Rue LW: **Management of colon wounds in the setting of damage control laparotomy: a cautionary tale.** *J Trauma* 2009, **67**(5):929–935.
20. Kashuk JL, Cothren CC, Moore EE, Johnson JL, Biffl WL, Barnett CC: **Primary repair of civilian colon injuries is safe in the damage control scenario.** *Surgery* 2009, **146**(4):663–668. discussion 668–70.
21. Ott MM, Norris PR, Diaz JJ, Collier BR, Jenkins JM, Gunter OL, Morris JA Jr: **Colon anastomosis after damage control laparotomy: recommendations from 174 trauma colectomies.** *J Trauma* 2011, **70**(3):595–602.
22. Collard CD, Gelman S: **Pathophysiology, clinical manifestations, and prevention of ischemia-reperfusion injury.** *Anesthesiology* 2001, **94**(6):1133–1138.
23. Aydin C, Teke Z, Aytekin F, Yenisey C, Kabay B, Simsek NG, Tekin K: **Tempol prevents harmful effects of remote ischemia reperfusion injury on healing of experimental colonic anastomoses.** *Int J Colorectal Dis* 2007, **22**(3):325–331.
24. Colak T, Turkmenoglu O, Dag A, Polat A, Comelekoglu U, Bagdatoglu O, Polat G, Kanik A, Akca T, Aydin S: **The effect of remote ischemic preconditioning on healing of colonic anastomoses.** *J Surg Res* 2007, **143**(2):200–205.
25. Murthy S, Hui-Qi Q, Sakai T, Depace DE, Fondacaro JD: **Ischemia/reperfusion injury in the rat colon.** *Inflammation* 1997, **21**(2):173–190.
26. Posma LA, Bleichrodt RP, van Goor H, Hendriks T: **A prolonged interval between deep intestinal ischemia and anastomotic construction does not impair wound strength in the rat.** *Int J Colorectal Dis* 2007, **22**(12):1485–1491.
27. Posma LA, Bleichrodt RP, van Goor H, Hendriks T: **Ischemia and prolonged reperfusion before anastomotic construction do not reduce wound strength in the rat intestine.** *Surgery* 2006, **139**(5):671–677.
28. Rolim MF, Riger CJ, Eleutherio EC, Colao Cda F, Pereira GC, Schanaider A: **Colonic healing after portal ischemia and reperfusion: an experimental study with oxidative stress biomarkers.** *Redox Rep* 2007, **12**(6):267–274.
29. Teke Z, Aytekin FO, Kabay B, Yenisey C, Aydin C, Tekin K, Sacar M, Ozden A: **Pyrrolidine dithiocarbamate prevents deleterious effects of remote ischemia/reperfusion injury on healing of colonic anastomoses in rats.** *World J Surg* 2007, **31**(9):1835–1842.
30. Holzner PA, Kulemann B, Kuesters S, Timme S, Hoeppner J, Hopt UT, Marjanovic G: **Impact of remote ischemic preconditioning on wound healing in small bowel anastomoses.** *World J Gastroenterol* 2011, **17**(10):1308–1316.

31. Kosmidis C, Efthimiadis C, Anthimidis G, Basdanis G, Apostolidis S, Hytiroglou P, Vasiliadou K, Prousalidis J, Fahantidis E: **Myofibroblasts and colonic anastomosis healing in Wistar rats.** *BMC Surg* 2011, **11**:6-2482-11-6.
32. Moore-Olufemi SD, Kozar RA, Moore FA, Sato N, Hassoun HT, Cox CS Jr, Kone BC: **Ischemic preconditioning protects against gut dysfunction and mucosal injury after ischemia/reperfusion injury.** *Shock* 2005, **23**(3):258–263.
33. Diepenhorst GM, van Gulik TM, Hack CE: **Complement-mediated ischemia-reperfusion injury: lessons learned from animal and clinical studies.** *Ann Surg* 2009, **249**(6):889–899.
34. Kabali B, Girgin S, Gedik E, Ozturk H, Kale E, Buyukbayram H: **N-acetylcysteine prevents deleterious effects of ischemia/reperfusion injury on healing of colonic anastomosis in rats.** *Eur Surg Res* 2009, **43**(1):8–12.
35. Teke Z, Bostanci EB, Yenisey C, Sacar M, Simsek NG, Akoglu M: **Caffeic acid phenethyl ester alleviates mesenteric ischemia/reperfusion injury.** *J Invest Surg* 2012, **25**(6):354–365.
36. Ersoy YE, Ayan F, Himmetoglu S: **Trace element levels in ischemia-reperfusion injury after left colonic anastomosis in rats and effects of papaverine and pentoxiphylline on vascular endothelial growth factor in anastomosis healing.** *Acta Gastroenterol Belg* 2011, **74**(1):22–27.
37. Chu WW, Nie L, He XY, Yan AL, Zhou Y, Wu GL, Wang DH: **Change of cytochrome c in postconditioning attenuating ischemia-reperfusion-induced mucosal apoptosis in rat intestine.** *Sheng Li Xue Bao* 2010, **62**(2):143–148.
38. Wen SH, Li Y, Li C, Xia ZQ, Liu WF, Zhang XY, Lei WL, Huang WQ, Liu KX: **Ischemic postconditioning during reperfusion attenuates intestinal injury and mucosal cell apoptosis by inhibiting JAK/STAT signaling activation.** *Shock* 2012, **38**(4):411–419.
39. Wen SH, Ling YH, Li Y, Li C, Liu JX, Li YS, Yao X, Xia ZQ, Liu KX: **Ischemic postconditioning during reperfusion attenuates oxidative stress and intestinal mucosal apoptosis induced by intestinal ischemia/reperfusion via aldose reductase.** *Surgery* 2013, **153**(4):555–564.

Thoracic hyperextension injury with complete "bony disruption" of the thoracic cage: Case report of a potentially life-threatening injury

James Bailey[1], Todd VanderHeiden[2], Clay Cothren Burlew[3], Sarah Pinski-Sibbel[2], Janeen Jordan[3], Ernest E. Moore[3] and Philip F. Stahel[2*]

Abstract

Background: Severe chest wall injuries are potentially life-threatening injuries which require a standardized multidisciplinary management strategy for prevention of posttraumatic complications and adverse outcome.

Case presentation: We report the successful management of a 55-year old man who sustained a complete "bony disruption" of the thoracic cage secondary to an "all-terrain vehicle" roll-over accident. The injury pattern consisted of a bilateral "flail chest" with serial segmental rib fractures, bilateral hemo-pneumothoraces and pulmonary contusions, bilateral midshaft clavicle fractures, a displaced transverse sternum fracture with significant diastasis, and an unstable T9 hyperextension injury. After initial life-saving procedures, the chest wall injuries were sequentially stabilized by surgical fixation of bilateral clavicle fractures, locked plating of the displaced sternal fracture, and a two-level anterior spine fixation of the T9 hyperextension injury. The patient had an excellent radiological and physiological outcome at 6 months post injury.

Conclusion: Severe chest wall trauma with a complete "bony disruption" of the thoracic cage represents a rare, but detrimental injury pattern. Multidisciplinary management with a staged timing for addressing each of the critical injuries, represents the ideal approach for an excellent long-term outcome.

Background

Blunt chest injuries represent a major cause of preventable mortality after trauma [1-3]. Serial rib fractures or a flail chest, in conjunction with a fractured sternum and unstable fractures of the thoracic spine, can lead to a complete "bony disruption" of the thoracic cage [4]. This entails a discontinuation of the chest wall integrity and muscular support, which is, most importantly, required for breathing and sufficient ventilation. While such critical injuries are rare, they pose a potential life-threatening risk related to underlying pulmonary contusions, impaired ventilatory mechanics, and the risk of developing posttraumatic complications and adverse pathophysiological sequelae [2,4]. These include the development of ventilator-associated pneumonia, acute respiratory distress syndrome, and subsequent multiple organ failure and death [5]. Some authors advocate for early rib fixation in patients with a flail chest, in order to restore the physiological ventilation impaired by the "paradoxical breathing" associated with segmental rib fractures [6,7]. In addition, unstable thoracic spine fractures are associated with a high risk for neurologic injury, particularly in younger victims and high-energy trauma mechanisms [8,9]. Early spine fixation for patients with unstable thoracic spine fractures results in a decreased incidence of respiratory complications [10-13].

In the present case report, we describe a successful management strategy for a complete "bony disruption" of the thoracic cage, in conjunction with a displaced transverse sternum fracture and an unstable hyperextension injury of the thoracic spine.

Case report

A 55-year-old man was involved in a helmeted "all-terrain vehicle" (ATV) roll-over accident. He had a loss of consciousness and a prolonged extrication, since his

* Correspondence: philip.stahel@dhha.org
[2]Department of Orthopaedics, Denver Health Medical Center, University of Colorado School of Medicine, 777 Bannock Street, Denver, CO 80204, USA
Full list of author information is available at the end of the article

body was pinned to the ground by the ATV. The patient was found to be comatose and in respiratory arrest, with a Glasgow Coma Scale (GCS) score of 3. He was endotracheally intubated at the accident scene and transferred to a local hospital in the Rocky Mountain region. On arrival, he was found to be hypotensive and tachycardic, with a blood pressure of 82/54 mmHg, a heart rate of 136 bpm, and SO_2 of 96% (on 100% FiO_2). The initial laboratory work-up showed a hemoglobin level of 8.2 g/dL, INR of 1.2, PTT of 30.1 s, pO_2 of 35 mmHg, base excess of 1.1 mEq/L, and lactate of 1.6 mmol/L. Chest radiograph revealed bilateral pneumo-hemothoraces, which were managed by placement of bilateral chest tubes, prior to airlift evacuation to our level 1 trauma center. After initial assessment and management by ATLS® protocol in our emergency department [14], the patient was transferred to the surgical intensive care unit (SICU) for ongoing resuscitation and ventilatory management. After radiologic workup by conventional films and "total body" computed tomography (CT) scan, the patient was diagnosed with the following injury pattern (Figures 1,2,3):

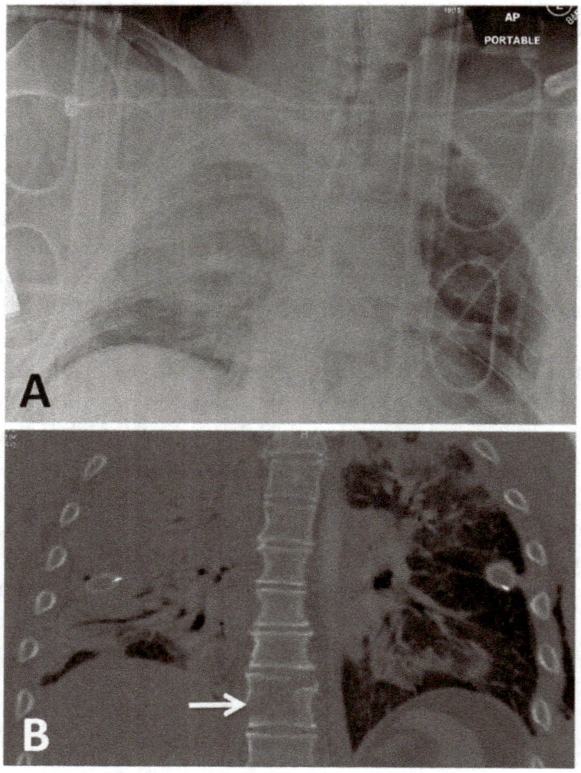

Figure 1 Initial chest radiograph (A) and coronal CT scan reconstruction (B) on arrival in the emergency department. Despite placement of bilateral chest drains, there is a persistent, extensive hemothorax on the right side, and signs of bilateral lung contusions. The arrow in **panel B** points out the T9 hyperextension injury in the coronal plane.

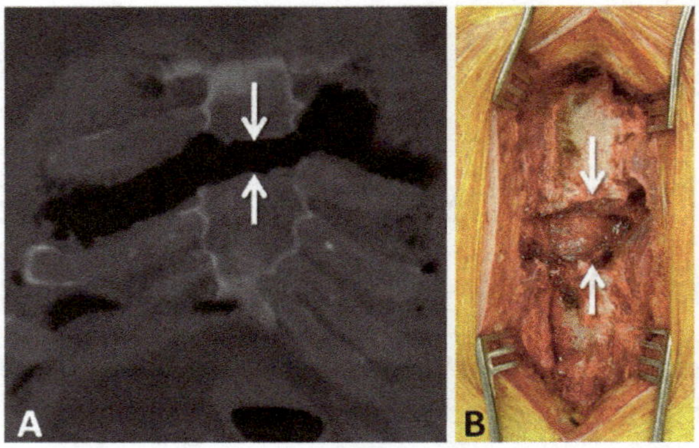

Figure 2 Displaced transverse sternal fracture in coronal CT scan (A) and operative site (B) after exposure for the sternal fracture fixation procedure. The arrows point out the impressive fracture diastasis of about 3 cm, with the retrosternal pericardium exposed in **panel B**.

Severe chest trauma with bilateral "flail chest" with serial segmental rib fractures (C1-8 on right side, C1-10 on left side), bilateral pulmonary contusions, and bilateral hemo-pneumothoraces, a displaced transverse sternum fracture with 3 cm diastasis, bilateral midshaft clavicle fractures, and an unstable T9 hyperextension injury.

The unstable T9 fracture was associated with a chronic hyperostotic ankylosing condition ("diffuse idiopathic skeletal hyperostosis"; DISH) of the thoracic spine, as revealed in the sagittal CT scan reconstruction (Figure 3A). An MRI of the T-spine was obtained to further assess for an associated disc or ligamentous injury, and to rule out the presence of an epidural hematoma, any of which may alter the surgical plan and modality of spinal fixation or fusion.

After resuscitation in the SICU, and adequate thoracic pain control by epidural anesthesia, the patient was taken to the OR on day 4 for fracture fixation. A

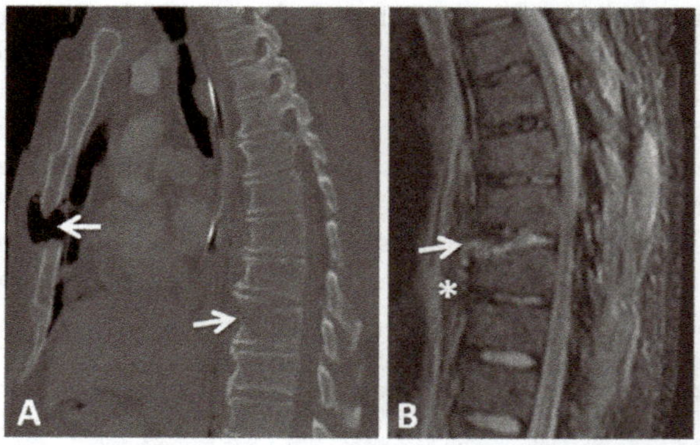

Figure 3 Sagittal CT scan (A) and STIR sequence in MRI (B) of the T9 hyperextension injury (arrows). The asterisk in **panel B** alludes to the extensive prevertebral hematoma.

decision was made for surgical fixation of bilateral clavicle fractures, the sternal fracture, and the T9 spine fracture, in order to achieve adjunctive stability of the thoracic cage and to allow early functional rehabilitation without restrictions. The patient was placed on a radiolucent flat-top operating table in supine position. The technique of positioning, preparation and draping, aimed at addressing both clavicle fractures and the sternum fracture in one session, are depicted in Figure 4.

The bilateral comminuted clavicle fractures were fixed through an S-shaped subclavicular approach, using two 10-hole 3.5 mm reconstruction plates (Synthes, West Chester, PA), which were applied in bridging technique (Figure 5). This was followed by a median approach to the transverse sternal fracture. The sternum had a diastasis of about 3 cm through which the mediastinal fat pad and pericardium was evident (Figure 2B). The video clip in the Additional file 1 shows the beating heart behind the sternal fracture. A 2.5 mm unicortical hole was drilled on each side of the fracture, to allow placement of a pointed reduction tenaculum for anatomic reduction of the sternal fracture (Figure 6A). The fracture was then fixed with two 8-hole 3.5 mm third-tubular locking plates (Synthes), using unicortical locking head screws. This technique was used to avoid screw penetration across the far cortex, with the risk of a delayed arrosion of the pericardium (Figure 6B).

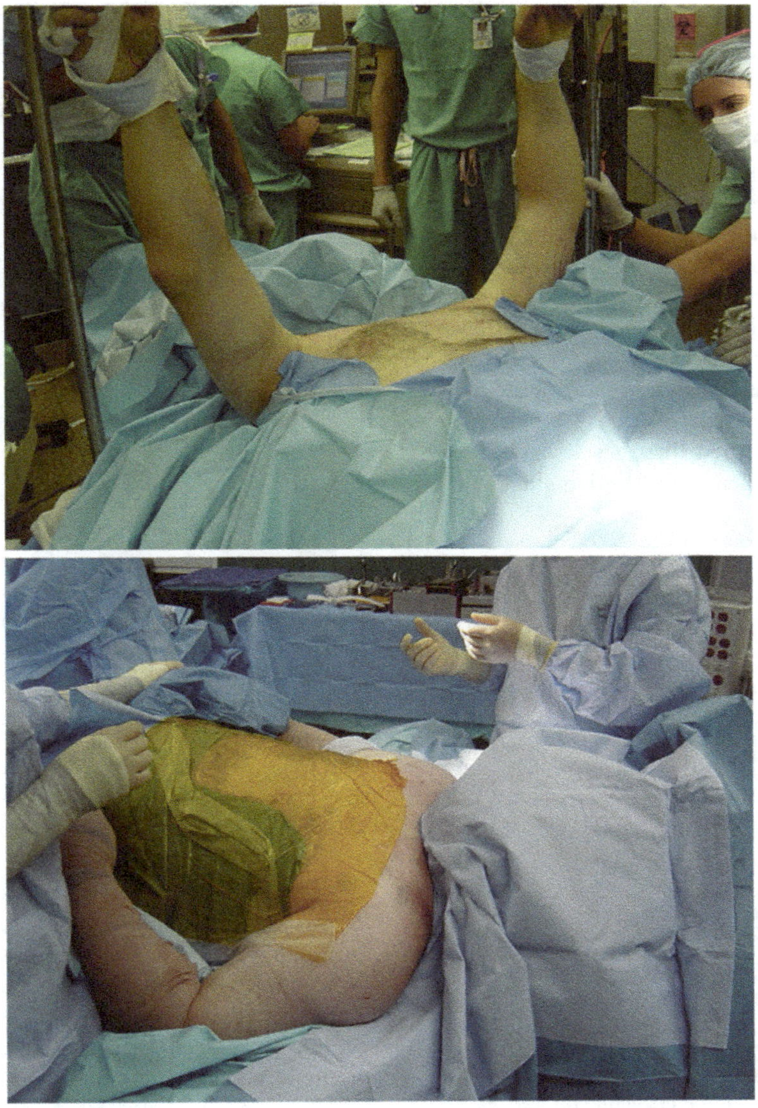

Figure 4 Technique of patient positioning and draping for surgical fixation of the bilateral clavicle fractures and the displaced sternal fracture.

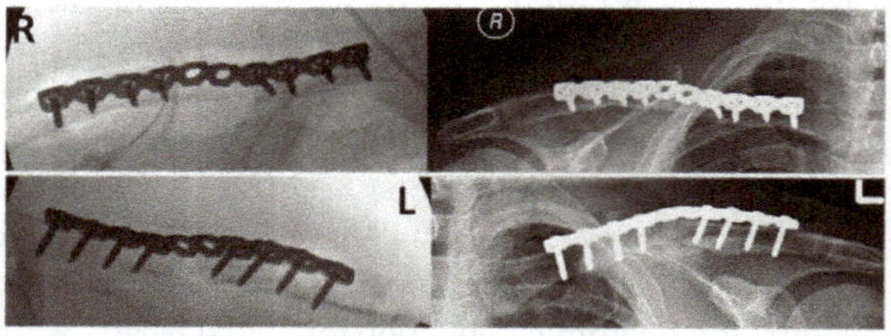

Figure 5 Intraoperative fluoroscopy films of bilateral clavicle fracture fixation in bridging technique (left panels), and follow-up radiographs at 6 months, demonstrating the bilateral healed fractures (right panels).

After wound closure, the patient was carefully log-rolled into a right lateral decubitus position on a pre-positioned beanbag, for operative fixation of the unstable T9 vertebral fracture. Two-level spinal fixation from T8-T10 was performed using a titanium locking plate system (THOR™, Stryker, Allendale, NJ), through a less-invasive postero-lateral approach, as previously described [15]. A tracheostomy was performed in the same session, due to the requirement of prolonged ventilation in the SICU. The postoperative chest radiographs demonstrates the plate fixation of bilateral clavicles, sternum, and thoracic spine (Figure 7A). The patient tolerated the surgical procedures well and remained hemodynamically stable throughout the case. He was weaned from mechanical ventilation, and the chest tubes were appropriately removed. The patient was transferred to an acute rehabilitative facility on postoperative day 16.

The patient was readmitted three weeks later, 6 weeks post injury, for acute fever, chills, and night sweats, in

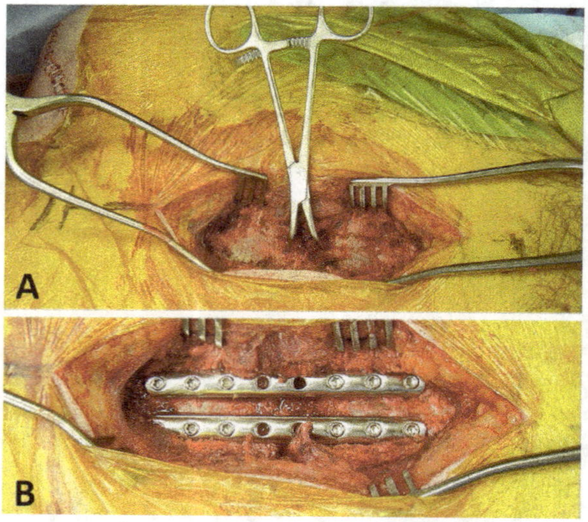

Figure 6 Intraoperative view of the technique for fracture reduction (A) and locked plating (B) of the displaced transverse sternum fracture. See text for details.

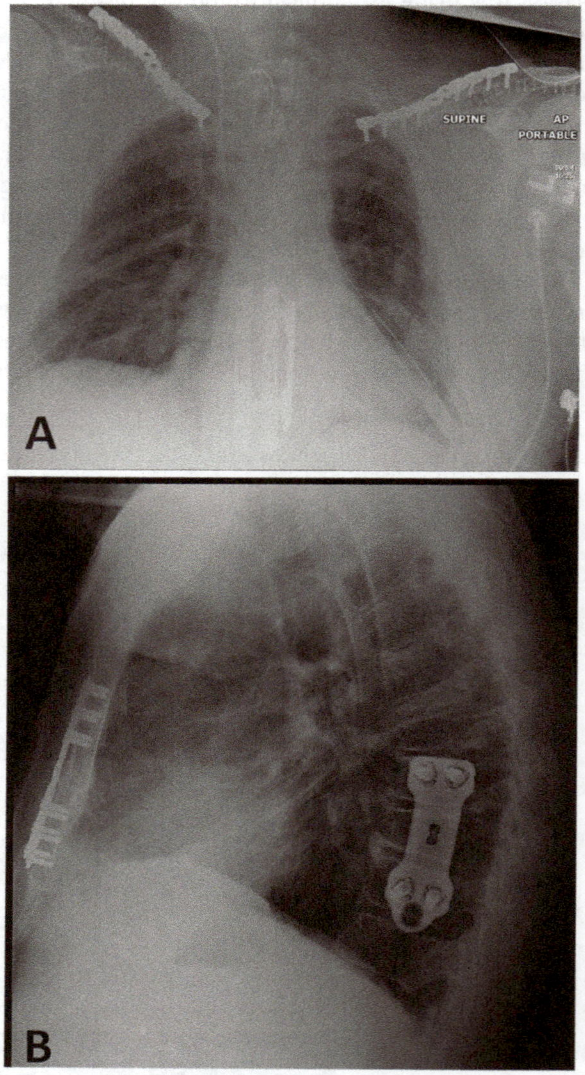

Figure 7 Radiographic documentation demonstrating the sternal fracture and T9 spine fixation in antero-posterior chest X-ray (A), and in the lateral plane at 6 months follow-up (B).

conjunction with increased oxygen requirement. A right-side chest drain was placed which showed purulent drainage, and the patient was diagnosed with a pleural empyema, likely related to a retained hemothorax. He underwent a video-assisted thoracoscopic pleural decortication. Two 32 French pleural chest drains were placed intraoperatively. The patient recovered well from the procedure, and he was treated with adjunctive antibiotics. The chest drains were removed prior to discharge within a week of surgery. The patient was discharged home in good condition.

All surgical wounds healed uneventfully, and there were no further complications. Within three months after the accident, the patient had returned to exercising without restrictions and was able to hike a mountain with altitude above 14,000 ft, with minimal subjective shortness of breath. At 6 months follow-up, X-rays revealed a fully healed sternal fracture, T9 vertebral fracture (Figure 7B), and bilateral clavicle fractures (Fig. 5). The patient had a full range of motion in bilateral shoulders and in the T- and L-spine, and a normal neurovascular status in all four extremities. He was released to full activity without restrictions, and scheduled to follow-up as needed.

Discussion

The structural support of the thoracic cage is provided by the sternum in conjunction with the rib cage and the thoracic spine [16,17]. The adjunctive anterior support for the thoracic spine by the sternum has been accurately described as "the 4th spinal column" by Berg in 1993 [18], in modification of Denis' classic "three column model" of spinal stability [19]. The thoracic cage stability is further bolstered by clavicular strut attachments to the sternum and a complex interplay between the clavicles and the scapulae as they attach to the posterior thorax [20]. High-energy trauma mechanisms to the chest and thoracic spine can result in critical injuries, including pulmonary and cardiac contusions, aortic injuries, and acute spinal cord injuries [21]. Unstable thoracic spine injuries typically result from flexion/distraction or hyperextension injuries in association with a sternal fracture, representing the classic "4-column thoracic spine fracture" [18,22-24]. These combined fractures often occur in high-energy, multi-system trauma, and can be easily overlooked on initial evaluation [25,26].

The present case reports describes the successful management of a severe chest trauma in a 55 year-old patient who sustained a complete "bony disruption" of the thoracic cage, consisting of bilateral segmental serial rib fractures ("flail chest"), bilateral comminuted clavicle fractures, an unstable T9 hyperextension injury, and a displaced transverse sternal fracture. The combination of early fracture fixation, in conjunction with modern ventilatory and pain management strategies in the SICU, allowed for an excellent long-term outcome.

The "ideal" timing and modality of managing a complete "bony disruption" of the chest wall remains controversial. The surgeon in charge should consider (1) the acute life-threatening aspects of the injury, related to airway compromise and ventilatory management; (2) the timing of definitive surgical fracture fixation in relation to the acute hyperinflammatory response, taking into account the risk of sustaining a "2nd hit" injury related to a prolonged surgical intervention [27]; (3) the anatomic and functional relation of the rib cage with the shoulder girdle and the thoracic spinal column, which provide the underlying rationale for the specific modality of surgical fracture fixation [8,17,20].

The primary objective of the initial management of multiply injured patients is *survival*. The acute management by "damage control" procedures will limit the extent of the operative and interventional burden, and allow early patient transfer to the SICU, for full resuscitation [14]. The pathophysiological disturbances of the immune and clotting systems render multiply injured patients vulnerable to "2nd hit" insults related to inadequate timing and modality of surgical procedures [27]. The ideal timing for definitive fracture fixation lies in a limited physiological "time-window of opportunity", somewhere around day 4 to 10 after trauma [11,14].

From a biomechanical perspective, the surgeon must take into consideration the "four-column model" of thoracic stability [18,28,29] provided by the rib-cage and the thoracic spine, in conjunction with the shoulder balance provided by clavicular strut integrity [16,17,22,30,31]. The present case report outlines the biomechanical importance of the integrity of the "upper transthoracic cage" [4], based on the functional interaction between the shoulder girdle, the rib cage, and the thoracic spine.

Notably, sternal fractures are frequently missed in the trauma bay, since dedicated sternum radiographs are not part of the standard trauma work-up. Based on the important biomechanical aspects related to thoracic cage integrity outlined above, missed sternal fractures in conjunction with upper thoracic spine injuries can have significant adverse effects, including respiratory distress and pulmonary complications, neurological compromise to the spinal cord, chronic pain, malunion, and progressive kyphotic deformity [4,8,23,26,32,33].

Multiple technical modalities for sternal fixation have been described in the literature [34], including wiring, conventional plating, threaded pin fixation, flexible intramedullary nailing [33]. Locked plating of sternal fractures and sternal nonunions has been previously described, by the use of designated sternal locking plates, anterior cervical locking plates, and mandibular locking plates [35-37]. However, the technique of using two parallel stainless-steel tubular locking plates applied in the present case has not been previously described in the literature, to our knowledge [34]. We believe that this represents a feasible, safe, and cost-effective strategy which results in excellent outcome, as reflected by this case report.

In conclusion, we present a safe and successful strategy for managing a highly unstable and potentially life-threatening disruption of the chest wall, associated with a "four-column" hyperextension injury of the thoracic spine in conjunction with a displaced transverse sternal fracture. A standardized multidisciplinary resuscitation protocol [14], in conjunction with modern ventilatory management strategies in the SICU [2,38] and a pro-active surgical fixation of the "bony disruption" of the chest wall during the physiological time-window of opportunity [11,14], likely contributed to the excellent long-term outcome of this critically injured patient.

Competing interests
The authors declare that they have no competing interests.

Authors' contributions
PFS, TVH, and CCB designed the case report. PFS, CCB, SSP, and JJ performed the surgical procedures in this patient. JB drafted the first version of the manuscript. PFS and EEM critically revised this paper. All authors contributed and approved the final version of the manuscript.

Disclosures
PFS has obtained occasional speaker's honoraria from Stryker Spine (Allendale, NJ) within the past 5 years. The authors declare no other competing interests related to this manuscript. The views expressed in this article are those of the authors and do not reflect the official policy or position of the Department of the Navy, Department of Defense, or the United States Government.

Acknowledgments
The patient agreed with publication of this case report, including the publication of medical data, radiological imaging, intraoperative pictures and video materials. Written informed consent is available to the Editor-in-Chief upon request.

Author details
[1]Department of Orthopaedics, Naval Medical Center, San Diego, CA 92134, USA. [2]Department of Orthopaedics, Denver Health Medical Center, University of Colorado School of Medicine, 777 Bannock Street, Denver, CO 80204, USA. [3]Department of Surgery, Denver Health Medical Center, University of Colorado School of Medicine, 777 Bannock Street, Denver, CO 80204, USA.

References
1. Battle CE, Hutchings H, Evans PA: **Expert opinion of the risk factors for morbidity and mortality in blunt chest wall trauma: Results of a national postal questionnaire survey of Emergency Departments in the United Kingdom.** *Injury* 2012, in press.
2. Haenel JB, Moore FA, Moore EE: **Pulmonary consequences of severe chest trauma.** *Respir Care Clin N Am* 1996, **2**(3):401–424.
3. Stahel PF, Schneider P, Buhr HJ, Kruschewski M: **Emergency management of thoracic trauma.** *Orthopäde* 2005, **34**(9):865–879.
4. Labbe JL, Peres O, Leclair O, Goulon R, Scemama P, Jourdel F: **Fractures of the upper transthoracic cage.** *J Bone Joint Surg Br* 2009, **91**(1):91–96.
5. Dewar D, Moore FA, Moore EE, Balogh Z: **Postinjury multiple organ failure.** *Injury* 2009, **40**(9):912–918.
6. Bottlang M, Helzel I, Long WB, Madey S: **Anatomically contoured plates for fixation of rib fractures.** *J Trauma* 2010, **68**(3):611–615.
7. Althausen PL, Shannon S, Watts C, Thomas K, Bain MA, Coll D, O'mara TJ, Bray TJ: **Early surgical stabilization of flail chest with locked plate fixation.** *J Orthop Trauma* 2011, **25**(11):641–647.
8. Vioreanu MH, Quinlan JF, Robertson I, O'Byrne JM: **Vertebral fractures and concomitant fractures of the sternum.** *Int Orthop* 2005, **29**(6):339–342.
9. Huang Z, Yi B, Liu H, Chen F, Huang J, Gong H, Xu T, Jian G, Wang B, Chen R, *et al*: **Treatment and classification of thoracic fracture accompanied by sternum fracture.** *Zhong Nan Da Xue Xue Bao Yi Xue Ban* 2011, **36**(12):1199–1205.
10. Frangen TM, Ruppert S, Muhr G, Schinkel C: **Respiratory failure in thoracic spine injuries: Does the timing of dorsal stabilization have any effect on the clinical course in multiply injured patients?.** *Orthopäde* 2007, **36**(4):365–371.
11. Stahel PF, Flierl MA, Moore EE, Smith WR, Beauchamp KM, Dwyer A: **Advocating "spine damage control" as a safe and effective treatment modality for unstable thoracolumbar fractures in polytrauma patients: a hypothesis.** *J Trauma Manag Outcomes* 2009, **3**:6.
12. Croce MA, Bee TK, Pritchard E, Miller PR, Fabian TC: **Does optimal timing for spine fracture fixation exist?.** *Ann Surg* 2001, **233**(6):851–858.
13. Rutges JP, Oner FC, Leenen LP: **Timing of thoracic and lumbar fracture fixation in spinal injuries: a systematic review of neurological and clinical outcome.** *Eur Spine J* 2007, **16**(5):579–587.
14. Stahel PF, Smith WR, Moore EE: **Current trends in resuscitation strategy for the multiply injured patient.** *Injury* 2009, **40**(Suppl 4):S27–35.
15. Weckbach S, Flierl MA, Blei M, Burlew CC, Moore EE, Stahel PF: **Survival following a vertical free fall from 300 feet: the crucial role of body position to impact surface.** *Scand J Trauma Resusc Emerg Med* 2011, **19**:63.
16. Oda I, Abumi K, Lu D, Shono Y, Kaneda K: **Biomechanical role of the posterior elements, costovertebral joints, and rib cage in the stability of the thoracic spine.** *Spine (Phila Pa 1976)* 1996, **21**(12):1423–1429.
17. Watkins Rt, Watkins R 3rd, Williams L, Ahlbrand S, Garcia R, Karamanian A, Sharp L, Vo C, Hedman T: **Stability provided by the sternum and rib cage in the thoracic spine.** *Spine (Phila Pa 1976)* 2005, **30**(11):x1283–1286.
18. Berg EE: **The sternal-rib complex. A possible fourth column in thoracic spine fractures.** *Spine (Phila Pa 1976)* 1993, **18**(13):1916–1919.
19. Denis F: **The three column spine and its significance in the classification of acute thoracolumbar spinal injuries.** *Spine (Phila Pa 1976)* 1983, **8**(8):817–831.
20. Gottschalk HP, Browne RH, Starr AJ: **Shoulder girdle: patterns of trauma and associated injuries.** *J Orthop Trauma* 2011, **25**(5):266–271.
21. Demetriades D, Velmahos GC, Scalea TM, Jurkovich GJ, Karmy-Jones R, Teixeira PG, Hemmila PG, O'Connor JV, McKenney MO, Moore FA, *et al*: **Diagnosis and treatment of blunt thoracic aortic injuries: changing perspectives.** *J Trauma* 2008, **64**(6):1415–1418.
22. el-Khoury GY, Whitten CG: **Trauma to the upper thoracic spine: anatomy, biomechanics, and unique imaging features.** *AJR Am J Roentgenol* 1993, **160**(1):95–102.
23. Lund JM, Chojnowski A, Crawford R: **Multiple thoracic spine wedge fractures with associated sternal fracture; an unstable combination.** *Injury* 2001, **32**(3):254–255.
24. Elgafy H, Bellabarba C: **Three-column ligamentous extension injury of the thoracic spine: a case report and review of the literature.** *Spine (Phila Pa 1976)* 2007, **32**(25):E785–788.
25. Gopalakrishnan KC: **el Masri WS: Fractures of the sternum associated with spinal injury.** *J Bone Joint Surg Br* 1986, **68**(2):178–181.
26. van Beek EJ, Been HD, Ponsen KK, Maas M: **Upper thoracic spinal fractures in trauma patients - a diagnostic pitfall.** *Injury* 2000, **31**(4):219–223.
27. Stahel PF, Smith WR, Moore EE: **Role of biological modifiers regulating the immune response after trauma.** *Injury* 2007, **38**(12):1409–1422.
28. Casey R, Emde K: **Displaced fractured sternum following blunt chest trauma.** *J Emerg Nurs* 2008, **34**(1):83–85.
29. Jones HK, McBride GG, Mumby RC: **Sternal fractures associated with spinal injury.** *J Trauma* 1989, **29**(3):360–364.
30. Andriacchi T, Schultz A, Belytschko T, Galante J: **A model for studies of mechanical interactions between the human spine and rib cage.** *J Biomech* 1974, **7**(6):497–507.
31. Oda I, Abumi K, Cunningham BW, Kaneda K, McAfee PC: **An in vitro human cadaveric study investigating the biomechanical properties of the thoracic spine.** *Spine (Phila Pa 1976)* 2002, **27**(3):E64–70.
32. Klaase JM, Zimmerman KW, Veldhuis EF: **Increased kyphosis by a combination of fractures of the sternum and thoracic spine.** *Eur Spine J* 1998, **7**(1):69–71.
33. Regauer M, Huber-Wagner S, Oedekoven T, Mutschler W, Euler E: **Flexible intramedullary nailing of a displaced transverse sternal fracture associated with a flexion-compression injury of the thoracic spine.** *Spine (Phila Pa 1976)* 2010, **35**(12):E553–558.
34. Harston A, Roberts C: **Fixation of sternal fractures: a systematic review.** *J Trauma* 2011, **71**(6):1875–1879.
35. Wu LC, Renucci JD, Song DH: **Sternal nonunion: a review of current treatments and a new method of rigid fixation.** *Ann Plast Surg* 2005, **54**(1):55–58.
36. Ciriaco P, Casiraghi M, Negri G, Gioia G, Carretta A, Melloni G, Zannini P: **Early surgical repair of isolated traumatic sternal fractures using a cervical plate system.** *J Trauma* 2009, **66**(2):462–464.

12

WSES Guidelines for the management of acute left sided colonic diverticulitis in the emergency setting

Massimo Sartelli[1*], Fausto Catena[2], Luca Ansaloni[3], Federico Coccolini[4], Ewen A. Griffiths[5], Fikri M. Abu-Zidan[6], Salomone Di Saverio[7], Jan Ulrych[8], Yoram Kluger[9], Ofir Ben-Ishay[9], Frederick A. Moore[10], Rao R. Ivatury[11], Raul Coimbra[12], Andrew B. Peitzman[13], Ari Leppaniemi[14], Gustavo P. Fraga[15], Ronald V. Maier[16], Osvaldo Chiara[17], Jeffry Kashuk[18], Boris Sakakushev[19], Dieter G. Weber[20], Rifat Latifi[21], Walter Biffl[22], Miklosh Bala[23], Aleksandar Karamarkovic[24], Kenji Inaba[25], Carlos A. Ordonez[26], Andreas Hecker[27], Goran Augustin[28], Zaza Demetrashvili[29], Renato Bessa Melo[30], Sanjay Marwah[31], Sanoop K. Zachariah[32], Vishal G. Shelat[33], Michael McFarlane[34], Miran Rems[35], Carlos Augusto Gomes[36], Mario Paulo Faro[37], Gerson Alves Pereira Júnior[38], Ionut Negoi[39], Yunfeng Cui[40], Norio Sato[41], Andras Vereczkei[42], Giovanni Bellanova[43], Arianna Birindelli[7], Isidoro Di Carlo[44], Kenneth Y Kok[45], Mahir Gachabayov[46], Georgios Gkiokas[47], Konstantinos Bouliaris[48], Elif Çolak[49], Arda Isik[50], Daniel Rios-Cruz[51], Rodolfo Soto[52] and Ernest E. Moore[22]

Abstract

Acute left sided colonic diverticulitis is one of the most common clinical conditions encountered by surgeons in acute setting. A World Society of Emergency Surgery (WSES) Consensus Conference on acute diverticulitis was held during the 3rd World Congress of the WSES in Jerusalem, Israel, on July 7th, 2015. During this consensus conference the guidelines for the management of acute left sided colonic diverticulitis in the emergency setting were presented and discussed. This document represents the executive summary of the final guidelines approved by the consensus conference.

Background

Acute left sided colonic diverticulosis is common in Western countries, however its prevalence is increasing throughout the world, probably because of changes in lifestyle [1]. Although left sided colonic diverticulosis is more common amongst elderly patients, a dramatic rise of its incidence has been seen in the younger age groups in recent years [2]. Data from Western populations suggest that up to one fifth of patients with acute diverticulitis are under the age of 50 years of age [3–5]. Recent evidence suggests that lifetime risk of developing acute left sided colonic diverticulitis (ALCD) is only about 4 % among patients with diverticulosis [6].

ALCD is a common problem encountered by surgeons in the acute setting. It encompasses a variety of conditions, ranging from localized diverticular inflammation to perforation and fecal peritonitis. Daily decisions in the diagnosis and treatment of acute diverticulitis generally depend on clinicians' personal preferences rather than evidence-based medicine. There is generally a lack of well conducted randomized clinical trials in ALCD and a large amount of evidence in the literature is low quality and conflicting.

Methods

A World Society of Emergency Surgery (WSES) working group published in 2015 a proposal for a new CT based classification for ALCD [7]. This has been extended and developed into guidelines for the management of acute diverticulitis in an emergency setting. A literature search, using the PubMed database, was performed without

* Correspondence: m.sartelli@virgilio.it; massimosartelli@gmail.com
[1]Department of Surgery, Macerata Hospital, Via Santa Lucia 2, 62019 Macerata, Italy
Full list of author information is available at the end of the article

restriction of time or type of manuscript. The search was limited to English language publications. The final grade of recommendation was performed by using the Grades of Recommendation, Assessment, Development, and Evaluation (GRADE) system (Table 1) [8, 9].

A World Society of Emergency Surgery (WSES) Consensus Conference on acute diverticulitis was held during the 3rd World Congress of the WSES in Jerusalem, Israel, on July 7th, 2015. During this consensus conference the guidelines were presented and debated. This document represents the executive summary of the final guidelines approved by the consensus conference.

Results

Classification systems

ALCD ranges in severity from uncomplicated inflammatory diverticulitis to complicated diverticulitis (abscess formation or perforation). For the past three decades, the Hinchey classification has been the most commonly used classification for complicated ALCD in international literature [10].

Based on the surgical findings of abscesses and peritonitis, Hinchey et al. classified the severity of acute diverticulitis into four grades:

Stage 1 Pericolic abscess
Stage 2 Pelvic, intra-abdominal, or retroperitoneal abscess
Stage 3 Generalized purulent peritonitis
Stage 4 Generalized fecal peritonitis

The management of ALCD has recently changed dramatically in recent years, due to better radiological imaging and availability of non-surgical treatment options. Computer tomography (CT) imaging has become a primary diagnostic tool in the diagnosis and staging of patients with acute diverticulitis and more detailed information provided by CT scans led to several modifications of the Hinchey classification [4, 11–17]. For example, in 1989 Neff et al. presented a new classification based on CT findings. It consisted of five stages, ranging from radiological diagnosis of uncomplicated AD (Stage 0) to pneumoperitoneum with abundant free liquid (Stage 4) [11]:

Table 1 Grading of recommendations from Guyatt and colleagues [8, 9]

rade of recommendation	Clarity of risk/benefit	Quality of supporting evidence	Implications
1A			
Strong recommendation, high-quality evidence	Benefits clearly outweigh risk and burdens, or vice versa	RCTs without important limitations or overwhelming evidence from observational studies	Strong recommendation, applies to most patients in most circumstances without reservation
1B			
Strong recommendation, moderate-quality evidence	Benefits clearly outweigh risk and burdens, or vice versa	RCTs with important limitations (inconsistent results, methodological flaws, indirect analyses or imprecise conclusions) or exceptionally strong evidence from observational studies	Strong recommendation, applies to most patients in most circumstances without reservation
1C			
Strong recommendation, low-quality or very low-quality evidence	Benefits clearly outweigh risk and burdens, or vice versa	Observational studies or case series	Strong recommendation but subject to change when higher quality evidence becomes available
2A			
Weak recommendation, high-quality evidence	Benefits closely balanced with risks and burden	RCTs without important limitations or overwhelming evidence from observational studies	Weak recommendation, best action may differ depending on the patient, treatment circumstances, or social values
2B			
Weak recommendation, moderate-quality evidence	Benefits closely balanced with risks and burden	RCTs with important limitations (inconsistent results, methodological flaws, indirect or imprecise) or exceptionally strong evidence from observational studies	Weak recommendation, best action may differ depending on the patient, treatment circumstances, or social values
2C			
Weak recommendation, Low-quality or very low-quality evidence	Uncertainty in the estimates of benefits, risks, and burden; benefits, risk, and burden may be closely balanced	Observational studies or case series	Very weak recommendation; alternative treatments may be equally reasonable and merit consideration

Stage 0 Uncomplicated diverticulitis; Diverticula, thickening of the wall, increased density of the pericolic fat
Stage 1 Locally complicated with local abscess
Stage 2 Complicated with pelvic abscess;
Stage 3 Complicated with distant abscess
Stage 4 Complicated with other distant complications

In 1997, Sher et al. [12] introduced a modification of Hinchey classification. This classification divided abscesses into pericolic abscesses (stage I), distant abscesses amendable for percutaneous drainage (stage IIa), and complex abscesses associated with a possible fistula (stage IIb). This classification implied the use of new treatment strategies, such as CT-guided percutaneous drainage of abscesses.

In 2002 Ambrosetti et al. [13] classified diverticulitis into severe or moderate disease. In this classification, the CT scan determined the grade of severity guiding the physician in the treatment of acute complications. Moderate diverticulitis was defined by wall thickening of ≥ 5 mm and signs of inflammation of pericolic fat. Severe diverticulitis was defined by wall thickening accompanied by abscess formation, extraluminal air or extraluminal contrast leak:

Moderate diverticulitis	Localized sigmoid wall thickening Pericolic fat stranding
Severe diverticulitis	Abscess Extraluminal air Extraluminal contrast

In 2005 Kaiser et al. [14] modified Hinchey classification according to specific CT findings:

Stage 0 mild clinical diverticulitis
Stage 1a confined pericolic inflammation,
Stage 1b confined pericolic abscess
Stage 2 pelvic or distant intra-abdominal abscess
Stage 3 generalized purulent peritonitis
Stage 4 fecal peritonitis at presentation.

In 2013 Mora Lopez et al. proposed [15] a modification of the previous Neff classification dividing Neff stage 1 into stage 1 a (localized pneumoperitoneum in the form of air bubbles) and 1 b abscess (<4 cm):

Stage 0 Uncomplicated diverticulitis. Diverticula, thickening of the wall, increased density of the pericolic fat
Stage 1 Locally complicated diverticulitis
Stage 1a Localized pneumoperitoneum in the form of air bubbles
Stage 1b Abscess (<4 cm)
Stage 2 Complicated diverticulitis with pelvic abscess. Abscess > 4 cm in pelvis
Stage 3 Complicated diverticulitis with distant abscess. Abscess in abdominal cavity (outside pelvis)
Stage 4 Complicated diverticulitis with other distant complications. Abundant pneumoperitoneum and/or intra-abdominal free liquid

Recently Sallinen at al. [16] published an interesting retrospective study of patients treated for diverticulitis, setting the stage for the treatment of acute diverticulitis based on clinical, radiologic and physiologic parameters. They included 5 stages:

Stage 1 Uncomplicated diverticulitis
Stage 2 Complicated diverticulitis with small abscess (<6 cm)
Stage 3 Complicated diverticulitis with large abscess (≥6 cm) or distant intraperitoneal or retroperitoneal air
Stage 4 Generalized peritonitis without organ dysfunction
Stage 5 Generalized peritonitis with organ dysfunction

Finally a proposal for a CT guided classification of left colon acute diverticulitis was published in 2015 by the WSES acute diverticulitis working group [7]. It is a simple classification system of acute diverticulitis based on CT scan findings. It may guide clinicians in the management of acute diverticulitis and may be universally accepted for day to day practice. The WSES classification divides acute diverticulitis into 2 groups: uncomplicated and complicated.

In the event of uncomplicated acute diverticulitis, the infection does not extend to the peritoneum. In the event of complicated acute diverticulitis, the infectious process proceeds beyond the colon. Complicated acute diverticulitis is divided into 4 stages, based on the extension of the infectious process:

Uncomplicated

Stage 0 Diverticula, thickening of the colonic wall or increased density of the pericolic fat
Complicated
Stage 1a Pericolic air bubbles or little pericolic fluid without abscess (within 5 cm from inflamed bowel segment)
Stage 1b Abscess ≤ 4 cm
Stage 2a Abscess > 4 cm
Stage 2b Distant air (>5 cm from inflamed bowel segment)

Stage 3 Diffuse fluid without distant free air (no hole in colon)
Stage 4 Diffuse fluid with distant free air (persistent hole in colon)

Diagnosis

1) An accurate assessment of the patients using clinical signs, laboratory inflammation markers and radiological findings is recommended to identify the best treatment for each patient with ALCD (Recommendation 1 C).
2) The clinical diagnosis of ALCD alone is not sufficiently accurate for patients with suspected diverticulitis (Recommendation 1 C).
3) Pain in the lower left abdomen on physical examination and C-reactive protein (CRP) 50 mg/l or more suggests a diagnosis of ALCD (Recommendation 1 C).

Clinical findings of patients having ALCD include acute pain or tenderness in the left lower quadrant which may be associated with increased inflammatory markers including C-reactive protein (CRP) and white blood cell count (WBC). Clinical diagnosis of ALCD usually lacks accuracy. In a prospective analysis [17] conducted on 802 consecutive patients that presented with abdominal pain to the emergency department, positive and negative predictive values of clinical diagnosis were 0.65 and 0.98 respectively. Additional cross-sectional imaging had a positive and negative predictive value of more 0.95 and 0.99 respectively. Additional radiology examinations improved the diagnostic accuracy in 37 % of the patients, but changed the management in only 7 %. Ultrasound and CT had superior diagnostic accuracy, however these examinations rarely changed the initial management proposal.

Using logistic regression analysis, Lameris et al. [18] in 2010, developed a clinical decision rule for diagnosis of diverticulitis, based on 3 criteria: direct tenderness in the left lower quadrant, 2) CRP > 50 mg/l and 3) absence of vomiting. Of 126 clinically suspected patients enrolled in this prospective study, 30 patients had all 3 features (24 %), of whom 29 had a final diagnosis of acute diverticulitis (97 %; 95 % CI: 83 %-99 %). Of the 96 patients without all 3 features, 45 (47 %) did not have diverticulitis. In a quarter of patients with suspected diverticulitis, the diagnosis could be made clinically based on a combination of the three criteria.

Andeweg et al. in 2011 [19], using retrospective data from 287 patients, developed a clinical scoring system for the diagnosis of ALCD that had a diagnostic accuracy of 86 %. It was based on the independent predictors of ALCD and included patients' age, one or more previous episodes, localization of symptoms in the lower left abdomen, aggravation of pain on movement, the absence of vomiting, localization of abdominal tenderness in the lower left abdomen, and C-reactive protein 50 or more.

CRP has been identified as a useful biomarker of inflammation and it may be useful in the prediction of the clinical severity of acute diverticulitis as demonstrated by several recent studies [20–22]. To investigate the value of C-reactive protein (CRP) and of other laboratory parameters of the patients in the prediction of the clinical severity of acute diverticulitis a retrospective study was published in 2014 [20]. A CRP cutoff value of 170 mg/L significantly discriminated severe from mild diverticulitis (87.5 % sensitivity, 91.1 % specificity, area under the curve 0.942, $P < 0.00001$). The author concluded that CRP is a useful tool in the prediction of the clinical severity of acute diverticulitis. A mild episode is very likely in patients with CRP less than 170 mg/L. Those with higher CRP values have a greater probability of undergoing surgery or radiological drainage.

In another study, the diagnostic value of serological infection markers and body temperature in discriminating complicated from uncomplicated diverticulitis was assessed [21]. A total of 426 patients were included in this study of which 364 (85 %) presented with uncomplicated and 62 (15 %) with complicated diverticulitis. Only CRP was of sufficient diagnostic value (area under the curve 0.715). The median CRP in patients with complicated diverticulitis was significantly higher than in patients with uncomplicated disease (224 mg/l, range 99–284 vs 87 mg/l, range 48–151). Patients with a CRP of 25 mg/l had a 15 % chance of having complicated diverticulitis. This increased from 23 % at a CRP value of 100 mg/l to 47 % for 250 mg/l or higher. The optimal threshold was reached at 175 mg/l with a positive predictive value of 36 %, negative predictive value of 92 %, sensitivity of 61 % and a specificity of 82 %.

Recently Makela et al. [22] published a study which compared the CRP values of 350 patients who presented first time with symptoms of acute diverticulitis with the CT findings and clinical parameters by means of both univariate and multivariate analyses. CRP cut-off value of 149.5 mg/l significantly discriminated acute uncomplicated diverticulitis from complicated diverticulitis (specificity 65 %, sensitivity 85 %, area under the curve 0.811, $p = 0.0001$). In multivariate analysis, a CRP value over 150 mg/l and old age were independent risk factors for acute complicated diverticulitis. The mean CRP value was significantly higher in the patients who died (mean CRP of 207) than in those who survived (mean CRP of 139). In addition, a CRP value over 150 mg/l and free abdominal fluid in CT were independent variables predicting postoperative mortality. The study confirmed that CRP is useful for the predicting the severity of acute diverticulitis on admission. The authors concluded that patients with a CRP value higher than 150 mg/l have an increased risk of complicated diverticulitis and should always undergo a CT examination.

4) Computed tomography (CT) scan of the abdomen and pelvis is indicated for all patients with suspected ALCD. It has high sensitivity and specificity and can assess the severity of diverticulitis guiding clinicians in planning treatment (Recommendation 1 C).
5) Ultrasound (US) may be a useful alternative in the initial evaluation of patients with suspected ALCD. It has wide availability and easy accessibility. It may have satisfactory sensitivity and specificity when performed by an expert operator. A step-up approach with CT performed after an inconclusive or negative US may be a safe approach for patients suspected of acute diverticulitis (Recommendation 1 C).

Radiological imaging techniques that are used for diagnosing acute diverticulitis in the emergency setting are computed tomography (CT) and ultrasound (US). CT imaging is becoming by now the gold standard in the diagnosis and staging of patients with ALCD. CT imaging with intravenous contrast has excellent sensitivity and specificity [23–25]. CT findings in patients with ALCD may include diverticulosis with associated colon wall thickening, fat stranding, phlegmon, extraluminal gas, abscess formation or intra-abdominal diffuse fluid. CT imaging can go beyond accurate diagnosis of ALCD; CT criteria may be also used to determine the grade of severity and may drive treatment planning of patients [7]. US is a real-time dynamic examination with wide availability and easy accessibility [26] and may be useful in diagnosing and managing critically ill patients who cannot be moved to CT. Its limitations include operator-dependency, poor assessment in obese patients, difficulty in the detection of free air and deeply located abscesses [27].

A systematic review and meta-analysis of studies [28] that reported diagnostic accuracy of the clinical diagnosis and diagnostic modalities in patients with suspected diverticulitis was published in 2014. Summary sensitivity estimates for US were 90 % (95 % CI: 76-98 %) versus 95 % (95 % CI: 91-97 %) for CT ($p = 0.86$). Summary specificity estimates for US were 90 % (95 % CI: 86-94 %) versus 96 % (95 % CI: 90-100 %) for CT ($p = 0.04$).

Although CT is the most sensitive imaging investigation for patients with suspected acute diverticulitis, a step-up approach with CT performed after an inconclusive or negative US, has been proposed as safe and alternative approach for patients with suspected acute diverticulitis [28, 29]. Magnetic resonance imaging, which is not constrained by the operator dependency limitation of ultrasound [30, 31], until now is difficult to perform at the emergency department.

Immunocompromised patients

6) Immunosuppression can increase the complication rate in patients with ALCD. Elective sigmoid resection after an episode of ALCD should be recommended in immunocompromised patients (Recommendation 1 C).

Immunocompromised patients, including patients with kidney failure, organ transplant patients and patients using corticosteroids are at increased risk to have complicated diverticulitis requiring emergency surgery [32–35]. Immunocompromised patients may fail standard, nonoperative treatment. As such, most of these patients require urgent surgical intervention, and this is associated with a significantly higher mortality rate [36].

A recent study by Biondo et al. [37] analyzed the relationship between the different causes of immunosuppression (IMS) and diverticulitis. Immunocompromised patients were divided in 5 groups according to the causes of IMS: group I, chronic corticosteroid therapy; group II, transplant patients; group III, malignant neoplasm disease; group IV, chronic renal failure; group V, others immunosuppressant treatment. The rate of emergency surgery was high (39.3 %). It was needed more frequently in group I. Overall, postoperative mortality was of 31.6 % and recurrence rate after successful nonoperative management occurred in 30 patients (27.8 %).

Treatment of uncomplicated acute diverticulitis

7) Antimicrobial therapy can be avoided in immunocompetent patients with uncomplicated diverticulitis without systemic manifestations of infection (Recommendation 1 A).
8) If patients need antimicrobial therapy, oral administration may be acceptable (Recommendation 1 B).

The utility of antimicrobial therapy in acute uncomplicated diverticulitis has been a point of controversy in the international medical community. In the last few years several studies demonstrated that antimicrobial treatment was not superior to withholding antibiotic therapy in patients with mild unperforated diverticulitis, in terms of clinical resolution [38].

The current consensus is that uncomplicated diverticulitis may be a self-limiting condition in which local host defenses' can manage the bacterial inflammation without antibiotics in immunocompetent patients. In this context antibiotics may, therefore, not be necessary in the treatment of uncomplicated disease.

A multi-centre randomized trial involving ten surgical departments in Sweden and one in Iceland recruited 623 patients with computed tomography-verified acute uncomplicated left-sided diverticulitis was published in 2012 by Chabok et al. [39]. Patients were randomized to treatment with (314 patients) or without (309 patients) antibiotics. Antibiotic treatment for acute uncomplicated diverticulitis neither accelerated recovery nor prevented complications or recurrence. It should therefore be reserved for the treatment of complicated diverticulitis.

A recent prospective single-arm study analyzed [40] the safety and efficacy of symptomatic (nonantibiotic) treatment for CT-proven uncomplicated diverticulitis during a 30-day follow-up period. Overall, 161 patients were included in the study, and 153 (95 %) completed the 30-day follow-up. A total of 14 (9 %) patients had pericolic air. Altogether, 140 (87 %) patients were treated as outpatients, and 4 (3 %) of them were admitted to the hospital during the follow-up. None of the patients developed complicated diverticulitis or required surgery, but, 2 days (median) after inclusion, antibiotics were given to 14 (9 %, 6 orally, 8 intravenously) patients.

However the high mortality associated with sepsis, requires clinicians to maintain a high index of clinical suspicion, in the conditions that predispose to sepsis. WSES expert panel suggests antimicrobial therapy covering Gram negative and anaerobes in patients with radiological documented uncomplicated acute diverticulitis associated with systemic manifestations of infection.

An appropriate antimicrobial regimen administered for an adequate duration has minimal impact on the emergence of antimicrobial resistance [41].

If antimicrobial therapy is necessary oral administration of antibiotics may be equally as effective as intravenous administration.

A randomized controlled trial of oral versus intravenous therapy for clinically diagnosed acute uncomplicated diverticulitis was published in 2009 [42]. Oral and intravenous regimens utilizing ciprofloxacin and metronidazole were compared. There were 41 patients in the oral arm and 38 in the IV arm ($n = 79$). No patients had to be converted to intravenous antibiotics from the oral group. There was a complete resolution of symptoms in both groups.

In immunocompromised patients antibiotics with a broader-spectrum should be used. No studies have examined the value of dietary restriction or bed rest [43].

9) Outpatient management is suggested for patients with uncomplicated acute diverticulitis, with no comorbidities. These patients should be clinically monitored as outpatients and re-evaluated within 7 days to assess for resolution of the inflammatory processes. Earlier revaluation is necessary if the clinical condition deteriorates (Recommendation 1 B).

Patients with uncomplicated diverticulitis symptoms without significant comorbidities, who are able to take fluids orally and manage themselves at home, can be treated as outpatients. They should be re-evaluated within 7 days. However if the clinical condition deteriorates, re-evaluation should be carried out earlier. Patients with significant comorbidities and unable to take fluids orally should be treated in hospital with intravenous fluid.

Etzioni et al. [44] in 2010 published a retrospective analysis, demonstrating that outpatient treatment was effective for the vast majority (94 %) of patients suffering from acute diverticulitis. A systematic review on outpatient management of acute uncomplicated diverticulitis was recently published in 2014 [45]. Jackson et al. concluded that current evidence suggested that a more progressive, ambulatory-based approach to the majority of cases of acute uncomplicated diverticulitis was justified. Rodríguez-Cerrillo et al. [46] have recently shown that elderly patients with co-morbidities can be safely treated at home avoiding hospital admission.

The DIVER trial [47] has recently demonstrated that outpatient treatment may be safe and effective in selected patients with uncomplicated acute diverticulitis and can reduces the costs without negatively influencing the quality of life of these patients. This multicenter, randomized controlled trial included patients older than 18 years with acute uncomplicated diverticulitis. All the patients underwent abdominal CT. The first dose of antibiotic was given intravenously to all patients in the emergency department and then patients were either admitted to hospital or discharged. Among a total of 132 patients, four patients in those admitted to hospital and three patients in those discharged to home management developed treatment failure (there was no differences between the groups ($P = 0.62$). The overall health care cost per episode was 3 times less in the outpatient treated group, with significant costs savings of €1124.70 per patient. No differences were observed between the groups in terms of quality of life.

Treatment of localized complicated diverticulitis

10) Patients with CT findings of pericolic air or small fluid collection should be managed by antimicrobial therapy. (Recommendation 1 C).

High mortality associated with sepsis, requires maintaining a high index of clinical suspicion for deterioration and more aggressive management. WSES expert panel routinely recommends antimicrobial therapy in patients with pericolic air or small fluid collection. CT findings of pericolic air in the form of air bubbles or little pericolic fluid without abscess and distant air indicates a complicated acute diverticulitis and antimicrobial therapy should always recommended [7].

Treatment of diverticular abscesses

11) Patients with small diverticular abscesses (<4-5 cm) may be treated by antibiotics alone (Recommendation 1 C).
12) Patients with large abscesses (>4–5 cm) can best be treated by percutaneous drainage combined with antibiotic treatment (Recommendation 1 C).
13) Whenever percutaneous drainage of the abscess is not feasible or not available, based on the clinical conditions patients with large abscesses can be initially treated by antibiotic therapy alone. However careful clinical monitoring is mandatory. (Recommendation 1 C).

Approximately 15–20 % of patients admitted with acute diverticulitis have an abscess on CT scan [48]. The size of 3–6 cm has been generally accepted as (all of low level of evidence), to be a reasonable limit between antimicrobial versus percutaneous drainage in the management of diverticular abscesses [48–53]. The size of 4–5 cm may be a reasonable limit between antibiotic treatment alone versus percutaneous drainage combined with antibiotic treatment in the management of diverticular abscesses. Based on the clinical conditions also patients with large abscesses can be initially treated by antibiotic therapy alone. However careful clinical monitoring is mandatory. A CT scan should be repeated if the patient fails to show clinical and laboratory improvement.

A retrospective study assessing the effectiveness of antibiotics as sole initial therapy in patients with large diverticular abscess was published in 2015 by Elagili et al. [54]. Thirty-two patients were treated with antibiotics alone because of either technically impossible percutaneous drainage or surgeon preference, while 114 underwent percutaneous drainage. Urgent surgery was required in 8 patients with persistent symptoms during treatment with antibiotics alone (25 %) and in 21 patients (18 %) after initial percutaneous drainage (p = 0.21). Patients treated with antibiotics had a significantly smaller abscess diameter (5.9 vs. 7.1 cm, $p = 0.001$) and shorter interval from initial treatment to sigmoidectomy (mean 50 vs. 80 days, $p = 0.02$). The Charlson comorbidity index, initial treatment failure rates, postoperative mortality, overall morbidity, length of hospital stay during treatments, and overall and permanent stoma rates were comparable in the two groups. Postoperative complications following antibiotics alone were significantly less severe than after percutaneous drainage based on the Clavien-Dindo classification ($p = 0.04$).

In patient displaying an appropriate clinical improvement, drainage catheter can be removed when the output has ceased and the patient has improved clinically. In doubtful cases a fistulogram can be performed with water-soluble contrast via the percutaneous drainage catheter prior to drain removal. If no identifiable cavity remains the catheter should be removed.

14) In patients with diverticular abscesses treated conservatively early colonic evaluation (4–6 weeks) should be planned (Recommendation 1 C).
15) In patients with CT-proven uncomplicated diverticulitis treated conservatively (without other risk factors) early follow-up colonoscopy is not required. Patients aged 50 years or older should participate in colorectal cancer screening programs (Recommendation 1 C).

Colonic localized abscess is an uncommon but possible presentation of colon cancer, and it may mimic complicated diverticular disease [55, 56]. It has been demonstrated that the risk of malignancy after a CT-proven uncomplicated diverticulitis is low and in the absence of other indications, routine colonoscopy may not be necessary. A systematic review investigating the rate of colorectal cancer (CRC) found by colonoscopy after an episode of uncomplicated diverticulitis was published in 2014 [57]. Nine studies met the inclusion criteria and included a total number of 2,490 patients with uncomplicated diverticulitis. Subsequent colonoscopy after an episode of uncomplicated diverticulitis was performed in 1,468 patients (59 %). Seventeen patients were diagnosed with CRC, having a prevalence of 1.16 % (95 % confidence interval 0.72-1.9 % for CRC). Hyperplastic polyps were seen in 156 patients (10.6 %), low-grade adenoma in 90 patients (6.1 %), and advanced adenoma was reported in 32 patients (2.2 %). The results of this review demonstrates that unless colonoscopy is regarded for screening in individuals aged 50 years and older, routine colonoscopy in the absence of other clinical signs of CRC is not required in patients following an episode of acute uncomplicated diverticulitis.

Another systematic review and meta-analysis on the role of routine colonic evaluation after radiologically confirmed acute diverticulitis was published in 2014 [58]. Eleven studies from 7 countries were included in the analysis. Among 1970 patients, cancer was only found in 22 (0.01 %) cases.

The risk of malignancy after a radiologically proven episode of acute uncomplicated diverticulitis was low. Patients with complicated diverticulitis had a significant risk of colorectal cancer at subsequent colonic evaluation.

A retrospective study of 633 patients with acute diverticulitis diagnosed by CT was published in 2014 [59]. Of 663, 97 underwent emergency resection, whereas 536 were treated conservatively, 394 of whom underwent colonoscopy. The findings showed 17 cancers (2.7 %) in patients with an initial diagnosis of acute diverticulitis. As shown by CT, 16 cancer patients (94 %) had abscess, whereas one patient had pericolic extraluminal air but no abscess. Of the patients with abscess, 11.4 % had cancer mimicking acute diverticulitis. No cancer was found in the patients with uncomplicated diverticulitis.

Treatment of diffuse peritonitis

Although most patients hospitalized for acute diverticulitis can be managed by non-operative treatment, up to 25 % may require urgent operative intervention [60]. Patients with diffuse peritonitis are typically critical ill patients and require prompt fluid resuscitation, antibiotic administration, and surgery without delay.

Although the absolute prevalence of perforated diverticulitis complicated by generalized peritonitis is low, it has a significant postoperative mortality, regardless of selected surgical strategy.

A critical issue may be the CT presence of distant free air without diffuse fluids (fluids in 2 or >2 abdominal quadrants) because distant pneumoperitoneum is pathognomonic for sigmoid perforation even in absence of CT findings of diffuse peritoneal fluid.

16) Patients with CT findings of distant air without diffuse fluid may be treated by conservative treatment in selected cases. However, there is a risk of treatment failure and emergency surgery may be required. Careful monitoring is mandatory. A CT scan should be repeated early on the basis of the clinical and laboratory evaluation (Recommendation 1 C).
17) If the conservative treatment fails in patients with distant air without diffuse fluid, surgical resection and anastomosis with or without stoma or Hartmann resection is suggested according to the patient clinical conditions and comorbidities (Recommendation 1 B).

Although CT findings of distant free air (a known predictor of failure of non-operative treatment [25]), Dharmarajan et al. [61] described a high success rate for non-operative management in patients with acute diverticulitis and a pneumoperitoneum, excluding those with hemodynamic instability. Sallinen et al. [62] reported results of non-operative management in patients with CT verified extra-luminal air. The study showed that non operative treatment was feasible therapy only for hemodynamic stable patients with pericolic extraluminal air or with small amount of distant intraperitoneal air in the absence of clinical diffuse peritonitis or fluid in the fossa Douglas. Occurrence of large amount of distant intraperitoneal air or distant retroperitoneal air even in the absence of clinical generalised peritonitis was associated with high failure rate (57 %–60 %) of non-operative management. Moreover nearly 60 % patients with distant intraperitoneal air were primary treated by surgery.

Highly selected group of patients at this stage may be treated by conservative treatment. However it may be associated with failure and a careful clinical and CT monitoring is mandatory [7]. Suggested intervention for patients at this stage should be surgical resection and anastomosis with or without stoma in stable patients without co-morbidities and Hartmann resection in unstable patients or in patients with multiple co-morbidities [7].

18) Laparoscopic peritoneal lavage and drainage should not be considered the treatment of choice in patients with generalized peritonitis. (Recommendation 1 A).

A conservative approach using laparoscopic peritoneal lavage and drainage has been debated in recent years as an alternative to colonic resection [63]. It can potentially avoid a stoma in patients with diffuse peritonitis. It consists of the laparoscopic aspiration of pus followed by abdominal lavage and the placement of abdominal drains, which remain for many days after the procedure.

In 2013 a Dutch retrospective analysis of 38 patients [64] treated by laparoscopic lavage was published highlighting some doubts about this procedure to treat critically ill patients. In seven patients laparoscopic lavage did not control abdominal sepsis, two died of multiple organ failure and five required further surgical interventions (three Hartmann resection, one diverting stoma and one perforation closure). One of these died from aspiration and the remaining four experienced prolonged complicated recovery. Multiple co-morbidities, immunosuppression, a high CRP level and/or a high Mannheim Peritonitis Index were also predictors of a high risk of failure. The authors concluded that patient selection was of utmost importance and identification of an overt sigmoid perforation is of critical importance.

Great debate is still open on this topic, mainly due to the discrepancy and sometime disappointing results of the latest prospective trials such as SCANDIV, Ladies, and DILALA trials [65–67]

In 2014 the first results from the randomized controlled trial DILALA were published [65]. Initial diagnostic laparoscopy showing Hinchey III disease was followed by randomization between laparoscopic lavage and colon resection and stoma. Morbidity and mortality after laparoscopic lavage did not differ when compared with the Hartmann procedure. Laparoscopic lavage resulted in shorter operating time, shorter time in the recovery unit, and shorter hospital stay with the avoidance of a stoma. In this trial, laparoscopic lavage as treatment for patients with perforated diverticulitis Hinchey III disease was feasible and safe in the short-term.

In 2015 the results of SCANDV study were published [66]. Among patients with likely perforated diverticulitis and undergoing emergency surgery, the use of laparoscopic lavage vs primary resection did not reduce severe postoperative complications and led to worse outcomes in secondary end points. These findings do not support laparoscopic lavage for treatment of perforated diverticulitis. In the same year, the result of LADIES Study was published. This showed that laparoscopic lavage was not superior to sigmoidectomy for the treatment of purulent perforated diverticulitis [67].

19) Hartmann resection is still advised for managing diffuse peritonitis in critically ill patients and in patients with multiple comorbidities. However in clinically stable patients with no co-morbidities primary resection with anastomosis with or without a diverting stoma may be performed (Recommendation 1 B).

Hartmann resection has been considered the procedure of choice in patients with generalized peritonitis and remains a safe technique for emergency colectomy in diverticular peritonitis, especially in critically ill patients and in patients with multiple co-morbidities. However restoration of bowel continuity after a Hartmann procedure has been associated with significant morbidity [68]. Many patients cannot undergo reversal surgery due to comorbidities; therefore, they remain with a permanent stoma [69].

Common use of Hartmann's resection in treating diverticular perforation worldwide is confirmed by a recent Australian study analyzing administrative data of patients with acute diverticulitis admitted, from 2009 to 2013, in eight tertiary referral centres with specialist colorectal services [70]. Among 2829 emergency admissions for AD across 4 years in eight hospitals, 724 were for complicated acute diverticulitis. The emergency operative intervention rate was 10.4 %, with one third of the admissions for complicated diverticulitis having an operation. Hartmann's procedure was the most commonly performed emergency operation, accounting for 72 % of resections.

Another population-based retrospective cohort study using administrative discharge data, conducted in Ontario (Canada) was published in 2014 [71]. Among 18,543 patients hospitalized with a first episode of diverticulitis, from 2002 to 2012, 3873 underwent emergency surgery. The use of laparoscopy increased (9 % to 18 %, $p < 0.001$), whereas the use of the Hartmann's procedure remained unchanged (64 %) and was the most frequently used urgent operative approach in patients with complicated AD.

In recent years, some authors have reported the role of primary resection and anastomosis with or without a diverting stoma, in the treatment of diverticulitis, even in the presence of diffuse peritonitis [72]. The decision regarding the surgical choice in patients with diffuse peritonitis is generally left to the judgment of the surgeon, who takes into account the clinical condition and the comorbidities of the patient. Studies comparing mortality and morbidity of Hartmann's procedure versus primary anastomosis did not show any significant differences. However, most studies had relevant selection bias as demonstrated by four systematic reviews [73–76].

A comparison of primary resection and anastomosis (PRA) with or without defunctioning stoma to Hartmann's procedure (HP) as the optimal operative strategy for patients presenting with Hinchey stage III-IV, was published by Constantinides et al. [76]. A total of 135 PRA, 126 primary anastomoses with defunctioning stoma (PADS), and 6619 Hartmann's procedures (HP) were considered in the study. Morbidity and mortality was 55 % and 30 % for PRA, 40 % and 25 % for PADS, and 35 % and 20 % for HP. Stomas remained permanent in 27 % of HP and in 8 % of PADS. The authors concluded that primary anastomosis with defunctioning stoma may be the optimal strategy for selected patients with diverticular peritonitis and may represent a good compromise between postoperative adverse events, long-term quality of life and risk of permanent stoma.

A small randomized trial of primary anastomosis with ileostomy vs Hartmann's procedure in patients with diffuse diverticular peritonitis was published by Oberkofler et al. in 2012 [77]. Sixty-two patients with acute left-sided colonic perforation (Hinchey III and IV) from 4 centers were randomized to Hartmann procedure (n = 30) and to primary anastomoses with diverting ileostomy (n = 32). A planned stoma reversal operation was performed after 3 months in both groups. The study reported no difference in initial mortality and morbidity (mortality 13 % vs 9 % and morbidity 67 % vs 75 % in Hartmann procedure vs primary anastomosis), but a reduction in length of stay, lower costs, fewer serious complications and greater stoma reversal rates in the primary anastomosis group.

20) Emergency laparoscopic sigmoidectomy for the treatment of perforated diverticulitis with

generalised peritonitis is feasible in selected patients provided they are handled by experienced hands (Recommendation 2 C).

Laparoscopic sigmoidectomy for diverticulitis has initially been confined to the elective setting however in stable patients, laparoscopic sigmoidectomy may be feasible in purulent and fecal diverticular peritonitis in the emergency setting. In 2015 a systematic review on laparoscopic sigmoidectomy for diverticulitis in the emergency setting was published [78].

The review included 4 case series and one cohort study (total of 104 patients) out of 1,706 references. Hartmann's procedure (HP) was performed in 84 patients and primary anastomosis in 20. The mean operating time varied between 115 and 200 min. The conversion rate varied from 0 to 19 %. The mean length of hospital stay ranged between 6 and 16 days. Surgical re-intervention was necessary in 2 patients. In 20 patients operated upon without defunctioning ileostomy, no anastomotic leakage was reported. Three patients died during the postoperative period. Stoma reversal after HP was performed in 60 out of 79 evaluable patients (76 %).

These guidelines are limited by the low quality evidence which showed that emergency laparoscopic sigmoidectomy for the treatment of perforated diverticulitis with generalised peritonitis is feasible. These studies occurred in selected patients and in experienced units and are not generalizable to all centers. High-quality prospective or randomised studies are needed to demonstrate benefits of acute laparoscopic sigmoidectomy compared to open sigmoidectomy for perforated diverticulitis.

21) Damage control surgery strategy may be suggested for clinically unstable patients with diverticular peritonitis (severe sepsis/septic shock) (Recommendation 1 B).

In an unstable patients with diverticular peritonitis 'damage control surgery' has become a valuable technique in the last years [79]. Damage control with lavage, limited bowel resection, laparostomy, and scheduled second-look operation represents a feasible strategy in patients with perforated diverticulitis (Hinchey III and IV) to enhance sepsis control and improve rate of anastomosis.

Generalized diverticular peritonitis is a life-threatening condition requiring prompt emergency operation. To improve outcome and reduce the rate of colostomy formation, a new algorithm with damage control operation, lavage, limited closure of perforation, and second look surgery to restore intestinal continuity was developed in recent years [80, 81]. Critically ill patients (patients with severe sepsis and septic shock) present with hypotension and myocardial depression, combined with coagulopathy. These patients, who are hemodynamically unstable, are not optimal candidates for immediate complex operative interventions. After initial surgery, which should be limited to source control e.g. primary closure of the perforation, the patient is taken to the ICU for physiologic optimization. This strategy may delay bowel anastomosis [81] and potentially avoid stoma formation.

In the setting of diverticulitis several reports (with low level of evidence) were published. In 2010 a prospective observational study was published by Kafka-Ritsch et al. [79]. A total of 51 patients (28 female, 55 %) with a median age of 69 (range) 28–87 years, with perforated diverticulitis Hinchey III (n = 40, 78 %) or Hinchey IV ($n = 11$, 22 %) were prospectively enrolled in the study. Patients were initially managed with limited resection, lavage and temporary abdominal closure followed by second, reconstructive operation 24–48 h later, which are supervised by a colorectal surgeon. Bowel continuity was restored in 38 (84 %) patients, of which four were protected by a loop ileostomy. Five anastomotic leaks (13 %) were encountered requiring loop ileostomy in two patients or Hartmann procedure in remaining three patients. The overall mortality rate was 9.8 % and 35/46 (76 %) of the surviving patients left the hospital with reconstructed colon continuity. Fascial closure was achieved in all patients.

Planning elective surgery

22) Patient-related factors and not number of previous episodes of diverticulitis, should be considered in planning elective sigmoid resection in patients with ALCD treated conservatively (Recommendation 1 C).
23) After a conservatively treated episode of ALCD an elective sigmoid resection should be planned in high-risk patients, such as immunocompromised patients (Recommendation 1 C).

Recurrence of acute diverticulitis is lower than previously thought. It has been frequently reported that about one third of all patients with acute diverticulitis will have a recurrent attack, often within one year [82, 83]. Recurrence after an uncomplicated episode of diverticulitis, however, has recently been shown to be much lower, with one prospective study reporting a recurrence of only 1.7 % over five years of follow up [84, 85].

In 2014, a systematic review of studies reviewing the diagnosis and management of chronic and recurrent diverticulitis (from studies published between January 2000 to March 2013) was published [86]. The 68 studies included were almost exclusively observational and had limited certainty of treatment effect. The authors found that complicated recurrence after recovery from an uncomplicated episode of diverticulitis was rare (<5 %) and that age at onset younger than 50 years and 2 or more recurrences did not increase the risk of complications.

The authors concluded that the indication for elective colectomy following 2 episodes of diverticulitis is no longer accepted. Indication to colectomy should be made based on consideration of the risks of recurrent diverticulitis, the morbidity of surgery, ongoing symptoms, the complexity of disease, and operative risk.

Clear indications for elective sigmoid resections are complaints of stenosis, fistulas, or recurrent diverticular bleeding. Furthermore, an elective sigmoid resection should be justified in high-risk patients such as immunocompromised patients, after a conservatively treated episode of diverticulitis [87].

Antimicrobial therapy

24) The empirically designed antimicrobial regimen depends on the underlying clinical condition of the patient, the pathogens presumed to be involved, and the risk factors indicative of major resistance patterns (Recommendation 1 C).
25) Although discontinuation of antimicrobial treatment should be based on clinical and laboratory criteria, a 4–6 days period of postoperative antimicrobial therapy in complicated ALCD is suggested if source control has been adequate (Recommendation 1 A).

Antimicrobial therapy plays an important role in the management of complicated acute diverticulitis. It is typically empiric antibiotic treatment. The empirically designed antimicrobial regimen depends on the underlying severity of infection, the pathogens presumed to be involved, and the risk factors indicative of major resistance patterns [41]. Several recommendations have been recently published in literature [41, 88] in the setting of intra-abdominal infections. However consideration of local epidemiological data and regional resistance profiles is essential for antibiotic selection.

Considering intestinal microbiota of large bowel acute diverticulitis requires antimicrobial coverage for gram-positive and gram-negative bacteria, as well as for anaerobes. Most of the complicated acute diverticulitis is community acquired infection. The main resistance threat in intra-abdominal infections is posed by Extended-Spectrum Beta-Lactamase (ESBL)-producing *Enterobacteriaceae,* which are becoming increasingly common in community-acquired infections worldwide [41]. The most significant risk factors for ESBL producing infection include prior exposure to antibiotics and comorbidities requiring concurrent antibiotic therapy [41]. Anti-ESBL-producer coverage should be warranted for patients with these risk factors. Although discontinuation of antimicrobial treatment should be based on clinical and laboratory criteria such as fever and markers of inflammation, a period of 4–6 days for adult patients is generally sufficient to treat in patients with acute diverticulitis who have been treated with proper source control and prompt surgical intervention [41, 88].

The recent prospective trial by Sawyer et al. demonstrated that in patients with complicated intra-abdominal infections undergoing an adequate source-control procedure, the outcomes after approximately 4 days fixed-duration antibiotic therapy were similar to those after a longer course of antibiotics that extended until after the resolution of physiological abnormalities [89]. Patients who have signs of sepsis beyond 5 to 7 days of antibiotic treatment warrant aggressive diagnostic investigation to determine if an ongoing uncontrolled source of infection exists.

Conclusions

In appendix 1 WSES recommendations for the management of ALCD are illustrated.

Appendix 1

1) An accurate assessment of the patients using clinical signs, laboratory inflammation markers and radiological findings is recommended to identify the best treatment for each patient with ALCD (Recommendation 1 C).
2) The clinical diagnosis of ALCD alone is not sufficiently accurate for patients with suspected diverticulitis (Recommendation 1 C).
3) Pain in the lower left abdomen on physical examination and C-reactive protein (CRP) 50 mg/l or more suggests a diagnosis of ALCD (Recommendation 1 C).
4) Computed tomography (CT) scan of the abdomen and pelvis is indicated for all patients with suspected ALCD. It has high sensitivity and specificity and can assess the severity of diverticulitis guiding clinicians in planning treatment (Recommendation 1 C).
5) Ultrasound (US) may be a useful alternative in the initial evaluation of patients with suspected ALCD. It has wide availability and easy accessibility. It may have satisfactory sensitivity and specificity when performed by an expert operator. A step-up approach with CT performed after an inconclusive or negative US may be a

safe approach for patients suspected of acute diverticulitis (Recommendation 1 C).

6) Immunosuppression can increase the complication rate in patients with ALCD. Elective sigmoid resection after an episode of ALCD should be recommended in immunocompromised patients (Recommendation 1 C).
7) Antimicrobial therapy can be avoided in immunocompetent patients with uncomplicated diverticulitis without systemic manifestations of infection (Recommendation 1 A).
8) If patients need antimicrobial therapy, oral administration may be acceptable (Recommendation 1 B).
9) Outpatient management is suggested for patients with uncomplicated acute diverticulitis, with no comorbidities. These patients should be clinically monitored as outpatients and re-evaluated within 7 days to assess for resolution of the inflammatory processes. Earlier revaluation is necessary if the clinical condition deteriorates (Recommendation 1 B).
10) Patients with CT findings of pericolic air or small fluid collection should be managed by antimicrobial therapy. (Recommendation 1 C).
11) Patients with small diverticular abscesses (<4-5 cm) may be treated by antibiotics alone (Recommendation 1 C).
12) Patients with large abscesses (>4–5 cm) can best be treated by percutaneous drainage combined with antibiotic treatment (Recommendation 1 C).
13) Whenever percutaneous drainage of the abscess is not feasible or not available, based on the clinical conditions patients with large abscesses can be initially treated by antibiotic therapy alone. However careful clinical monitoring is mandatory. (Recommendation 1 C).
14) In patients with diverticular abscesses treated conservatively early colonic evaluation (4–6 weeks) should be planned (Recommendation 1 C).
15) In patients with CT-proven uncomplicated diverticulitis treated conservatively (without other risk factors) early follow-up colonoscopy is not required. Patients aged 50 years or older should participate in colorectal cancer screening programs (Recommendation 1 C).
16) Patients with CT findings of distant air without diffuse fluid may be treated by conservative treatment in selected cases. However, there is a risk of treatment failure and emergency surgery may be required. Careful monitoring is mandatory. A CT scan should be repeated early on the basis of the clinical and laboratory evaluation (Recommendation 1 C).
17) If the conservative treatment fails in patients with distant air without diffuse fluid, surgical resection and anastomosis with or without stoma or Hartmann resection is suggested according to the patient clinical conditions and comorbidities (Recommendation 1 B).
18) Laparoscopic peritoneal lavage and drainage should not be considered the treatment of choice in patients with generalized peritonitis. (Recommendation 1 A).
19) Hartmann resection is still advised for managing diffuse peritonitis in critically ill patients and in patients with multiple comorbidities. However in clinically stable patients with no co-morbidities primary resection with anastomosis with or without a diverting stoma may be performed (Recommendation 1 B).
20) Emergency laparoscopic sigmoidectomy for the treatment of perforated diverticulitis with generalised peritonitis is feasible in selected patients provided they are handled by experienced hands (Recommendation 2 C).
21) Damage control surgery strategy may be suggested for clinically unstable patients with diverticular peritonitis (severe sepsis/septic shock) (Recommendation 1 B).
22) Patient-related factors and not number of previous episodes of diverticulitis, should be considered in planning elective sigmoid resection in patients with ALCD treated conservatively (Recommendation 1 C).
23) After a conservatively treated episode of ALCD an elective sigmoid resection should be planned in high-risk patients, such as immunocompromised patients (Recommendation 1 C).
24) The empirically designed antimicrobial regimen depends on the underlying clinical condition of the patient, the pathogens presumed to be involved, and the risk factors indicative of major resistance patterns (Recommendation 1 C).
25) Although discontinuation of antimicrobial treatment should be based on clinical and laboratory criteria, a 4–6 days period of post-operative antimicrobial therapy in complicated ALCD is suggested if source control has been adequate (Recommendation 1 A).

Abbreviations

ALCD, acute left sided colonic diverticulitis; CT, computed tomography; US, ultrasound

Acknowledgements

Not applicable.

Funding

No funding sources to disclose.

Authors' contributions
MS wrote the first draft of the manuscript. All authors reviewed and approved the manuscript.

Competing interest
The authors declare that they have no competing interests.

Author details
[1]Department of Surgery, Macerata Hospital, Via Santa Lucia 2, 62019 Macerata, Italy. [2]Department of Surgery, Maggiore Hospital, Parma, Italy. [3]General Surgery Department, Papa Giovanni XXIII Hospital, Bergamo, Italy. [4]Department of Surgery, "Infermi" Hospital, Rimini, Italy. [5]General and Upper GI Surgery, Queen Elizabeth Hospital, Birmingham, UK. [6]Department of Surgery, College of Medicine and Health Sciences, UAE University, Al-Ain, United Arab Emirates. [7]Department of Surgery, Maggiore Hospital, Bologna, Italy. [8]1st Department of Surgery - Department of Abdominal, Thoracic Surgery and Traumatology, General University Hospital, Prague, Czech Republic. [9]Department of General Surgery, Division of Surgery, Rambam Health Care Campus, Haifa, Israel. [10]Department of Surgery, Division of Acute Care Surgery, and Center for Sepsis and Critical Illness Research, University of Florida College of Medicine, Gainesville, FL, USA. [11]Department of Surgery, Virginia Commonwealth University, Richmond, VA, USA. [12]Department of Surgery, UC San Diego Medical Center, San Diego, USA. [13]Department of Surgery, University of Pittsburgh School of Medicine, Pittsburgh, USA. [14]Abdominal Center, University Hospital Meilahti, Helsinki, Finland. [15]Division of Trauma Surgery, Department of Surgery, School of Medical Sciences, University of Campinas (Unicamp), Campinas, SP, Brazil. [16]Department of Surgery, University of Washington, Seattle, WA, USA. [17]Emergency Department, Niguarda Ca'Granda Hospital, Milan, Italy. [18]Assia Medical Group, Assuta Medical Center, Tel Aviv, Israel. [19]First Clinic of General Surgery, University Hospital/UMBAL/St George Plovdiv, Plovdiv, Bulgaria. [20]Department of Traumatology, John Hunter Hospital, Newcastle, NSW, Australia. [21]Department of Surgery, Trauma Research Institute, University of Arizona, Tucson, AZ, USA. [22]Department of Surgery, University of Colorado, Denver Health Medical Center, Denver, CO, USA. [23]Trauma and Acute Care Surgery Unit, Hadassah Hebrew University Medical Center, Jerusalem, Israel. [24]Clinic for Emergency Surgery, Faculty of Medicine, University of Belgrade, Belgrade, Serbia. [25]Department of Surgery, Division of Acute Care Surgery and Surgical Critical Care, Los Angeles County and University of Southern California Medical Center, Los Angeles, CA, USA. [26]Department of Surgery, Fundación Valle del Lili, Hospital Universitario del Valle, Universidad del Valle, Cali, Colombia. [27]Department of General and Thoracic Surgery, University Hospital Giessen, Giessen, Germany. [28]Department of Surgery, University Hospital Center Zagreb and School of Medicine, University of Zagreb, Zagreb, Croatia. [29]Department of Surgery, Tbilisi State Medical University, Kipshidze Central University Hospital, Tbilisi, Georgia. [30]Department of General Surgery, Centro Hospitalar São João, Faculdade de Medicina da Universidade do Porto, Porto, Portugal. [31]Department of Surgery, Pt BDS Post-graduate Institute of Medical Sciences, Rohtak, India. [32]Department of Surgery, Mosc Medical College, Kolenchery, Cochin, India. [33]Department of General Surgery, Tan Tock Seng Hospital, Tan Tock Seng, Singapore, Singapore. [34]Department of Surgery, Radiology, Anaesthetics and Intensive Care, University Hospital of the West Indies, Kingston, Jamaica. [35]Surgical Department, General Hospital Jesenice, Jesenice, Slovenia. [36]Federal University of Juiz de Fora (UFJF) AND Faculdade de Ciências Médicas e da Saúde de Juiz de Fora (SUPREMA), Juiz de Fora, MG, Brazil. [37]Department of General Surgery, Trauma and Emergency Surgery Division, ABC Medical School, Santo André, SP, Brazil. [38]Emergency Surgery and Trauma Unit, Department of Surgery, University of Ribeirão Preto, Ribeirão Preto, Brazil. [39]Emergency Hospital of Bucharest, University of Medicine and Pharmacy Carol Davila Bucharest, Bucharest, Romania. [40]Department of Surgery, Tianjin Nankai Hospital, Nankai Clinical School of Medicine, Tianjin Medical University, Tianjin, China. [41]Department of Primary Care & Emergency Medicine, Kyoto University Graduate School of Medicine, Kyoto, Japan. [42]Department of Surgery, Medical School University of Pécs, Pécs, Hungary. [43]Department of Surgery, S.S. Annunziata Hospital, Taranto, Italy. [44]Department of Surgical Sciences, Organs Transplantation and Advanced Technologies, "G.F. Ingrassia" University of Catania, Cannizzaro Hospital, Catania, Italy. [45]Department of Surgery, The Brunei Cancer Centre, Jerudong Park, Brunei. [46]Department of Surgery, Clinical Hospital of Emergency Medicine, Vladimir City, Russian Federation. [47]2nd Department of Surgery, Aretaieion University Hospital, National and Kapodistrian University of Athens, Athens, Greece. [48]Department of General Surgery, University Hospital of Larissa, Larissa, Greece. [49]Department of Surgery, Samsun Education and Research Hospital, Samsun, Turkey. [50]Department of Surgery, Mengucek Gazi Training Research Hospital, Erzincan, Turkey. [51]Department of Surgery, Hospital de Alta Especialidad de Veracruz, Veracruz, Mexico. [52]Department of Emergency Surgery and Critical Care, Centro Medico Imbanaco, Cali, Colombia.

References
1. Weizman AV, Nguyen GC. Diverticular disease: epidemiology and management. Can J Gastroenterol. 2011;25:385–9.
2. Schoetz DJ. Diverticular disease of the colon: a century-old problem. Dis Colon Rectum. 1999;42:703–9.
3. Collins D, Winter DC. Modern concepts in diverticular disease. J Clin Gastroenterol. 2015;49:358–69.
4. Warner E, Crighton EJ, Moineddin R, Mamdani M, Upshur R. Fourteen-year study of hospital admissions for diverticular disease in Ontario. Can J Gastroenterol. 2007;21:97–9.
5. Jamal Talabani A, Lydersen S, Endreseth BH, Edna TH. Major increase in admission- and incidence rates of acute colonic diverticulitis. Int J Colorectal Dis. 2014;29:937–45.
6. Shahedi K, Fuller G, Bolus R, Cohen E, Vu M, Shah R, et al. Long-term risk of acute diverticulitis among patients with incidental diverticulosis found during colonoscopy. Clin Gastroenterol Hepatol. 2013;11:1609–13.
7. Sartelli M, Moore FA, Ansaloni L, Di Saverio S, Coccolini F, Griffiths EA, et al. A proposal for a CT driven classification of left colon acute diverticulitis. World J Emerg Surg. 2015;10:3.
8. Guyatt G, Gutterman D, Baumann MH, Addrizzo-Harris D, Hylek EM, Phillips B, et al. Grading strength of recommendations and quality of evidence in clinical guidelines: Report from an American College of Chest Physicians task force. Chest. 2006;129:174–81.
9. Brozek JL, Akl EA, Jaeschke R, Lang DM, Bossuyt P, Glasziou P, et al. Grading quality of evidence and strength of recommendations in clinical practice guidelines: Part 2 of 3. The GRADE approach to grading quality of evidence about diagnostic tests and strategies. Allergy. 2009;64:1109–16.
10. Hinchey EJ, Schaal PH, Richards MB. Treatment of perforated diverticular disease of the colon. Adv Surg. 1978;12:85–109.
11. Neff CC. vanSonnenberg E. CT of diverticulitis. Diagnosis and treatment. Radiol Clin North Am. 1989;27:743–52.
12. Sher ME, Agachan F, Bortul M, Nogueras JJ, Weiss EG, Wexner SD. Laparoscopic surgery for diverticulitis. Surg Endosc. 1997;11:264–7.
13. Ambrosetti P, Becker C, Terrier F. Colonic diverticulitis: impact of imaging on surgical management - a prospective study of 542 patients. Eur Radiol. 2002;12:1145–9.
14. Kaiser AM, Jiang JK, Lake JP, Ault G, Artinyan A, Gonzalez-Ruiz C, et al. The management of complicated diverticulitis and the role of computed tomography. Am J Gastroenterol. 2005;100:910–7.
15. Mora Lopez L, Serra Pla S, Serra-Aracil X, Ballesteros E, Navarro S. Application of a modified Neff classification to patients with uncomplicated diverticulitis. Colorectal Dis. 2013;15:1442–7.
16. Sallinen VJ, Leppäniemi AK, Mentula PJ. Staging of acute diverticulitis based on clinical, radiologic, and physiologic parameters. J Trauma Acute Care Surg. 2015;78:543–51.
17. Toorenvliet BR1. Colonic diverticulitis: a prospective analysis of diagnostic accuracy and clinical decision-making. Colorectal Dis. 2010;12:179–86.
18. Laméris W, van Randen A, van Gulik TM, Busch OR, Winkelhagen J, Bossuyt PM, et al. A clinical decision rule to establish the diagnosis of acute diverticulitis at the emergency department. Dis Colon Rectum. 2010;53:896–904.
19. Andeweg CS, Knobben L, Hendriks JC, Bleichrodt RP, van Goor H. How to diagnose acute left-sided colonic diverticulitis: proposal for a clinical scoring system. Ann Surg. 2011;253:940–6.

20. Kechagias A, Rautio T, Kechagias G, Mäkelä J. The role of C-reactive protein in the prediction of the clinical severity of acute diverticulitis. Am Surg. 2014;80:391–5.
21. Van de Wall BJ, Draaisma WA, van der Kaaij RT, Consten EC, Wiezer MJ, Broeders IA. The value of inflammation markers and body temperature in acute diverticulitis. Colorectal Dis. 2013;15:621–6.
22. Mäkelä JT, Klintrup K, Takala H, Rautio T. The role of C-reactive protein in prediction of the severity of acute diverticulitis in an emergency unit. Scand J Gastroenterol. 2015;50:536–41.
23. Laméris W, van Randen A, Bipat S, Bossuyt PM, Boermeester MA, Stoker J. Graded compression ultrasonography and computed tomography in acute colonic diverticulitis: meta- analysis of test accuracy. Eur Radiol. 2008;18:2498–511.
24. Liljegren G, Chabok A, Wickbom M, Smedh K, Nilsson K. Acute colonic diverticulitis: a systematic review of diagnostic accuracy. Colorectal Dis. 2007;9:480–8.
25. Ambrosetti P, Jenny A, Becker C, Terrier TF, Morel P. Acute left colonic diverticulitis–compared performance of computed tomography and water-soluble contrast enema: prospective evaluation of 420 patients. Dis Colon Rectum. 2000;43:1363–7.
26. Mazzei MA, Cioffi Squitieri N, Guerrini S, Stabile Ianora AA, Cagini L, Macarini L, et al. Sigmoid diverticulitis: US findings. Crit Ultrasound J. 2013;5:5.
27. Puylaert JB. Ultrasound of colon diverticulitis. Dig Dis. 2012;30:56–9.
28. Andeweg CS, Wegdam JA, Groenewoud J, van der Wilt GJ, van Goor H, Bleichrodt RP. Toward an evidence-based step-up approach in diagnosing diverticulitis. Scand J Gastroenterol. 2014;49:775–84.
29. Laméris W, van Randen A, van Es HW, van Heesewijk JP, van Ramshorst B, Bouma WH, et al. OPTIMA study group: Imaging strategies for detection of urgent conditions in patients with acute abdominal pain: diagnostic accuracy study. BMJ. 2009;338:b2431.
30. Heverhagen JT, Sitter H, Zielke A, Klose KJ. Prospective evaluation of the value of magnetic resonance imaging in suspected acute sigmoid diverticulitis. Dis Colon Rectum. 2008;51:1810–5.
31. Halpenny DF, McNeil G, Snow A, Geoghegan T, Torreggiani WC. Prospective evaluation of the value of magnetic resonance imaging in suspected acute sigmoid diverticulitis. Dis Colon Rectum. 2009;52:1030–1.
32. Hwang SS, Cannom RR, Abbas MA, Etzioni D. Diverticulitis in transplant patients and patients on chronic corticosteroid therapy: a systematic review. Dis Colon Rectum. 2010;53:1699–707.
33. Dalla Valle R, Capocasale E, Mazzoni MP, Busi N, Benozzi L, Sivelli R, et al. Acute diverticulitis with colon perforation in renal transplantation. Transplant Proc. 2005;37:2507–10.
34. Qasabian RA, Meagher AP, Lee R, Dore GJ, Keogh A. Severe diverticulitis after heart, lung, and heart-lung transplantation. J Heart Lung Transplant. 2004;23:845–9.
35. Lederman ED, Conti DJ, Lempert N, Singh TP, Lee EC. Complicated diverticulitis following renal transplantation. Dis Colon Rectum. 1998;41:613–8.
36. Bordeianou L, Hodin R. Controversies in the surgical management of sigmoid diverticulitis. J Gastrointest Surg. 2007;11:542–8.
37. Biondo S, Trenti L, Elvira J, Golda T, Kreisler E. Outcomes of colonic diverticulitis according to the reason of immunosuppression. Am J Surg. 2016. doi: 10.1016/j.amjsurg.2016.01.038
38. Shabanzadeh DM, Wille-Jørgensen P. Antibiotics for uncomplicated diverticulitis. Cochrane Database Syst Rev. 2012;11:CD009092.
39. Chabok A, Påhlman L, Hjern F, Haapaniemi S, Smedh K, AVOD Study Group. Randomized clinical trial of antibiotics in acute uncomplicated diverticulitis. Br J Surg. 2012;99:532–9.
40. Mali JP, Mentula PJ, Leppäniemi AK, Sallinen VJ. Symptomatic Treatment for Uncomplicated Acute Diverticulitis: A Prospective Cohort Study. Dis Colon Rectum. 2016;59(6):529–34.
41. Sartelli M, Viale P, Catena F, Ansaloni L, Moore E, Malangoni M, et al. 2013 WSES guidelines for management of intra-abdominal infections. World J Emerg Surg. 2013;8:3.
42. Ridgway PF, Latif A, Shabbir J, Ofriokuma F, Hurley MJ, Evoy D, et al. Randomized controlled trial of oral vs intravenous therapy for the clinically diagnosed acute uncomplicated diverticulitis. Colorectal Dis. 2009;11:941–6.
43. Fozard JB, Armitage NC, Schofield JB, Jones OM. Association of Coloproctology of Great Britain and Ireland. ACPGBI position statement on elective resection for diverticulitis. Colorectal Dis. 2011;13:1–11.
44. Etzioni DA, Chiu VY, Cannom RR, Burchette RJ, Haigh PI, Abbas MA. Outpatient treatment of acute diverticulitis: rates and predictors of failure. Dis Colon Rectum. 2010;53:861–5.
45. Jackson JD, Hammond T. Systematic review: outpatient management of acute uncomplicated diverticulitis. Int J Colorectal Dis. 2014;29:775–81.
46. Rodrìguez-Cerrillo M, Poza-Montoro A, Fernandez-Diaz E, Matesanz-David M, Inurrieta RA. Treatment of elderly patients with uncomplicated diverticulitis, even with comorbidity, at home. Eur J Intern Med. 2013;24:430–2.
47. Biondo S, Golda T, Kreisler E, Espin E, Vallribera F, Oteiza F, et al. Outpatient versus hospitalization management for uncomplicated diverticulitis: a prospective, multicenter randomized clinical trial (DIVER Trial). Ann Surg. 2014;259:38–44.
48. Andersen JC, Bundgaard L, Elbrønd H, Laurberg S, Walker LR, Støvring J. Danish Surgical Society. Danish national guidelines for treatment of diverticular disease. Dan Med J. 2012;59:C4453.
49. Ambrosetti P, Chautems R, Soravia C, Peiris-Waser N, Terrier F. Long-term outcome of mesocolic and pelvic diverticular abscesses of the left colon: a prospective study of 73 cases. Dis Colon Rectum. 2005;48:787–91.
50. Brandt D, Gervaz P, Durmishi Y, Platon A, Morel P, Poletti PA. Percutaneous CT scan guided drainage versus antibiotherapy alone for Hinchey II diverticulitis: a case–control study. Dis Colon Rectum. 2006;49:1533–8.
51. Siewert B, Tye G, Kruskal J, Sosna J, Opelka F, Raptopoulos V, Goldberg SN. Impact of CT-guided drainage in the treatment of diverticular abscesses: size matters. AJR Am J Roentgenol. 2006;186:680–6.
52. Singh B, May K, Coltart I, Moore NR, Cunningham C. The long-term results of percutaneous drainage of diverticular abscess. Ann R Coll Surg Engl. 2008;90:297–301.
53. Kumar RR, Kim JT, Haukoos JS, Macias LH, Dixon MR, Stamos MJ, Konyalian VR. Factors affecting the successful management of intra-abdominal abscesses with antibiotics and the need for percutaneous drainage. Dis Colon Rectum. 2006;49:183–9.
54. Elagili F, Stocchi L, Ozuner G, Kiran RP. Antibiotics alone instead of percutaneous drainage as initial treatment of large diverticular abscess. Tech Coloproctol. 2015;19(2):97–103.
55. Tsai HL, Hsieh JS, Yu FJ, Wu DC, Chen FM, Huang CJ, et al. Perforated colonic cancer presenting as intra-abdominal abscess. Int J Colorectal Dis. 2007;22:15–9.
56. Yeo ES, Ng KH, Eu KW. Perforated colorectal cancer: an important differential diagnosis in all presumed diverticular abscesses. Ann Acad Med Singapore. 2011;40:375.
57. de Vries HS, Boerma D, Timmer R, van Ramshorst B, Dieleman LA, van Westreenen HL. Routine colonoscopy is not required in uncomplicated diverticulitis: a systematic review. Surg Endosc. 2014;28(7):2039–47.
58. Sharma PV, Eglinton T, Hider P, Frizelle F. Systematic review and meta-analysis of the role of routine colonic evaluation after radiologically confirmed acute diverticulitis. Ann Surg. 2014;259:263–72.
59. Sallinen V, Mentula P, Leppäniemi A. Risk of colon cancer after computed tomography-diagnosed acute diverticulitis: is routine colonoscopy necessary? Surg Endosc. 2014;28:961.
60. Feingold D, Steele SR, Lee S, Kaiser A, Boushey R, Buie WD, Rafferty JF. Practice parameters for the treatment of sigmoid diverticulitis. Dis Colon Rectum. 2014;57:284–94.
61. Dharmarajan S, Hunt SR, Birnbaum EH, Fleshman JW, Mutch MG. The efficacy of nonoperative management of acute complicated diverticulitis. Dis Colon Rectum. 2011;54:663–71.
62. Sallinen VJ, Mentula PJ, Leppäniemi AK. Nonoperative management of perforated diverticulitis with extraluminal air is safe and effective in selected patients. Dis Colon Rectum. 2014;57:875–81.
63. Rossi GL, Mentz R, Bertone S, Ojea Quintana G, Bilbao S, et al. Laparoscopic Peritoneal Lavage for Hinchey III Diverticulitis: is it as effective as it is applicable? Dis Colon Rectum. 2014;57:1384–90.
64. Swank HA, Mulder IM, Hoofwijk AG, Nienhuijs SW, Lange JF, Bemelman WA. Dutch Diverticular disease collaborative study G. Early experience with laparoscopic lavage for perforated diverticulitis. Br J Surg. 2013;100:704–10.
65. Angenete E, Thornell A, Burcharth J, Pommergaard HC, Skullman S, Bisgaard T, et al. Laparoscopic lavage is feasible and safe for the treatment of perforated diverticulitis with purulent peritonitis: the first results from the randomized controlled trial DILALA. Ann Surg. 2016;263:117–22.

66. Schultz JK, Yaqub S, Wallon C, Blecic L, Forsmo HM, Folkesson J, et al. Laparoscopic Lavage vs Primary Resection for Acute Perforated Diverticulitis: The SCANDIV Randomized Clinical Trial. JAMA. 2015;314:1364–75.
67. Vennix S, Musters GD, Mulder IM, Swank HA, Consten EC, Belgers EH, et al. Laparoscopic peritoneal lavage or sigmoidectomy for perforated diverticulitis with purulent peritonitis: a multicentre, parallel-group, randomised, open-label trial. Lancet. 2015;386(10000):1269–77.
68. McCafferty MH, Roth L, Jorden J. Current management of diverticulitis. Am Surg. 2008;74:1041–9.
69. Fleming FJ, Gillen P. Reversal of Hartmann's procedure following acute diverticulitis: is timing everything? Int J Colorectal Dis. 2009;24:1219–25.
70. Hong MK, Tomlin AM, Hayes IP, Skandarajah AR. Operative intervention rates for acute diverticulitis: a multicentre state-wide study. ANZ J Surg. 2015;85:734–8.
71. Li D, Baxter NN, McLeod RS, Moineddin R, Wilton AS, Nathens AB. Evolving practice patterns in the management of acute colonic diverticulitis: a population-based analysis. Dis Colon Rectum. 2014;57:1397–405.
72. Chandra V, Nelson H, Larson DR, Harrington JR. Impact of primary resection on the outcome of patients with perforated diverticulitis. Arch Surg. 2004;139:1221–4.
73. Salem L, Flum DR. Primary anastomosis or Hartmann's procedure for patients with diverticular peritonitis? A systematic review. Dis Colon Rectum. 2004;47:1953–64.
74. Abbas S. Resection and primary anastomosis in acute complicated diverticulitis, a systematic review of the literature. Int J Colorectal Dis. 2007;22:351–7.
75. Cirocchi R, Trastulli S, Desiderio J, Listorti C, Boselli C, Parisi A, et al. Treatment of Hinchey stage III-IV diverticulitis: a systematic review and meta-analysis. Int J Colorectal Dis. 2013;28:447–57.
76. Constantinides VA, Heriot A, Remzi F, Darzi A, Senapati A, Fazio VW, Tekkis PP. Operative strategies for diverticular peritonitis: a decision analysis between primary resection and anastomosis versus Hartmann's procedures. Ann Surg. 2007;245:94–103.
77. Oberkofler CE, Rickenbacher A, Raptis DA, Lehmann K, Villiger P, Buchli C, et al. A multicenter randomized clinical trial of primary anastomosis or Hartmann's procedure for perforated left colonic diverticulitis with purulent or fecal peritonitis. Ann Surg. 2012;256:819–26.
78. Vennix S, Boersema GS, Buskens CJ, Menon AG, Tanis PJ, Lange JF, Bemelman WA. Emergency Laparoscopic Sigmoidectomy for Perforated Diverticulitis with Generalised Peritonitis: A Systematic Review. Dig Surg. 2016;33:1–7.
79. Kafka-Ritsch R, Birkfellner F, Perathoner A, Raab H, Nehoda H, Pratschke J, Zitt M. Damage control surgery with abdominal vacuum and delayed bowel reconstruction in patients with perforated diverticulitis Hinchey III/IV. J Gastrointest Surg. 2012;16:1915–22.
80. Perathoner A, Klaus A, Mühlmann G, Oberwalder M, Margreiter R, Kafka-Ritsch R. Damage control with abdominal vacuum therapy (VAC) to manage perforated diverticulitis with advanced generalized peritonitis–a proof of concept. Int J Colorectal Dis. 2010;25:767–74.
81. Ordóñez CA, Sánchez AI, Pineda JA, Badiel M, Mesa R, Cardona U, et al. Deferred primary anastomosis versus diversion in patients with severe secondary peritonitis managed with staged laparotomies. World J Surg. 2010;34:169–76.
82. Rafferty J, Shellito P, Hyman NH, Buie WD. Standards committee of the american society of colon and rectal surgeons. Practice parameters for sigmoid diverticulitis. Dis Colon Rectum. 2006;49:939–44.
83. Hall JF, Roberts PL, Ricciardi R, Read T, Scheirey C, Wald C, et al. Long-term follow-up after an initial episode of diverticulitis: what are the predictors of recurrence? Dis Colon Rectum. 2011;54:283–8.
84. Humes DJ, West J. Role of acute diverticulitis in the development of complicated colonic diverticular disease and 1-year mortality after diagnosis in the UK: population-based cohort. Gut. 2012;61:95–100.
85. Salem TA, Molloy RG, O'Dwyer PJ. Prospective, five-year follow up study of patients with symptomatic uncomplicated diverticular disease. Dis Colon Rectum. 2007;50:1–5.
86. Regenbogen SE, Hardiman KM, Hendren S, Morris AM. Surgery for diverticulitis in the 21st Century: a systematic review. JAMA Surg. 2014;149:292–303.
87. Klarenbeek BR, Samuels M, van der Wal MA, van der Peet DL, Meijerink WJ, Cuesta MA. Indications for elective sigmoid resection in diverticular disease. Ann Surg. 2010;251:670–4.
88. Solomkin JS, Mazuski JE, Bradley JS, Rodvold KA, Goldstein EJ, Baron EJ, et al. Diagnosis and management of complicated intra-abdominal infection in adults and children: guidelines by the surgical infection society and the infectious diseases society of America. Surg Infect (Larchmt). 2010;11:79–109.
89. Sawyer RG, Claridge JA, Nathens AB, Rotstein OD, Duane TM, Evans HL, et al. Trial of short-course antimicrobial therapy for intraabdominal infection. N Engl J Med. 2015;372:1996–2005.

13

Colorectal emergencies associated with penetrating or retained foreign bodies

Selim Yigit Yildiz[1*], Murat Kendirci[2], Serkan Akbulut[3], Ali Ciftci[1], Hamdi Taner Turgut[1] and Suleyman Hengirmen[4]

Abstract

Background: Foreign bodies in rectum and colon is an uncommon problem in surgical practice. Anal eroticism leads amongst etiologic factors. In some patients accidents or forceful application of foreign bodies are causative factors. This study was designed to describe our experience in diagnosis and treatment of this exciting clinical problem.

Methods: Data were collected prospectively from 1998 to 2013 in 30 patients. Patient demographics, diagnostic findings, location, type, extraction method, and postextraction period were reviewed.

Results: All the 30 patients were their first admission in emergency service of a hospital. On admission high alcohol intake was determined in 15(50%) patients. All the patients were hospitalized. Most of the rectal foreign bodies (23 of 25) was located distal 2/3 of the rectum. Colorectal perforation was diagnosed in 5 patients who had not any retained foreign body. Under adequate anesthesia transanal extraction was implemented in 23 (92%) patients in the operating room. In the patients with proximal located rectal foreign bodies (2/25), grade III and IV rectal injury or colonic perforation (7/30) laparotomy was carried out.

Conclusion: A careful physical and rectal examination is essential for correct diagnosis and localization of retained foreign bodies. Forceful and repeated efforts without sphincter relaxation is gives rise to proximal migration of objects and unwanted complications such as rectal perforation. The operating room provides adequate anaesthesia for muscle relaxation and technical advantages in transanal extraction of rectal foreign bodies. Therefore, nonoperative success rate improves. If the objects are large and proximally migrated and if the patients suffer from peritonitis due to rectal or colon perforation or pelvic sepsis, laparatomy is performed witout much delay.

Keywords: Rectum, Foreign bodies, Erotica, Wounds and injuries, Operating rooms

Background

The insertion of foreign bodies (FB) into the anus is an uncommon clinical problem. Most patients are present to emergency rooms when their own efforts to remove the retained object have failed [1]. The most common etiology is anal eroticism, followed by blunt or penetrating trauma by an accident or forceful action [2,3]. Because of the late admission of the patient to the hospital the management can be difficult and may be associated with the complications. This clinical review reports our experience to this rare situation and associated complications.

* Correspondence: selimyigit2002@yahoo.com
[1]Department of General Surgery, Kocaeli Derince Training and Research Hospital, Kocaelı, Izmit, Turkey

Materials and methods

Clinical datas of the emergency department of Ankara Numune and Kocaeli Derince Training and Research Hospital between November 1998 and April 2013 was reviewed prospectively. Separate files was constituted for every patient on admission. Patient demographics, findings of physical examinations and the results of diagnostic and therapothic interventions were recorded. The cases of anally introduced foreign bodies and patients with a history of colorectal foreign bodies and serious symptoms were free have been included in this review. Patients with orally ingested foreign materials have been excluded. A total of 30 patients who were diagnosed with retained colorectal foreign bodies and cases with complication of forcefull access via anus.

After their medical history were taken, all the patients were evaluated in the emergency room with help of physical and rectal examination by surgeons. Abdominal and chest x-rays of each patient were taken for the localization of foreign body and to rule out pneumoperitomeum inthe case of rectal or colonic perforation. Computed tomography was performed in case of perforation and proximally located foreign bodies. Endoscopic asssesment was not carried out in the emergency room. After full evaluation, all the patients were hospitalized. Extraction of the foreign bodies were performed in the operating room. Transanal route was the first choice for extraction of rectal FB. Anaesthesia was implemented according to the need of sphincter relaxation, choice of various instruments, and laparatomy.

After the extraction procedure, rectosigmoidoscopy was performed routinely. In the patients with large and angular foreign bodies, extraction procedure which had a long duration and difficulties were controlled more carefully after extraction procedure. When traumatic rectal injuries were determined, Rectal Organ Injury Scale (ROIS) was used to classify. Rectal lesions were classified as Grade I(simple contusion) to Grade V (devascularization of rectal segment). This grade system was used to define the lesions only. Objects that can not be removed transanal route and patients with severe colorectal injuries or perforation laparotomy was carried out.

Results

A total of 30 patients, 26 men and 4 women, were admitted with retained rectal foreign body or associated complications. The mean age of the patients were 43 (range, 20–63) years. As for the reason of insertion, 12 patients reported sexual activity, 2 reported an accident in the house and 5 reported that the objects were forcefully introduced into the anus. 11 patients had been unable to state description. Fifteen patients (50%) had high alcohol intake and 3 patients (10%) had psychiatric disease at admission. The most common complaint among the patients was perianal (90%) and abdominal pain (70%). Abdominal X-rays were helpful diagnosis and localization of FB (Figure 1). After the first evaluation in the emergency service, all the patients were hospitalized and evaluation for extraction was carried out in the operating room. Characteristics, localization, type of extraction of foreign bodies were detailed in Table 1. Most of the foreign bodies (23 of 25) were located in the 2/3 distal rectum; remaining 2 FB were located in rectosigmoid junction. Transanal route was the first choice for extraction and it was performed in 23 patients (92%) succesfully. Various surgical techniques such as anal dilatation and digital extraction in 8 (40%) patients, surgical forceps and foley catheters in 10 (50%) patients, and in 2 (10%) patients by means of rectosigmoidoscopy for extraction of rectal FB, have been applied. Figure 2 shows various extracted bodies. Regional anaesthesia was the most common technique for muscle relaxation and it was preferred in 12 (40%) patients. Anal block and intravenous sedation was undertaken in the first 8 (26.6%) and in the remaining 10 (33.4%) patients general anaesthesia was carried out. Seven patients needed emergent laparatomy. Fife of these patients with perforation or severe rectal injury and the remaining 2 patients with failure of transanal extraction. On laparatomy, colotomy, loop colostomy, Hartmann's procedure and rectal suturation were applied in different patients.

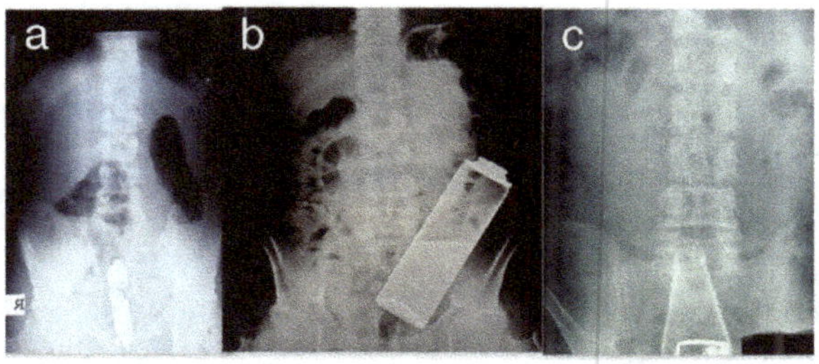

Figure 1 Abdominal X-rays of patients with rectal FB. (a) Vibrator, **(b)** shaving foam bottle, **(c)** bottle.

On evaluation with rectal examination and rectosigmoidoscopy, most of rectal injuries (10 patients,%33) are classified as grade I and II. When local treatment was apllied in grade I and II, diverting colostomy was implemented in 2 patients with Grage III injuries (Table 2).

The patients were hospitalized for 1 to 7 days (median 4 days) postoperatively. On postoperative period 2 patent with wound infection and 1 patient with mild perianal infection was observed.

Table 1 Characteristics, localization, type of extraction of rectal foreign bodies

	Patient (n=30)	Transanal extraction (n = 23)	Laparatomy (n = 7)
Type of foreign body			
Glass	8	8	1
Bottle	6	5	1
Metal object	5	5	1
Vibrator	2	2	
Toilet Bush	1		1
Localisation in rectum			
Proximal (%)	2 (8)	-	2
Distal (%)	23 (92)	23	3
Other*	5		3

*: Patients are free of FB but existence of colorectal injury and history of FB access.

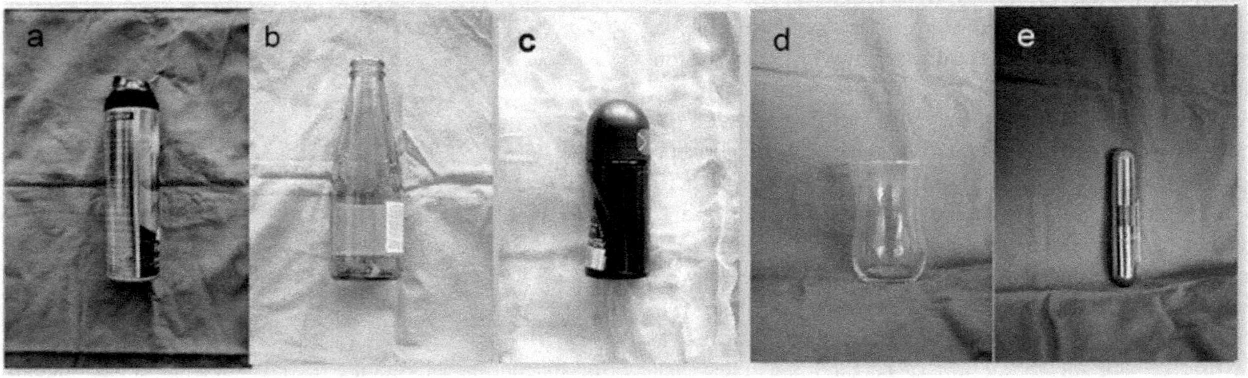

Figure 2 Photographs of extracted foreign bodies. **(a)** shaving foam bottle, **(b)** bottle, **(c)** deodorant, **(d)** glass, **(e)** metal object.

Discussion

Rectal FB are seen less commonly in surgical practice especially in emergency department. This phenomenon is most commonly associated with anal eroticisim. Accidental or iatrogenic events, ingestion of animal bones and foreign bodies, psychiatric diseases and drug trafficking are other reasons [4-6]. Foreign bodies that are retained in rectum have various shapes, numbers, and sizes. Amongst the objects encountered are different types such as bottles, cup, glasses, bananas, carrots, vibrators, metal objects, bulbs, pieces of wood and shaving foam cups, etc. [5-7].

After emergency or hospital admission, patients must be evaluated by surgeons with both a detailed history and physical examination. Digital rectal examination is essential. Patient's complaints usually vary from obscure anal pain and abdominal discomfort and pain, to constipation and anal hemorrhage. Patients can even present with acute abdomen with peritoneal irritation and pelvic sepsis [2,3,8]. The first complaint of 15% of our patients was retained rectal FB. Abdominal X-rays should be undertaken to identify the location, size and the shape of the subject. Chest X-ray should be undertaken to identify the perforation, as there might be free air under the diaphgram. Before admission many of the patients attempted to extract the FB. Unsuccesful attemps are the main reason of delayed hospital admission and rectal FB related complications such as rectal or colonic perforation, peritonitis, perirectal or perianal sepsis [3,9].

Table 2 Type of rectal injuries, treatment and postoperative complications

			Treatment	
	N	%	Local	Colostomy
Colorectal injuries				
Grade I	6	(20)	6	
Grade II	4	(13.3)	4	
Grade III	4	(13.3)	2	2
Perforation	3	(10)		3
Complication				
Wound infection	2			
Perianal infection	1			

Following the diagnosis and to localize the rectal FB, transanal route is the first choice for extraction especially in low lying objects. Before transanal interventions, acute abdomen due to rectal or colonic perforation should be excluded. In various literature attempts to remove FB in the emergency room or at bedside is initially preferred [10,11]. The succes rate of bedside or emergency room attempts are about 16 to 75% in some literatures [12]. Repeated and vigorous efforts to remove rectal FB cause distress, pain and profound involuntary anorectal spazm; it is the main source of this reduced succes rate. In this study all the efforts to extract the rectal FB was carried out in the operating room. Patient personal privacy, Turkish sociocultural assets, and technical and medical requirements cause surgeons to choose this method. In the operating room adequate anesthesia is applied and various instruments are used depending on the foreign bodies characteristics and this improves the nonoperative success rate [12-15]. Adequate anal dilatation by way of caudal or anal block and intravenous sedation is essential for succesful transanal extraction. Sphincter function, tone and contractilitiy and continence should be evaluated. Bimanual pressure on anterior abdominal wall, grasping with forceps, manuplation with foley catheter,magnets for metal objects and rectosigmoidoscopy is complementary techniques for transanal removal of the FB [16]. These methods can be more effectively used only in the operating room.

Prolonged retain period and unsuccessful attempts to remove rectal foreign body by the patient are two important factors that reduce transanal achievement. In our series the success rate of transanal extraction is up to 90 percent. It is related to advantages of operating room and short admission time of our patients. Objects larger than 10cm and those located in the proximal rectum are most likely to require surgical intervention in literature [10]. In our study proximal rectal localization of foreign bodies were more affected laparatomy requirement.

When endoscopic or manual transanal extraction fails or complications are present, laparatomy is necessary [17-19]. Different operative techniques can also be used for the removal of the foreign body and treatment of the complications. The decision to perform colostomy to primary rectal suturing only depends on various factors such as intraabdominal contamination, grade of rectal injury, extend of perianal trauma and chronicity of the case. On laparatomy milking the objects towards the rectum or anus enables the surgeon to extract FB without colotomy. Laparascopic asistance can be used in transanal extraction of proximally migrated FB. It allows for easy removal and direct visualization of the rectum to evaluate for injury. Laparascopic primary suturing, resection and diverting colostomy could be realised [20].

After difficult extraction procedure rectal and distal colonic mucosa is have to evaluate with rectosigmoidoscopy that determine extend of injury and exclude possible perforation. In postextraction rectosigmoidoscopy most of the rectal injuries are in grade I and II as in our series [11].

Surgeons must be aware, in patients with chronicity, of serious anorectal injuries, possibility of perirectal sepcis, and important sequelae such as anal incontinence, fistulas and stenosis in the follow-up period [21].

Our clinical algorithm was showed in Figure 3. This treatment guide was developed in the light of our clinical experiences. This sequential management system which we use in our clinical practice of colorectal FB, have helped transanal extraction rate to reach over 90%.

All the patients should be evaluated psychologically. Patients presented with foreign bodies in the rectum should be asked for different sexual behaviours such as homosexuality. Most of the patients reject the abnormal sexual activities. Additionally, the patients should be examined for the use of alcohol and narcotic drugs. 50% of our cases reported high level intake of alcoholic beverages before rectal FB introduction.

Conclusions

Retained rectal foreign bodies are usually related to improper anal sexual behaviour. Patients should be evaluated with a careful physical and rectal examination and plain radiograms for correct diagnosis and

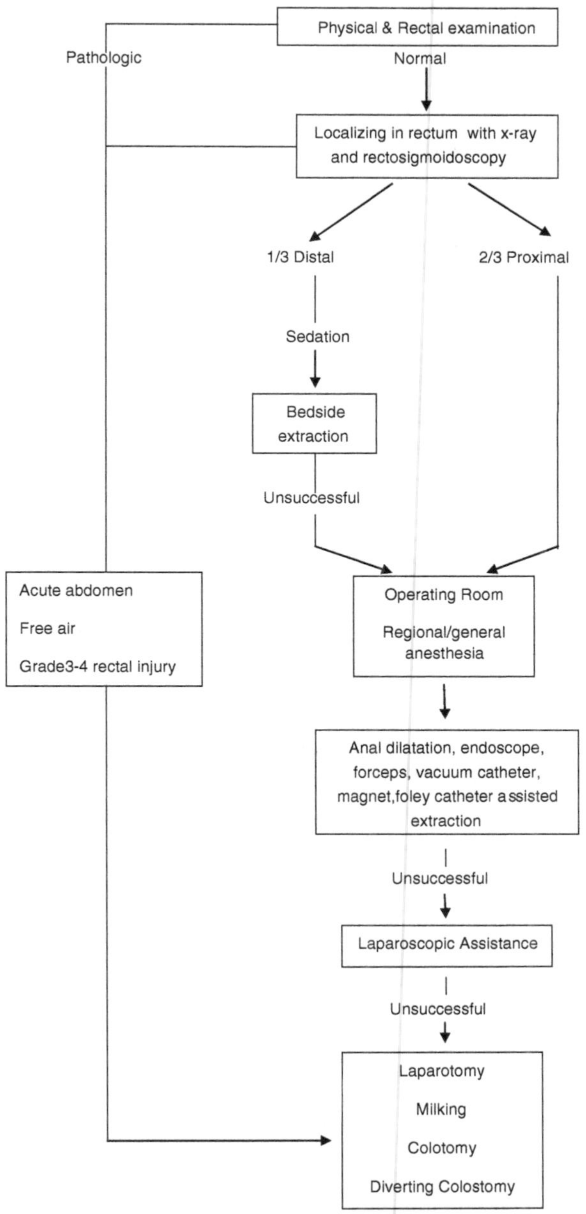

Figure 3 Management algorithm of colorectal foreign body.

localization. Small, low lying rectal foreign bodies may be extracted at bedside and in the emergency room. Forceful and repeated efforts without sphincter relaxation gives rise to proximal migration of objects and unwanted complications such as rectal perforation. The operating room serves appropiate anaesthesia for muscle relaxation and tecnical advantages especially in transanal extraction. If the objects are large and proximally migrated and if the patients suffer from peritonitis due to rectal or colon perforation or pelvic sepsis, laparatomy is performed witout much delay.

Competing interests
The authors declare that they have no competing interests.

Authors' contributions
SYY: conception and design, or acquisition of data, or analysis and interpretation of data, have given final approval of the version to be published. MK: conception and design, or acquisition of data, or analysis and interpretation of data. SA: revising it critically for important intellectual content; AC: revising it critically for important intellectual content; HTT: have made substantial contributions to conception and design. SH: have made substantial contributions to conception and design. All authors read and approved the final manuscript.

Author details
[1]Department of General Surgery, Kocaeli Derince Training and Research Hospital, Kocaelı, Izmit, Turkey. [2]General Surgery, Edirne State Hospital, Edirne, Turkey. [3]Department of Surgical Oncology, Ankara University Medical School, Ankara, Turkey. [4]Department of General Surgery, Ankara Numune Training and Research Hospital, Ankara, Turkey.

References
1. Turner B: **Management of retained foreign bodies and rectal sexual trauma.** *Nur Times* 2004, **100**:30–32.
2. Hellinger MD: **Anal trauma and foreign bodies.** *Surg Clin N Am* 2002, **82**:1253–1260.
3. Yaman M, Deitel M, Burul CJ, Shahi B, Hadar B: **Foreign bodies in the rectum.** *Can J Surg* 1993, **36**:173–177.
4. Cohen JS, Sackier JM: **Management of colorectal foreign bodies.** *J R Coll Surg Edinb* 1996, **41**:312–315.
5. Rodrígues-Her mosa JI, Codina A, Alayrach J, *et al*: **Foreign bodies in the rectum and sigmoid colon.** *Cir Esp* 2001, **69**:404–407.
6. Lledó S, Roig JV: **Anorectal trauma and their sequelae.** *Cir Esp* 1991, **50**:472–479.
7. Coulson CJ, Brammer RD, Stonelake PS: **Extraction of a rectal foreign body using an electromagnet.** *Int J Colorectal Dis* 2005, **20**:194–195.
8. Kouraklis G, Misiakos E, Dovas N, Karatzas G, Gogas J: **Management of foreign bodies of the rectum;report of 21 cases.** *J R Coll Surg Edinb* 1997, **42**:246–247.
9. Delikoukos S, Zacharoulis D, Hatzytheofilou C: **Perianal abscesses due to ingested foreign bodies.** *Int J Clin Pract* 2005, **59**:856–857.
10. Lake JP, Essani R, Petrone P, Kasier AM, Asensio J, Beart RW Jr: **Management of retained colorectal foreign bodies: predictors of operative intervention.** *Dis Colon Rectum* 2004, **47**:1694–1698.
11. Rodrígues-Hermosa JI, Codina-Cazador A, *et al*: **Management of foreign bodies in rectum.** *Colorectal Dis* 2006, **9**:543–548.
12. Clarke DL, Buccimazza I, Anderson FA, Thomson SR: **Colorectal foreign bodies.** *Colorectal Dis* 2005, **7**:98–103.
13. Huang WC, Jiang JK, Wang HS, *et al*: **Retained Foreign bodies.** *J Chin Med Assoc* 2003, **66**:606–611.
14. Ooi BS, Ho YH, Eu KW, *et al*: **Management of anorectal foreign bodies: a cause of obscure anal pain.** *Aust N Z J Surg* 1998, **68**:852–855.
15. Cirocco WC: **Anesthesia facilitates the extraction of rectal foreign bodies.** *Gastrointest Endosc* 2000, **52**:452–453.
16. Kantarian JC, Riether RD, Sheets JA, Stasik JJ, Rosen L, Khubchandani IT: **Endoscopic retrieval of foreign bodies from the rectum.** *Dis Colon Rectum* 1987, **30**:902–904.
17. Hoitzma HF, Meije S, De Jong D: **The transsphincteric approach for removal of a huge foreign body from the rectum.** *Neth J Surg* 1984, **36**:83–84.
18. Ruiz J, Sellés R, Millán M, Zummárraga P, Asencio F: **Colorectal trauma caused by foreign bodies introduced during sexual activity: diagnosis and management.** *Rev Esp Enferm Dig* 2001, **93**:631–634.
19. Thomson SR, Fraser M, Stupp C, Baker LW: **Iatrogenic and accidental colon injuries – what to do?** *Dis Colon Rectum* 1994, **37**:496–502.
20. Berghoff KR, Franklin ME Jr: **Laparoscopic-assisted rectal foreign body removal: report of a case.** *Dis Colon Rectum* 2005, **48**:1975–1977.
21. Agnew J: **Some anatomical and physiological aspects of anal sexual practices.** *J Homosex* 1985, **12**:75–96.

14

Correlation of serum C-reactive protein, white blood count and neutrophil percentage with histopathology findings in acute appendicitis

Shefki Xharra[1], Lumturije Gashi-Luci[2], Kumrije Xharra[3], Fahredin Veselaj[4], Besnik Bicaj[5], Fatos Sada[6] and Avdyl Krasniqi[5*]

Abstract

Background: Acute appendicitis is one of the most common surgical emergencies. Accurate diagnosis of acute appendicitis is based on careful history, physical examination, laboratory and imaging investigation. The aim of the study is to analyze the role of C-reactive protein (CRP), white blood count (WBC) and Neutrophil percentage (NP) in improving the accuracy of diagnosis of acute appendicitis and to compare it with the intraoperative assessment and histopathology findings.

Materials and methods: This investigation was a prospective double blinded clinical study. The study was done on 173 patients surgically treated for acute appendicitis. The WBC, NP, and measurement of CRP were randomly collected pre-operatively from all involved patients. Macroscopic assessment was made from the operation. Appendectomy and a histopathology examination were performed on all patients. Gross description was compared with histopathology results and then correlated with CRP, WBC, and NP.

Results: The observational accuracy was 87,3%, as compared to histopathological accuracy which was 85.5% with a total of 173 patients that were operated on. The histopathology showed 25 (14.5%) patients had normal appendices, and 148 (85.5%) patients had acutely inflamed, gangrenous, or perforated appendicitis. 52% were male and 48% were female, with the age ranging from 5 to 59 with a median of 19.7. The gangrenous type was the most frequent (52.6%). The WBC was altered in 77.5% of the cases, NP in 72.3%, and C-reactive protein in 76.9% cases. In those with positive appendicitis, the CRP and WBC values were elevated in 126 patients (72.8%), whereas NP was higher than 75% in 117 patients (67.6%). Out of 106 patients with triple positive tests, 101 (95.2%) had appendicitis. The sensitivity, specificity, and positive predictive values of the 3 tests in combination were 95.3%, 72.2%, and 95.3%, respectively.

Conclusion: The raised value of the CRP was directly related to the severity of inflammation (p-value <0.05). CRP monitoring enhances the diagnostic accuracy of acute appendicitis. The diagnostic accuracy of CRP is not significantly greater than WBC and NP. A combination of these three tests significantly increases the accuracy. We found that elevated serum CRP levels support the surgeon's clinical diagnosis.

Keywords: Acute appendicitis, CRP correlation, White blood count, Neutrophil percentage, Histopathology findings

* Correspondence: avdyl.krasniqi@yahoo.com
[5]Department of Abdominal Surgery, University Clinical Center of Kosovo, Prishtina, Kosovo
Full list of author information is available at the end of the article

Introduction

Acute appendicitis is one of the most common surgical emergencies and the most common source of infection in community-acquired intra-abdominal infections [1-3]. Its diagnosis is usually made depending on the presenting history, clinical evaluation, and physical examination [1,2,4]. It is further reinforced by laboratory investigations, such as white blood cells, differential counts (the percentage of neutrophil granulocytes and band neutrophil granulocytes), and C-reactive protein (CRP) that were the only diagnostic tools for many years [4-10]. It has been estimated that the accuracy of the clinical diagnosis of acute appendicitis is only between 76 percent and 92 percent [9,11]. Thus, accurate diagnosis of acute appendicitis is still difficult [1,12,13]. The perforation rate is high, as well as the number of negative appendectomies [9,14]. Following the introduction of ultrasound scans during the last two decades and computed tomography (CT) in the last decade, the rate of negative appendectomies has decreased [4,15-17], but the perforation rate has remained high (22%-62%) [4,18,19]. Negative appendectomies are one of the burdens facing not only the general surgeon but also the patient her/himself and society as a whole, since appendectomy, as any other operation, results in socio-economic impacts in the form of lost working days and declined productivity.

CRP is a non-specific inflammatory marker that is used routinely in many hospitals as an aid in the diagnosis of patients with an acute abdomen [9,10,14]. An acute phase protein is produced in the liver. Normal serum concentration is less than 10 mg/l 8–12 hours after infection or trauma; the increase of acute phase protein in liver the CRP is more important in clinical practice. Production of CRP is controlled by Interleukin-6 and in a few minutes increases from 10 to 1,000 times. CRP is increased in infections, inflammatory arthritis, autoimmune disorders, neoplasia, pregnancy, and aging [9,10,20-24].

Many reports have investigated the value of the raised serum CRP measurement in improving the diagnosis of acute appendicitis [9,10,25].

Additional tests that would improve the diagnostic accuracy and reduce the number of unnecessary operations are needed. This is particularly important these days when health planning is driven by cost containment. The C-reactive protein (CRP), together with other acute-phase proteins, increased in response to tissue injury [26].

The aim of this study was to analyze the role of C-reactive protein (CRP) values, in accuracy of diagnosis of acute appendicitis in comparison with WBC, NP, the surgeon's clinical diagnosis, and the histopathologic findings.

Patients and methods

Patients

The study included randomly all operated patients (173) suspected of acute appendicitis between November 2008 and February 2009 in the Department of Surgery.

Methods

Clinical signs of acute appendicitis determined by the surgeon and the duration of the symptoms were documented on admission. The clinical signs included direct tenderness in the right lower quadrant, percussion and rebound tenderness, localized rigidity, and diffuse rigidity of the abdominal wall. At least one clinical sign had to be present in order to consider the patient positive for clinical signs. In all operated patients, in-hospital observation time until the surgical procedure was performed was recorded. The surgeons were aware of the routine laboratory and ultrasound findings.

Blood samples for routine laboratory tests (white blood cell count, differential count), and C-reactive protein were obtained on admission. White blood cell and differential counts were measured by the Hematology Analyzer (HARIBA ABX Micros 60). The normal WBC value in our laboratory is 0–10 x 109/L. Levels above 10 x 109/L were considered as above normal. The percentage of neutrophils was considered elevated when >75%. The C-reactive protein concentration was quantified by a Latex agglutination slide test for the qualitative and semi-quantitative determination in Non-diluted serum (Humatex, Wiesbaden, Germany). For semi-quantitative determination, serum dilutions were prepared with the 0.9% sodium chloride, according to the instructions of the manufacturers. Each dilution was tested according to the qualitative procedure described above until no further agglutination was observed. The serum CRP concentration was then estimated by multiplying the dilution factor from the last dilution with visible agglutination (2, 4, 8, 16, 32) by the detection limit (6 mg/l). E.g. if the agglutination titer appears at 1:16, the approximate serum CRP level is 16 x 6 = 96 mg/l. The normal CRP level in our laboratory is 0–6 mg/L. Levels above 6 mg/L were considered as being above normal.

Serum CRP measurements were not taken into account for the decision of surgical intervention and to compare it with the surgeon's clinical diagnosis. Further, the laboratory staff was not informed about the clinical findings, decisions, and outcomes (double blind study).

Removed appendixes were fixed in 4% formalin, stained with hematoxylin and eosin (H&E) and analyzed histologically. Based on the histological features of the removed appendix, according to the criteria described by Shashtari M H S, 2006 (24), the patients were divided into three groups: Group A normal appendix, Group B inflamed appendix (simple appendicitis), and Group C perforated/gangrenous appendix (complicated appendicitis). The final diagnosis was based on the histology and, in the case of perforation, on the macroscopic evaluation by the surgeon. The pathologists were not informed of the patients' clinical and laboratory data, except for the surgical diagnosis.

Statistical analysis

All variables showing a significant difference between the groups were further analyzed. The receiver-operating characteristic (ROC) curves were drawn to define the optimum sensitivity, specificity, cut-off value, predictive values, and diagnostic accuracy, determined by the area under the ROC curve (AUC) of the studied laboratory markers.

Results

Out of a total of 173 patients, the histopathologic findings confirmed acute appendicitis in 148 (85.55%) patients. Normal appendixes were removed in the remaining 25 (14.45%) patients: males were 52.02% (N = 90), females 47.97% (N = 83), and children 39.3% (N = 68). The male female ratio was 1.09:1. The age range was from 5 to 59 years with the mean (SD) being 19.7 years (± 10,5), whereas 83.5% of patients were under 30 years old. According to the histopathology reports, Group A where normal appendix was found comprised 25 (14.45%) patients, whereas inflamed appendix was found in 148 (85.5%) patients. Among patients with a positive appendicitis, 36 (20.81%) belonged to group Group B with acute simple appendicitis and 112 (64.74%) had a ruptured/perforated/gangrenous appendix (Group-C, complicated appendicitis). The rate of perforated appendicitis was 12.1% (Table 1).

Among the patients in Group A, the most common diagnoses associated with primary negative appendectomy included nonspecific abdominal pain 15 (8.7%), ruptured ovarian cysts 4 (2.3%), mesenteric lymphadenitis 5 (2.9%), and urinary infection 1 (0.6%).

In Group A the CRP values ranged from 0 to 96 with a mean of 10.6 mg/l. In Group B these values were from 0 to 192 with a mean value of 37 mg/l, and in Group C from 0 to 192 with a mean of 79.2 mg/l. The serum CRP levels were normal in 22 patients with acute appendicitis. Thus, the false-negative rate of CRP was 12.71 percent. Of the 25 patients with normal appendectomy, serum CRP levels were slightly elevated in 7 patients. A false-positive rate of CRP was 4.05 percent. Further, based on the surgeons' clinical impression, the diagnosis was true in 87.28% (N = 151) and false in 12.72% (N = 22) patients. In the present study, the positive predictive value of the CRP was 94.7%, specificity 72%, sensitivity 85.1%, and accuracy 83.2%.

Similarly, when the WBC count was assessed, Group A varied from 5.3 to 14.7 (mean 8.8 $x10^9/l$), Group B from 5.0 to 28.0 (mean 12.6 $x10^9/l$), and Group C from 5.0 to 28.0 (mean 15.6 $x10^9/l$). The false positives were 4.62% and false negatives were 12.72% with a sensitivity of 85.1% and a specificity of 68%,; the positive predictive value was 94% and the accuracy was calculated to be 82.6%. The neutrophil percentage in Group A varied from 54.2 to 88.6 (mean 71.5), in Group B from 56.2 to 94.3 (mean 79.8) and in Group C from 60.7 to 96.6 (mean 84.0). The false positives were 4.62% and false negatives 17.92% with a sensitivity of 79.1% and the specificity 68%; the positive predictive value was 93.6% and the accuracy was calculated to be 77.5%.

The WBC and CRP were elevated in 126 (85.1%) cases with positive histopathology (Groups B and C). Seven patients had normal CRP and eight patients had normal WBC. In 25 patients with negative appendix, 18 had a normal CRP and 17 had normal WBC; only 5 patients had both CRP and WBC values increase. Again, in patients in Groups B and C, 113 (76.35%) had both WBC and CRP value increase and 9 patients had both values in the normal range. Combining all three parameters (WBC, CRP and percentage of neutrophil count) had positive results

Table 1 Distribution of histopathologic features of appendix by sex

Histopathology of Appendix		Female	Male	N	%
Group - A Normal appendix		20	5	25	14.5
Group - B	Catarrhal App.	2	0	2	1.2
(Non-complicated appendicitis)	Phlegmonous App.	23	11	34	19.7
Group - C	Gangrenous App.	31	60	91	52,6
(complicated appendicitis) Perforative App.		7	14	21	12,1
Total	**N**	83	90	173	100
	%	48	52	100	

for the appendicitis in 101 (68.24%) patients (Groups B and C), and only 5 patients had one or more values in the normal range. In Group A, only five patients had all the three values increase and 13 patients had one or more values in the normal range. The combined WBC and CRP had a sensitivity, specificity, and positive predictive value of 95.3%, 91.1%, and 95.8%, respectively. While the combined percentage of the neutrophil count and CRP had a sensitivity, the specificity and positive predictive value of 94.3%, 91.1%, and 95.2%, respectively. Combined all the three parameters (WBC, CRP, and percentage of neutrophil count) gave the sensitivity, and specificity of 95.3% and 91.9%, respectively. The positive predictive value was 95.3% (Table 2).

Discussion

The positive CRP is more accurate than the WBC and neutrophil counts and combined together it further improves diagnostic accuracy [10]. In a double blind study Asfar et al. (2000) reported a sensitivity and specificity of CRP as 86.6% and 93.6%, respectively. They concluded that a normal CRP value probably indicates a normal non-inflamed appendix [14]. It is a more sensitive test than the WBC and neutrophil counts and their combined usage significantly increases sensitivity and specificity. Erkassap (2000) in a positive study on 102 patients reported that sensitivity and specificity of the CRP were 96% and 78%, respectively; the positive predictive value was 100% [27]. In a retrospective study, Wu and coworkers (2005) concluded that the combined usage of the WBC, neutrophil count, and the CRP monitoring increased the positive predictive value [28]. Grönroos (1999) in his study concluded that when both the WBC and CRP are normal, acute appendicitis is very unlikely [29].

In our study, the rate of complicated appendicitis at admission to the hospital was very high (Table 1). 112 (64.7%) patients had a ruptured/perforated/gangrenous appendix. The rate of perforated appendicitis was 12.1%. The delayed treatment can be attributed to the fact that most of the rural patients either did not report to the medical practitioners during the early stages of the disease or were seen by sought expert medical care only when complicated. Misdiagnosis by qualified medical practitioners in rural places delayed the reporting of patients to surgery, treating them with as gastroenteritis, urinary infection, etc. In these regions, the primary healthcare systems are not well-established; missed and delayed diagnosis is a major factor in complicating appendicitis.

Table 2 Diagnostic accuracy, sensitivity, specificity, and positive (PPV) of white blood cell (WBC) count, C-reactive protein (CRP), percentage of neutrophil (PN) and combined WBC, CRP and PN in diagnosing acute appendicitis

	Indices of diagnostic values			
Diagnostic method	**Diagnostic accuracy**	**Sensitivity (%)**	**Specificity (%)**	**PPV (%)**
CRP	83.2	85.1	72	94.7
WBC	82.6	85.1	68	94
PN	77.5	79.1	68	93.6
CRP + LEU	90.1	92.6	75	95.8
CRP + PN	91.1	94.3	72	95.2
LEU + PN	87.1	89.9	71.4	94.7
CRP + LEU + PN	91.9	95.3	91.9	95.3

According to Shakhatreh (2000), CRP measurement is very useful in the diagnosis of acute appendicitis, but it does not replace the clinical judgment of a surgeon [11]. Accuracy of the CRP (83.2%) is not significantly greater than the WBC (82.6%) and NP (80%). A combination of these significantly increases the accuracy to 91.9%. Anderson (2000) in a prospective study on 420 patients with borderline diagnosis of appendicitis concluded that the WBC and neutrophil count are the better criteria for the subsequent examinations [23]. In our study, from 148 patients with acute appendicitis, 22 patients had CRP and WBC in the normal range (12.72%). Mean values of the CRP in simple acute appendicitis (Group-B) were significantly greater than in normal appendix (Group A) ($p < 0.001$), and also in complicated acute appendicitis (Group C) the CRP is significantly greater than in normal appendix and uncomplicated acute appendicitis ($p < 0.0001$). The WBC and neutrophil percentage are also increased in correlation with severity of inflammation ($p > 0.05$). None of these tests are 100% diagnostic. The CRP measurement or leukocyte count by itself is not completely preventive for negative appendectomy [30]. A study on 200 children showed that unlike the adult, normal leukocyte and CRP does not rule out acute appendicitis in pediatric cases [31]. Our results showed that the most affected age group was 10–19 years old (50.3%). A significant difference regarding CRP values as being diagnostic tools of acute appendicitis for different age groups and genders was not found.

In our study, the CRP values corresponds to the series with high percentage of complicated appendicitis, which is typical for rural hospitals and dysfunctional healthcare systems. But, the consistence of CRP level with the severity of appendicitis was reported by the other authors as well [32].

There are in use different clinical classification for the acute appendicitis [32,33], but, since the correlation of CRP values with histopathology findings were studied, we used the classification that combines the gross appearance of the appendix with pathologic stage [33]. Actually, the non-surgical initial management of acute appendicitis with catarrhalis changes (inflammation within the mucous membrane), or phlegmonous changes (inflammation in all layers) has been shown to be safe and effective [34,35].

Our results and other studies as well [32,36], clearly suggested that CRP leads to precise prediction of the severity of acute appendicitis. We think that CRP is not specific test for appendicitis, therefore, before diagnostic decision and indication for treatment, clinicians must depend on structural interpretation of their subjective experience, clinical information and modalities such as laboratory tests, ultrasonography and computed tomography where is available [37,38]. Finally, laboratory tests combined with imaging diagnostic procedures, remains the useful tools in establishing the diagnosis of acute appendicitis and excluding other causes of acute abdominal pain.

Conclusions

The diagnostic accuracy of the CRP is not significantly greater than the WBC and NP. The increased value of the CRP was directly related to the severity of the inflammation ($p < 0.05$). The combination of the CRP, the WBC, and the neutrophil percentage has greater diagnostic accuracy in acute appendicitis. This preoperative combination significantly decreases false positive and false negative diagnosis, but none of these is 100% diagnostic for acute appendicitis.

We found that elevated serum CRP levels support the surgeon's clinical diagnosis. We recommend CRP measurement as a routine laboratory test in patients with suspected diagnosis of acute appendicitis.

Competing interests

The authors declare that they have no competing interests.

Authors' contributions

SX designed the study, carried out acquisition, analysis, interpretation of the data, and drafting of the manuscript. LG-L analyzed histologically the removed appendixes. KX measured the Serum CRP. FV, BB, and FS participated in the study's design. AK designed the study, was involved in interpretation of the data, the drafting of the manuscript, and revised it critically for the intellectual content until the final version was reached. All authors read and approved the final manuscript.

Acknowledgements

The authors thank Mrs. Julie Kolgjinaj, professor of English language and literature at The American University in Kosovo for her English language proof of this manuscript.

Author details

[1]Department of Surgery, Regional Hospital, Prizren, Kosovo. [2]Institute of Pathology, Faculty of Medicine, University of Prishtina, Prishtina, Kosovo. [3]Department of Microbiology, National Institute of Public Health of Kosovo, Prishtina, Kosovo. [4]Department of Urology, University Clinical Center of Kosovo, Prishtina, Kosovo. [5]Department of Abdominal Surgery, University Clinical Center of Kosovo, Prishtina, Kosovo. [6]Department of Anesthesiology, University Clinical Center of Kosovo, Prishtina, Kosovo.

References

1. Kozar RA, Roslyn JJ: **The Appendix**. In *Principles of Surgery*. 7th edition. Edited by Schwartz SI, Shires GT, Spencer FC. New York-London: The McGraw-Hill Companies Inc; 1999:1383–1393.
2. Pal K, Khan A: **Appendicitis: a continuing challenge.** *J Pak Med Assoc* 1998, **48**(7):189–192.
3. Sartelli M, *et al*: **Complicated intra-abdominal infections in Europe: preliminary data from the first three months of the CIAO Study.** *World Journal of Emergency Surgery* 2012, **7**(1):15.
4. Khan MN, Davie E, Irshad K: **The role of white cell count and C-reactive protein in the diagnosis of acute appendicitis.** *J Ayub Med Coll Abbottabad* 2004, **16**(3):17–19.
5. Groselj-Grenc M, Repše S, Vidmar D, Derganc M: **Clinical and Laboratory Methods in Diagnosis of Acute Appendicitis in Children.** *Croat Med J* 2007, **48**:353–361.
6. Garcia Pena BM, Cook EF, Mandl KD: **Selective imaging strategies for the diagnosis of appendicitis in children.** *Pediatrics* 2004, **113**:24–28. Medline:14702442.
7. Teepen HJ, Zwinderman KA, *et al*: **Comparison of CT and sonography in the diagnosis of acute appendicitis: a blinded prospective study.** *AJR Am J Roentgenol* 2003, **181**:1355–1359.
8. Lau WY, Ho YC, Chu KW, Yeung C: **Leukocyte count and neutrophil percentage in appendicectomy for suspected appendicitis.** *Aust N Z J Surg* 1989, **59**(5):395–398.
9. Gurleyik E, Gurleyik G, Unalmişer S: **Accuracy of serum C-reactive protein measurements in diagnosis of acute appendicitis compared with surgeon's clinical impression.** *Dis Colon Rectum* 1995, **38**(12):1270–1274.
10. Mohammed AA, Daghman NA, Aboud SM, Oshibi HO: **The diagnostic value of C-reactive protein, white blood cell count and neutrophil percentage in childhood appendicitis.** *Saudi Med J* 2004, **25**(9):1212–1215.
11. Shakhatreh HS: **The accuracy of C-reactive protein in the diagnosis of acute appendicitis compared with that of clinical diagnosis.** *Med Arh* 2000, **54**(2):109–110.
12. Kim-Choy N, Shin-Wei L: **Clinical Analysis of the related factors in Acute Appendicitis.** *Yale J Biol Med* 2002, **75**:41–45.
13. Salem TA, Molloy RG, O'dwyer PJ: **Prospective study on the role of C-reactive protein (CRP) in patients with an acute abdomen.** *Ann R Coll Surg Engl* 2007, **89**:233–237.
14. Asfar S, Safar H, Khoursheed M, Dashti H, Al-bader A: **Would measurement of C-reactive protein reduce the rate of negative exploration for acute appendicitis?** *J R Coll Surg Edinb* 2000, **45**:21–24.
15. Kaiser S, Mesas-Burgos C, Soderman E, Frenckner B: **Appendicitis in children – impact of US and CT on the negative appendectomy rate.** *Eur J Pediatr Surg* 2004, **14**:260–264. Medline:15343467.
16. Rosengren D, Brown AF, Chu K: **Radiological imaging to improve the emergency department diagnosis of acute appendicitis.** *Emerg Med Australas* 2004, **16**:410–416. Medline:15537403.
17. Jones K, Pena AA, Dunn EL, Nadalo L, Mangram AJ: **Are negative appendectomies still acceptable?** *Am J Surg* 2004, **188**:748–754. Medline:15619494.
18. Ponsky TA, Huang ZJ, Kittle K, Eichelberger MR, Gilbert JC, Brody F, *et al*: **Hospital- and patient-level characteristics and the risk of appendiceal rupture and negative appendectomy in children.** *JAMA* 2004, **292**:1977–1982. Medline:15507583.
19. Nwomeh BC, Chisolm DJ, Caniano DA, Kelleher KJ: **Racial and socioeconomic disparity in perforated appendicitis among children: where is the problem?** *Pediatrics* 2006, **117**(3):870–875. March 1.
20. Albu E, Miller BM, Choi Y, Lakhanpal S, Murthy RN, Gerst PH: **Diagnostic value of C-reactive protein in acute appendicitis.** *Dis Colon Rectum* 1994, **37**:49–51.
21. Davies AH, Bernau F, Salisbury A, Souter RG: **C-reactive protein in right iliac fossa pain.** *J R Coll Surg Edinb* 1991, **36**:242–244.
22. Grönroos JM, Grönroos P: **A fertile-aged woman with right lower abdominal pain but unelevated leukocyte count and C-reactive protein: acute appendicitis is very unlikely.** *Langenbecks Arch Surg* 1999, **384**:437–440.
23. Andersson RE, Hugander A, Ravn H, Offenbartl K, Ghazi SH, Nyström PO, *et al*: **Repeated clinical and laboratory examinations in patients with an equivocal diagnosis of appendicitis.** *World J Surg* 2000, **24**:479–485.

24. Shoshtari MHS, Askarpour S, Alamshah M, Elahi A: **Diagnostic value of Quantitative CRP measurement in patients with acute appendicitis.** *Pak J Med Sci July - September* 2006, **22**(3):300–303.
25. Öztürk ZA, Köklü S, Erol MF, Ylmaz FM, Baar Ö, Yüksel O, Ylmaz G, Ksack Yüksel B: **Serum adenosine deaminase levels in diagnosis of acute appendicitis.** *Emerg Med J* 2008, **25:**583–585.
26. Pepys MB: **C-reactive protein fifty years on.** *Lancet* 1981, **i:**653–656.
27. Erkasap S, Ates E, Ustuner Z, Sahin A, Yilmaz S, Yasar B, *et al*: **Diagnostic value of interleukin-6 and Creactive protein in acute appendicitis.** *Swiss Surg* 2000, **6**(4):169–172.
28. Wu HP, Lin CY, Chang CF, Chang YJ, Huang CY: **Predictive value of C-reactive protein at different cutoff levels in acute appendicitis.** *Am J Emerg Med* 2005, **23**(4):449–453.
29. Gronroos JM, Gronroos P: **Leukocyte count and Creactive protein in the diagnosis of acute appendicitis.** *Br J Surg* 1999, **86**(4):501–504.
30. Eryilmaz R, Sahin M, Alimoglu O: **The value of C-reactive protein and leukocyte count in preventing negative appendectomies.** *Ulus Treuma Derg* 2001, **713:**142–145.
31. Grönroos JMJU: **Do normal leukocyte count and C-reactive protein value exclude acute in children?** *Acta Paediatr* 2001, **90**(6):649–5.
32. Yokoyama S, Takifuji K, Hota T, Matsuda K, Nasu T, Nakamori M, Hirabayashi N, Kinoshita H, Yamaue H: **C-Reactive protein is an independent surgical indication marker for appendicitis: a retrospective study.** *World J of Emergency Surgery* 2009, **4:**36.
33. Sinanan M, *et al*: **Acute Abdomen and Appendix.** In *Surgery; Scientific Principles and Practice*. 4th edition. Edited by Greenfield L. Philadelphia: J.B. Lippincot Company; 2005:1120–1142.
34. Eriksson S, Granstrom L: **Randomized controlled trial of appendicectomy versus antibiotic therapy for acute appendicitis.** *Br J Surg* 1995, **82:**166–169.
35. Styrud J, Eriksson S, Nilsson I, Ahlberg, Haapaniemi S, Neovius G, Rex L, Badume I, Granstrom L: **Appendectomy versus antibiotic treatment in acute appendicitis; a prospective multicenter randomized trial.** *World J Surg* 2006, **30:**133–137.
36. Exadactylos A, Sadowski-Cron C, Mader P, Weissmann M, Dinkel HP, Negri M, Zimmerman H: **Decision making in patients with acute abdominal pain at a university and at a rural hospital: does the value of abdominal sonography differ?** *World Journal of Emergency Surgery* 2008, **3:**29.
37. Leaper DJ, Horrocks JC, Staniland JR, De Dombal FT: **Computer-assisted diagnosis of abdominal pain using "estimates" provided by clinicians.** *Br Med J* 1972, **4:**350–354.
38. Kessler N, Cyteval C, Gallix B, Lesnik A, Blayac PM, Bruel JM, Taourel P: **Appendicitis: Evaluation of sensitivity, specificity, and predictive values of US, Doppler US, and laboratory findings.** *Radiology* 2004, **2:**474–478.

15

Triage using a self-assessment questionnaire to detect potentially life-threatening emergencies in gynecology

Cyrille Huchon[1,2*], Alexandre Dumont[2,3], Anne Chantry[4], Bruno Falissard[5] and Arnaud Fauconnier[1,2]

Abstract

Objective: Acute pelvic pain is a common reason for emergency room visits that can indicate a potentially life-threatening emergency (PLTE). Our objective here was to develop a triage process for PLTE based on a self-assessment questionnaire for gynecologic emergencies (SAQ-GE) in patients experiencing acute pelvic pain.

Methods: In this multicenter prospective observational study, all gynecological emergency room patients seen for acute pelvic pain between September 2006 and April 2008 completed the SAQ-GE after receiving appropriate analgesics. Diagnostic procedures were ordered without knowledge of questionnaire replies. Laparoscopy was the reference standard for diagnosing PLTE; other diagnoses were based on algorithms. In two-thirds of the population, SAQ-GE items significantly associated with PLTEs ($P < 0.05$) by univariate analysis were used to develop a decision tree by recursive partitioning; the remaining third served for validation.

Results: Of 344 derivation-set patients and 172 validation-set patients, 96 and 49 had PLTEs, respectively. Items significantly associated with PLTEs were vomiting, sudden onset of pain, and pain to palpation. Sensitivity of the decision tree based on these three features was 87.5% (95% confidence interval (95% CI), 81%-94%) in the derivation set and 83.7% in the validation set. Derivation of the decision tree provided probabilities of PLTE of 13% (95% CI, 6%-19%) in the low-risk group, 27% (95% CI, 20%-33%) in the intermediate-risk group and 62% (95% CI, 48%-76%) in the high-risk group, ruling out PLTE with a specificity of 92.3%; (95% CI, 89%-96%). In the validation dataset, PLTE probabilities were 16.3% in the low-risk group, 30.6% in the intermediate-risk group, and 44% in the high-risk group, ruling out the diagnosis of PLTE with a specificity of 88.6%.

Conclusion: A simple triage model based on a standardized questionnaire may assist in the early identification of patients with PLTEs among patients seen in the gynecology emergency room for acute pelvic pain.

Keywords: Gynecologic emergencies, Triage, Sensitivity, Questionnaire

Introduction

Acute pelvic pain is the leading reason for gynecological emergency room visits [1]. However, only a minority of these patients require emergency surgery. Thus, in a study of 205 patients seen at the gynecological emergency room of a French hospital in 2011, only 24 (12%) required hospital admission and 9 (4.5%) surgical treatment [2]. The early identification of patients with potentially life-threatening emergencies (PLTEs) requiring prompt surgical treatment is crucial [3].

In general emergency rooms, nurses typically prioritize patients to ensure that those with serious conditions are seen first by the emergency physicians. Triage scales such as the Emergency Severity Index [4] are used to determine whether medical care is required immediately, within a few minutes, within the next hour, or can be delayed. However, these scales are not well suited to gynecological emergencies [5], in which the main challenge consists in identifying patients with PLTEs, whose condition may not be immediately alarming but may

* Correspondence: cyrillehuchon@yahoo.fr
[1]Service de gynécologie & obstétrique, CHI Poissy-St-Germain, 10 rue du champ Gaillard, BP 3082 78303, Poissy CEDEX, France
[2]Equipe d'accueil EA 7285 « Risques, cliniques et sécurité en santé des femmes et en santé périnatale », Université Versailles-Saint-Quentin en Yvelines, 78000 Versailles, France

deteriorate rapidly [3]. Examples of these PLTEs, presenting with acute pelvic pain as a common signal precursor, include ectopic pregnancy [3,6], adnexal torsion [7] or tuboovarian abscess [8] which can lead to hemodynamic instability, organ failures, severe morbidity and death. Triage tools specifically designed for gynecological emergencies may be useful to rapidly identify patients in whom endovaginal ultrasonography by a gynecologist or radiologist may detect a condition requiring prompt treatment, thus protecting the patient from life-threatening or function-threatening events [6,8,9].

A self-assessment questionnaire for gynecological emergencies (SAQ-GE) recently developed by our group for the assessment of acute pelvic pain in women with gynecologic emergencies has been used to build clinical prediction rules for tubal rupture complicating ectopic pregnancy [10] and for adnexal torsion [11]. Our objective here was to develop and validate a clinical prediction rules for identifying PLTEs in emergency room patients with acute pelvic pain, based on SAQ-GE items.

Methods

Ethical aspects

The study was approved by the French Department of Higher Education and Research (n°06.336) and by the French National Committee for Information Technology and Individual Liberties (n°906253).

Study design and setting

We conducted a prospective multicenter study in five gynecology departments in the Paris metropolitan area, France. Four departments were in teaching hospitals (Poissy-Saint Germain en Laye, Créteil, Port-Royal, and Louis Mourier) and one was in a general hospital (Versailles).

Selection of Participants

From September 2006 to April 2008, all patients at least 18 years of age who presented to study-center gynecological emergency rooms with acute pelvic pain were eligible to complete the SAQ-GE on a voluntary basis. Exclusion criteria were a history of chronic pelvic pain, neurological or psychiatric disease, hemodynamic instability, and no knowledge of French. Patients with a verbal 11-point numerical rating scale (NRS) pain score lower than 1 and those with bartholinitis or breast pain were excluded.

Self-Assessment Questionnaire for Gynecological Emergencies (SAQ-GE)

The SAQ-GE was developed using a qualitative method [12] and advice from a panel of French experts, as reported in detail elsewhere [10,11]. The 89 items cover six domains: (i) qualitative description of pain, (ii) intensity of pain, (iii) location and (iv) time-course of pain, (v) vaginal bleeding, and (vi) other signs.

The SAQ-GE was completed by the patients after appropriate initial pain management and before diagnostic investigations or surgery. The nurses collected the completed questionnaires, which were not made available to the physicians. Thus, in this non-interventional study, all diagnostic and therapeutic decisions were made without knowledge of the questionnaire replies.

Methods and measurements

The final diagnosis was the diagnosis at hospital discharge established based on the physical examination, abdominal and endovaginal ultrasound, routine biology (if needed), computed tomography (CT) of the abdomen and pelvis (if needed), and surgical procedures (if needed: laparoscopy, dilatation and curettage, or diagnostic hysteroscopy). The diagnosis of ectopic pregnancy was based on laparoscopy or on an algorithm [13,14], with laparoscopy being performed when a complication was suspected (i.e., abundant hemoperitoneum with active bleeding and/or tubal rupture), as well as in patients with contraindications to medical treatment. Pelvic inflammatory disease was diagnosed based either on laparoscopy, if deemed necessary, or on noninvasive diagnostic models [15,16]. Other diagnoses based on surgical findings were abundant hemoperitoneum related to ovarian cyst rupture, adnexal torsion, appendicitis, and intestinal obstruction.

Among patients who did not undergo emergency laparoscopy, those who were pregnant were followed until a definitive diagnostic was made [17]. In nonpregnant patients, when the findings of all examinations were deemed normal and the pain subsided with appropriate analgesia by the end of the visit or hospitalization, a diagnosis of idiopathic acute pelvic pain was made. After discharge, patients were encouraged to return to the gynecological emergency room in the event of pain recurrence.

Outcomes

For the purpose of the study, patients were classified according to whether they had a prospectively recorded diagnosis of PLTE. PLTEs were defined as gynecological or nongynecological disorders causing acute pain and associated with a high risk of complications likely to cause residual impairments, severe morbidity, or death within a short period in the absence of appropriate emergency surgical or radiological treatment [3]. This definition included (i) ectopic pregnancy with tubal rupture or active bleeding or fetal cardiac activity or hemoperitoneum exceeding 300 mL [9,18]; (ii) complicated pelvic inflammatory disease with tuboovarian abscess or pelvic peritonitis [8,15,19]; (iii) adnexal torsion [11]; (iv) hemoperitoneum exceeding 300 mL due to rupture of hemorrhagic ovarian cysts or other gynecological causes (uterine rupture in the first trimester of pregnancy, rupture of a pedunculated uterine fibroid, rupture of an arteriovenous malformation, or uterine perforation); (v) appendicitis; and (vi) intestinal obstruction.

Analysis

We randomly assessed two-thirds of the patients to the derivation dataset and the remaining third to the validation dataset. All statistical tests were done using Stata 11.0 (Stata Corp., College Station, TX, USA).

SAQ-GE replies of patients with a final diagnosis of PLTE were compared to those of the other patients by univariate analysis using Pearson's chi-square test or Fisher's exact test. Variables significantly associated with PLTE with P values <0.05 were classified as possible predictors. For each of these variables, we computed sensitivity, specificity, the positive likelihood ratio (Lr+) and negative likelihood ratio (Lr-), and the crude diagnostic odds ratio with their 95% confidence interval (95% CI).

Variables significantly associated with PLTEs by univariate analysis were used for multivariable analysis by recursive partitioning to create a decision tree based on the best combination of variables. The decision tree identified groups at high, intermediate, and low risk for PLTEs based on the sequential Lr values [20]. When a data was missing for a patient, it was considered absent. For each of the three groups, we computed the probability of PLTE with the 95% CI. Sensitivity of the decision tree was defined as the number of patients with PLTEs in the high- and intermediate-risk groups over the total number of patients with PLTEs.

Finally, we assessed the performance of the decision tree in the validation dataset.

Results

Characteristics of the study patients

At the five study centers, 574 of about 992 eligible patients completed the SAQ-GE. Among them, 516 met our inclusion criteria and were entered into the study. A final diagnosis of PLTE was made in 145 (28.1%) patients. Table 1 lists the main patient characteristics and diagnoses in the overall population of 516 patients, of whom 344 were randomly allocated to the derivation dataset and 172 to the validation dataset. PLTEs were diagnosed in 96 (27.9%) derivation-dataset patients and 49 (28.5%) validation-dataset patients. Patient characteristics were not significantly different in the two datasets (data not shown).

Main results

Table 2 reports the results of the univariate analysis. None of the SAQ-GE items had Lr + values greater than 4 or Lr- values lower than 0.25.

Figure 1 shows the decision tree, in which three items are taken into account sequentially: vomiting, sudden onset of pain, and pain upon self-palpation. Patients with no vomiting or pain upon palpation are at low risk, with a probability of PLTE of 13% (95% CI, 6%-19%). The intermediate risk group is defined based on either no vomiting but pain upon self-palpation or vomiting but no sudden onset of pain; the probability of a PLTE is 27% (95% CI, 20%-33%). In the high-risk group, with both vomiting and sudden-onset pain, the probability of a PLTE is 62% (95% CI, 48%-76%), ruling out PLTE with a specificity of 92.3%; (95% CI, 89%-96%) (Figure 1). Sensitivity of the decision tree was 87.5% (95% CI, 81%-94%).

In the validation dataset, the diagnostic performance characteristics of our decision tree were similar to those in the derivation dataset, with most of the validation-dataset values being within the 95% CI for the derivation-dataset values. The PLTE probability was 16.3% in the low-risk group, 30.6% in the intermediate-risk group, and 44% in the high-risk group, ruling out the diagnosis of PLTE with a specificity of 88.6%. Sensitivity of the decision tree was 83.7% in the validation dataset.

Discussion

We built a decision tree for triaging women presenting to the emergency room with acute pelvic pain using a standardized yes/no items from a self-questionnaire. The decision tree relies on three simple items: vomiting, pain upon self-palpation, and sudden onset of pain. It separates three groups of patients, at low, intermediate, and high risk for PLTEs, respectively. Sensitivity of the decision tree was 87.5% (95% CI, 81%-94%).

The time to management of gynecological emergencies is the sum of four periods: time from symptom onset to arrival; time from arrival to the first medical assessment; time from the first medical assessment to the diagnosis, which usually required pelvic and endovaginal ultrasonography by a specialist [21]; (iv) and time from the diagnosis to the implementation of specific treatment, if any is needed. Our decision tree may diminish the time from arrival to the first medical assessment by helping the nurses to identify patients with suspected PLTEs. In a previous study, mean time from arrival to ultrasonography was 84 minutes in a gynecological emergency room, and far longer times were found in general emergency rooms [2]. Then, this decision tree can speed up the use of ultrasound examination that has proven to be reliable for the diagnosis of surgical emergencies [22].

Most triage tools use clinical decision rules that separate patients into five triage categories depending on the acceptable time to medical management [4,23]. These rules are usually established by consensus among experts, both for the triage category and for the acceptable time to medical management [23]. We used a different

Table 1 Characteristics and main diagnoses in the study patients

	Overall population N = 516	PLTE N = 145	Other N = 371
Age in years, mean ± SD	31.6 ± 7.7	30.7 ± 7.9	31.9 ± 7.6
Gravidity, median [range]	2 [0–11]	2 [0–9]	2 [0–11]
Parity, median [range]	1 [0–7]	1 [0–4]	1 [0–7]
Contraception, n/N (%)	136/504 (27.0)	40/141 (28.4)	96/363 (26.5)
NRS pain score at admission, mean ± SD	6.4 ± 2.7	6.8 ± 2.7	6.2 ± 2.7*
Diagnosis			
Ectopic pregnancy, n (%)	148 (28.7)	77 (53.1)	71 (19.1)
Pelvic inflammatory disease, n (%)	73 (14.1)	25 (17.2)	48 (12.9)
Uncomplicated ovarian cyst, n (%)	70 (13.6)	NA	70 (18.9)
Adnexal torsion, n (%)	31 (6.0)	31 (21.4)	NA
Appendicitis, n (%)	6 (1.2)	6 (4.1)	NA
Ruptured cyst with hemoperitoneum > 300 mL, n (%)	5 (1.0)	5 (3.5)	NA
Miscarriage, n (%)	79 (15.3)	NA	79 (21.3)
Myoma necrobiosis, n (%)	15 (2.9)	NA	15 (4.0)
Urologic disease, n (%)	10 (1.9)	NA	10 (2.7)
Ovarian hyperstimulation, n (%)	7 (1.4)	NA	7 (1.9)
Other diagnosis, n (%)	72 (13.9)	1 (0.7)‡	71 (19.1)

PLTE, potentially life-threatening emergencies; NRS, numerical rating scale for pain severity; NA, not applicable; SD, standard deviation.
*$P < 0.05$, Student's t test; ‡Intestinal obstruction.

approach, using statistical data to separate the patient groups and focusing on the diagnosis rather than on acceptable time to management. Our classification system could serve as a reference for classifying gynecological emergencies. Our next step will be to determine the acceptable time to medical management in each of the three groups, before validating the decision tree in other settings and evaluating its impact in clinical practice [23]. Moreover, our triage tool is not expensive. Then, it could be used, after scaling up, in developing countries where institutional and human resources are often low, in order to decrease women's severe morbidity.

Table 2 SAQ-GE items significantly associated ($P < 0.05$) with PLTE by univariate analysis in the derivation dataset

	Total, n/N* (%)	PLTE, n/N (%)	Other, n/N (%)	Se (%)	Sp (%)	LR+	LR-	DOR [95% CI]
Prior surgery for ovarian cyst	53/338 (15.6)	23/93 (24.7)	30/245 (12.2)	24.7	87.8	2.0	0.86	2.4 [1.3-4.4]
No history of pain of similar intensity	175/336 (52.1)	65/95 (58.4)	110/241 (45.6)	58.4	54.4	1.3	0.76	2.6 [1.5-4.3]
Pain on one side	184/337 (54.6)	69/92 (75.0)	115/245 (46.9)	75.0	53.1	1.6	0.47	3.4 [2.0-5.9]
Ovarian pain	210/337 (62.3)	69/92 (75.0)	141/245 (57.6)	75.0	42.4	1.3	0.59	2.2 [1.3-3.8]
Pain radiating to the stomach	59/336 (17.6)	23/93 (24.7)	36/243 (14.8)	24.7	85.2	1.7	0.88	1.9 [1.0-3.4]
Sudden onset of pain	170/333 (51.0)	61/94 (64.9)	109/239 (45.6)	64.9	54.4	1.4	0,64	2.2 [1.3-3.6]
Pain exacerbated by movements	248/337 (73.6)	81/94 (86.2)	167/243 (68.7)	86.2	31.3	1.3	0.44	2.8 [1.5-5.5]
Pain upon self-palpation	222/335 (66.3)	75/91 (82.4)	147/244 (60.3)	82.4	39.7	1.4	0.44	3.1 [1.7-5.7]
Vomiting	88/338 (26.0)	44/94 (46.8)	44/244 (18.0)	46.8	82.0	2.6	0.65	4.0 [2.3-6.9]
Radiating pain	35/309 (11.3)	19/87 (21.8)	16/222 (16.2)	21.8	83.8	1.3	0.93	3.6 [1.7-7.5]
Penetrating pain	114/329 (34.6)	44/92 (47.8)	70/237 (29.5)	47.8	70.5	1.6	0.74	2.2 [1.3-3.6]
Twisting pain	72/329 (21.9)	34/93 (36.6)	38/236 (16.1)	36.6	83.9	2.3	0.76	3.0 [1.7-5.3]
Pain leading to syncope	25/332 (7.5)	12/94 (12.8)	13/238 (5.5)	12.8	94.5	2.3	0.92	2.5 [1.1-5.8]
Pain with sensation of oppression	82/333 (24.6)	34/94 (36.2)	48/239 (20.1)	36.2	79.9	1.8	0.80	2.3 [1.3-3.8]
Torturous pain	68/333 (20.4	29/94 (30.8)	39/239 (16.3)	30.8	83.7	1.9	0.83	2.3 [1.3-4.0]

*Because of missing data, the total may be different from 344.
PLTE, potentially life-threatening emergency; Se, sensitivity; Sp, specificity; LR, likelihood ratio; DOR, diagnostic odds ratio; 95% CI, 95% confidence interval.

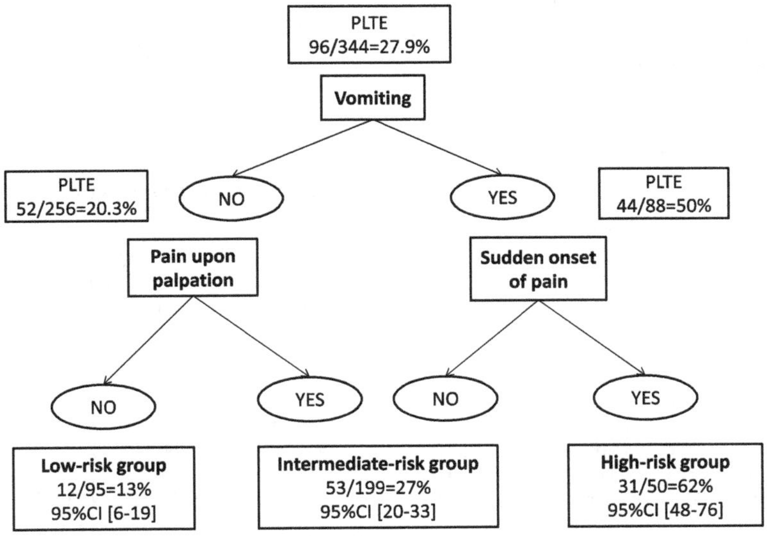

Figure 1 Decision tree for classifying the risk of potentially-life-threatening emergency in patients presenting to gynecological emergency rooms with acute pelvic pain.

A rigorous statistical approach was used to develop our decision tree, in contrast to the methods generally used by consensus panels [23]. Decision trees developed using recursive partitioning are simple to use. No computations are needed to determine the risk group to which a given patient belongs. In addition, recursive partitioning has been proven equivalent to logistic regression in terms of diagnostic efficiency [24,25]. We also found that recursive partitioning and logistic regression performed similarly in our datasets (data not shown).

The high predictive values of our model may seem surprising in the light of pathophysiological considerations. Our definition of PLTE encompassed a variety of conditions that differ regarding the pathophysiological mechanisms responsible for pain [26,27]. However, when we built the SAQ-GE, our main hypothesis was that words used by women to describe acute pelvic pain and concomitant symptoms reflect an underlying sensory experience shared by various pathological and anatomical abnormalities [27] and not the symptoms of a specific disease. For instance, vomiting strongly predicted both tubal rupture [10] and adnexal torsion [28]. Most gynecological emergencies may involve the same general protective mechanisms triggered in response to danger, such as activation of the autonomic nervous system [26,27]. Thus, acute pelvic pain and other symptoms as described by women may serve as warning signals that can provide diagnostic orientation.

Limitations

One limitation of our study is related to our definition of PLTE. This definition was not established by consensus among a panel of experts [29]. Nevertheless, our definition of PLTE is consistent with clinical reality in patients with gynecological emergencies. For instance, ectopic pregnancy can be life threatening in the event of tubal rupture with hemodynamic shock from massive intraabdominal bleeding. In this situation, substandard care is often related to misdiagnosis [3,6]. We extended this concept to all gynecological emergencies that may not pose an immediate threat but may worsen rapidly. We used acute pelvic pain as the warning signal for such situations. Our definition of PLTE is similar to that used pragmatically in general emergency rooms with the goal of identifying conditions likely to cause serious subsequent manifestations (http://www.acem.org.au/media/policies_and_guidelines/G24_Implementation__ATS.pdf). In patients with PLTEs as defined for our study, an earlier and more accurate diagnosis allows the rapid provision of appropriate care, thereby improving patient outcomes in terms of both morbidity and mortality.

Another limitation may be overfitting of the decision tree to our data. However, the validation study in the third of our population not used to build the decision tree showed similar diagnostic performance characteristics and substantial overfitting was also prevented by constructing the SAQ-GE in a preliminary study involving different patients and experts.

Conclusion

In summary, our decision tree is the first dedicated to the diagnosis of PLTEs with a 87.5% sensitivity. In addition, it relies on only three simple items of a self-questionnaire. We plan to study the extent to which our decision tree decreases time to appropriate management and improves outcomes in patients presenting with acute pelvic pain to crowded emergency rooms.

Competing interest

The authors declare that they have no competing interests.

Authors' contributions

CH and AF wrote the manuscript. AF, AD and BF designed the study. AAC, CH and AF collected the datas. CH, AD and AF performed the statistical analysis.

Funding

Assistance Publique-Hôpitaux de Paris (AP-HP).

Author details

[1]Service de gynécologie & obstétrique, CHI Poissy-St-Germain, 10 rue du champ Gaillard, BP 3082 78303, Poissy CEDEX, France. [2]Equipe d'accueil EA 7285 « Risques, cliniques et sécurité en santé des femmes et en santé périnatale », Université Versailles-Saint-Quentin en Yvelines, 78000 Versailles, France. [3]UMR 216, IRD Paris Descartes, 4 Avenue de l'Observatoire, Paris - Université, 75 006 Paris Descartes, France. [4]INSERM, UMR S953, Epidemiological Research Unit on Perinatal Health and Women's and Children's Health, Hôpital Cochin, Paris, France. [5]INSERM UMR S669, Université Paris Sud, Paris, France.

References

1. Kontoravdis A, Chryssikopoulos A, Hassiakos D, Liapis A, Zourlas PA: **The diagnostic value of laparoscopy in 2365 patients with acute and chronic pelvic pain.** *Int J Gynecol Obstet* 1996, **52**:243–248.
2. Alouini S, Mesnard L, Coly S, Dolique M, Lemaire B: **[Gynecological emergencies: etiology and degree of gravity.].** *J Gynecol Obstet Biol Reprod (Paris)* 2012, **41**:48–54.
3. Abbott J, Emmans LS, Lowenstein SR: **Ectopic pregnancy: ten common pitfalls in diagnosis.** *Am J Emerg Med* 1990, **8**:515–522.
4. Elshove-Bolk J, Mencl F, van Rijswijck BT, Simons MP, van Vugt AB: **Validation of the Emergency Severity Index (ESI) in self-referred patients in a European emergency department.** *Emerg Med J* 2007, **24**:170–174.
5. Gerdtz MF, Chu M, Collins M, *et al*: **Factors influencing consistency of triage using the Australasian Triage Scale: implications for guideline development.** *Emerg Med Australas* 2009, **21**:277–285.
6. van Mello NM, Zietse CS, Mol F, *et al*: **Severe maternal morbidity in ectopic pregnancy is not associated with maternal factors but may be associated with quality of care.** *Fertil Steril* 2012, **97**:623–629.
7. Huchon C, Fauconnier A: **Adnexal torsion: a literature review.** *Eur J Obstet Gynecol Reprod Biol* 2010, **150**:8–12.
8. Dewitt J, Reining A, Allsworth JE, Peipert JF: **Tuboovarian abscesses: is size associated with duration of hospitalization & complications?** *Obstet Gynecol Int* 2010, **2010**:847041.
9. Popowski T, Huchon C, Toret-Labeeuw F, Chantry AA, Aegerter P, Fauconnier A: **Hemoperitoneum assessment in ectopic pregnancy.** *Int J Gynaecol Obstet* 2012, **116**:97–100.
10. Huchon C, Panel P, Kayem G, *et al*: **Is a standardized questionnaire useful for tubal rupture screening in patients with ectopic pregnancy?** *Acad Emerg Med* 2012, **19**:24–30.
11. Huchon C, Panel P, Kayem G, Schmitz T, Nguyen T, Fauconnier A: **Does this woman have adnexal torsion?** *Hum Reprod* 2012, **27**:2359–2364.
12. Colaizzi PF: **Psychological Research as the Phenomenologist Views It.** In *Existential-Phenomenological Alternatives for Psychology.* Edited by Valle RS, King G. New York: Oxford University Press; 1978:48–71.
13. Ankum WM, Van der Veen F, Hamerlynck JV, Lammes FB: **Transvaginal sonography and human chorionic gonadotrophin measurements in suspected ectopic pregnancy: a detailed analysis of a diagnostic approach.** *Hum Reprod* 1993, **8**:1307–1311.
14. Mol BW, van Der Veen F, Bossuyt PM: **Implementation of probabilistic decision rules improves the predictive values of algorithms in the diagnostic management of ectopic pregnancy.** *Hum Reprod* 1999, **14**:2855–2862.
15. Kahn JG, Walker CK, Washington E, Landers DV, Sweet RL: **Diagnosing pelvic inflammatory disease. A comprehensive analysis and consideration for devellopping a new model.** *JAMA* 1991, **226**:2594–2604.
16. Soper DE: **Pelvic inflammatory disease.** *Infect Dis Clin* 1994, **4**:821–840.
17. Barnhart KT, Fay CA, Suescum M, *et al*: **Clinical factors affecting the accuracy of ultrasonography in symptomatic first-trimester pregnancy.** *Obstet Gynecol* 2011, **117**:299–306.
18. Fauconnier A, Mabrouk A, Salomon LJ, Bernard JP, Ville Y: **Ultrasound assessment of haemoperitoneum in ectopic pregnancy: derivation of a prediction model.** *World J Emerg Surg* 2007, **2**:23.
19. Soper DE: **Pelvic inflammatory disease.** *Obstet Gynecol* 2010, **116**:419–428.
20. Buckley RG, King KJ, Disney JD, Ambroz PK, Gorman JD, Klausen JH: **Derivation of a clinical prediction model for the emergency department diagnosis of ectopic pregnancy.** *Acad Emerg Med* 1998, **5**:951–960.
21. Bignardi T, Burnet S, Alhamdan D, *et al*: **Management of women referred to an acute gynecology unit: impact of an ultrasound-based model of care.** *Ultrasound Obstet Gynecol* 2010, **35**:344–348.
22. Toret-Labeeuw F, Huchon C, Popowski T, Chantry A, Dumont A, Fauconnier A: **Routine ultrasound examination by OB/GYN residents increase the accuracy of diagnosis for emergency surgery in gynecology.** *World J Emerg Surg* 2013, **8**(1):16.
23. Moll HA: **Challenges in the validation of triage systems at emergency departments.** *J Clin Epidemiol* 2010, **63**:384–388.
24. Rouzier R, Coutant C, Lesieur B, *et al*: **Direct comparison of logistic regression and recursive partitioning to predict chemotherapy response of breast cancer based on clinical pathological variables.** *Breast Cancer Res Treat* 2009, **117**:325–331.
25. Shariat SF, Karakiewicz PI, Suardi N, Kattan MW: **Comparison of nomograms with other methods for predicting outcomes in prostate cancer: a critical analysis of the literature.** *Clin Cancer Res* 2008, **14**:4400–4407.
26. Abbott J: **Pelvic pain: lesson from anatomy and physiology.** *J Emerg Med* 1990, **8**:441–447.
27. Lamvu G, Steege JF: **The anatomy and neurophysiology of pelvic pain.** *J Minim Invasive Gynecol* 2006, **13**:516–522.
28. Houry D, Abbott JT: **Ovarian torsion: a fifteen-year review.** *Ann Emerg Med* 2001, **38**:156–159.
29. Milholland AV, Wheeler SG, Heieck JJ: **Medical assessment by a Delphi group opinion technic.** *N Engl J Med* 1973, **288**:1272–1275.

Clinical value of total white blood cells and neutrophil counts in patients with suspected appendicitis

Zuhoor K Al-gaithy*

Abstract

Introduction: Acute appendicitis (AA) is common surgical problem associated with acute-phase reaction. Blood tests role in decision-making process is unclear. This retrospective study aimed to determine diagnostic value of preoperative evaluation of white blood cells (WBCs) and neutrophils and its value in predicting AA severity.

Methods: Medical records of 456 patients who underwent appendectomy during 4-years period were retrospectively reviewed. Patients were subdivided according to histological finding into: normal appendix (n = 29), uncomplicated inflamed appendix (n = 350), complicated appendicitis (n = 77). Diagnostic performances of WBCs and neutrophils were analyzed using receiver operating characteristic (ROC) curves.

Results: WBCs and neutrophils counts were higher in patients with inflamed and complicated appendix than normal appendix and in complicated than inflamed appendix. In patients, WBCs count 9.400 × 10^3/mL had sensitivity of 76.81%, specificity of 65.52%, positive predictive value (PPV) of 97.0%, negative predictive value (NPV) of 16.1%, positive likelihood ratio [LR(+)] of 2.23, negative LR(−) of 0.35. Neutrophil count 7.540 × 10^3/mL had sensitivity of 70.96%, specificity of 65.52%, PPV of 96.8%, NPV of 13.3%, LR(+) of 2.06, LR(−) of 0.44. Areas under ROC curve were 0.701, 0.680 for elevated WBCs and neutrophils count.

Conclusions: Clinicians should not rely on either elevated WBCs or neutrophils count as appendicitis indicator as clinical data are superior in decision-making appendectomy.

Keywords: Acute appendicitis, Diagnosis, White blood cells, Histological diagnosis, Neutrophil count, Receiver operating characteristic curves

Introduction

Acute appendicitis (AA) is one of the most common abdominal emergencies. Although patients with AA often present with a characteristic symptom complex and physical findings, atypical presentations are common. Missed or delayed diagnosis can lead to increased rates of perforation and morbidity [1]. The clinical diagnosis of AA is difficult, and management errors are frequent, with rates of negative explorations reaching 20% to 30% [2]. Despite the wide use of imaging techniques, appendicitis remains a challenging diagnosis [3].

Patients with suspected appendicitis are mainly managed on the basis of their disease history and physical examination; the value of laboratory examinations is controversial. Some works have assessed the diagnostic accuracy of different inflammatory markers in appendicitis with heterogeneous designs and results including: total white blood cells (WBCs), granulocytes, C-reactive protein, leukocyte elastase activity, D-lactate, phospholipase A2 and interleukine-6 [4-6]. Studies have shown inconsistent information regarding the use of WBCs count and differential in AA diagnosis. Although most studies show an association between elevated WBCs count in appendicitis diagnosis, its significance varies greatly [7-10]. Another question that has been raised is whether a normal WBCs count and differential can adequately rule out a diagnosis of appendicitis. There have been reports of high negative predictive values (NPVs >90%) for normal WBCs count and differential [7,9].

Correspondence: zkngaithy@hotmail.com
Department of Surgery, King Abdulaziz University, P.O. Box 80215, Jeddah 21589, Saudi Arabia

The aim of this retrospective study was to assess diagnostic value of total WBCs and neutrophils counts in patients who underwent appendectomy due to suspicious of AA. Using receiver-operating characteristic (ROC) curves, sensitivity, specificity, NPV, positive predictive value (PPV), and likelihood ratios (LR) were calculated by correlating the preoperative WBCs and neutrophil counts with histological diagnosis. In addition, this study will attempt to determine cutoff point for WBCs and neutrophils counts with best sensitivity and specificity for determination of acute appendicitis.

Material and methods

Four hundred and fifty six patients (273 male and 183 female) who underwent appendectomy with a clinical diagnosis of AA in Surgery Department at King Abdulaziz Medical Center, Jeddah, Saudi Arabia were recruited in this retrospective study between January 2003 and January 2007. The diagnosis of AA was established by history, clinical examination, and laboratory tests including WBCs and neutrophil counts. Demographic, symptoms, signs, surgical procedures, and histopathological results of appendix examination were recorded. Patients who underwent incidental appendectomy as part of another procedure, and patients on steroids or immunosuppressive medications excluded from the study. According to the results of histopathological examination of the removed appendix, patients were divided into 3 groups, group (1) normal appendix (no pathological diagnosis) (n = 29); group (2) with uncomplicated inflamed appendicitis (n = 350) and group (3) with complicated appendicitis (n = 77) (perforated and gangrenous). The ethical committee of King Abdelaziz University approved the study.

Laboratory tests were carried on admission to hospital before antibiotics administered. WBCs count and differential were measured by an automated hematology analyzer counter (SE-9000; Sysmex, Kobe, Japan). All the excised appendices were underwent histopathological examination.

Data analysis

The statistical analysis was performed using MedCalc for Windows, version 5.0 (MedCalc Software, Mariakerke, Belgium) and Statistical Package for the Social Sciences for Windows, version 12.0 (SPSS Inc., Chicago, IL, USA). The data were expressed as mean +/− stander deviation [SD] (range) or number (%) as appropriate. Statistical analysis was done with one-way analysis of variance to compare data between groups. For comparison of 2 groups unpaired Student "t test" and Chi square test were used for parametric and non-parametric parameters, respectively. For describing the diagnostic properties of WBCs and neutrophils counts, we used the area under ROC curve (AUC) and likelihood ratio (LR) [11]. AUC of 1.00 indicates perfect discriminating power while area of 0.50 indicates absence of discriminating power. LR (+) is the ratio of the frequency of a finding among the diseased patients (true-positive rate) and among the non-diseased patients (false-positive rate). A true diagnostic test usually has an LR >10, and an exclusion test has a LR < 0.1. All results were reported with 95% confidence intervals (95% CIs). A P value of < 0.05 was considered statistically significant.

Results

Table 1 showed patients' demographic characteristics. The number of males were significantly higher than females (273 versus 183, P < 0.0001). Regarding type of operation, 406 patients underwent opened appendectomy, 45 patients had laparoscopic appendectomy and 5 had laparoscopic converted to open with significant difference between them P < 0.0001.

Table 2 showed the clinical and laboratory characteristics of patients subgroups according to the hisopathological findings. In normal, inflamed and complicated appendix, the type of pain was mainly localized 88,2%, 82.7%, 68.8% than generalized 13.8%, 18.3%, 31.2% with significant difference between groups P < 0.026. In normal, inflamed and complicated appendix, the duration of pain was mainly >12 hours, 75.9%, 88.3%, 98.7% than ≤12 hours, 24.1%, 11.8%, 1.3% with significant difference between patients subgroups P < 0.002. Fever was significantly higher in complicated than normal or inflamed appendix (64.9% versus 24.1% and 47.7%, P < 0.0001). WBCs and neutrophils counts were higher in inflamed

Table 1 Demographic characteristics of the patients

Parameters	All patients (n = 456)
Age (years)	23.25 ± 9.80 (6.00-61.00)
Gender	
Male	273 (59.9%)
Female	183 (40.1%)
Significance	***P* < 0.0001**
Operation type	
Open	406 (89.0%)
Laparoscopic	45 (9.9%)
Laparoscopic converted to open	5 (1.1%)
Significance	***P* < 0.0001**

Data are expressed as mean +/− SD (range) or number (%). Significant between variables was made using non parametric Chi-Square test.

Table 2 Clinical and laboratory characteristics of patient subgroups

Parameters	Normal appendix (*n* = 29, 6.4%)	Appendicitis (*n*= 427, 93.6%)		*P* -Value
		Inflamed (n = 350, 76.8%)	Complicated (n = 77, 16.9%)	
Pain type				**0.026**
Localized	25 (88.2%)	286 (81.7%)	53 (68.8%)	
Generalized	4 (13.8%)	64 (18.3%)	24 (31.2%)	
Pain duration				**0.002**
≤12 hours	7 (24.1%)	41 (11.8%)	1 (1.3%)	
>12hours	22 (75.9%)	309 (88.3%)	76 (98.7%)	
Symptoms & signs				
Vomiting	18 (62.1%)	268 (76.6%)	64 (83.1%)	0.072
Anorexia	17 (58.6%)	261 (74.6%)	54 (70.1%)	0.151
Nausea	14 (48.3%)	193 (55.1%)	44 (57.1%)	0.713
Fever	7 (24.1%)	167 (47.7%)	50 (64.9%)	**0.0001**
Diarrhea	2 (6.9%)	17 (4.9%)	3(3.9%)	0.812
Dysurea	2 (6.9%)	8 (2.3%)	4 (5.2%)	0.190
Laboratory investigations				
WBCs count ($\times 10^3$/mm^3)	10.67 ± 7.56	13.03 ± 4.94	14.34 ± 5.25	
	(4.10-35.70)	(2.90-29.60)	(2.20-33.60)	
*Significance		***P* <0.019**	***P* <0.001, ***P* <0.045**	
Neutrophil count ($\times 10^3$/mm^3)	7.95 ± 6.67	9.92 ± 4.88	11.74 ± 4.88	
	(1.10-30.93)	(0.20-27.10)	(1.70-24.67)	
*Significance		***P* <0.045**	***P* <0.001, ***P* <0.004**	

Data are expressed as mean +/− SD (range) or number (%). Significant between subgroups was made using Chi-Square test (P) for non-parametric parameters and *ANOVA test for parametric parameters, *P* significance between all groups, **P* significance versus controls, ***P* significance versus inflamed appendix.

($P < 0.019$, $P < 0.045$) and complicated ($P < 0.001$, $P < 0.001$) than normal appendix and in complicated than inflamed appendix ($P < 0.045$, $P < 0.004$).

Cut-off values, at which the greatest sum of sensitivity and specificity was obtained, in WBCs and neutrophils counts were 9.400×10^3 and 7.540×10^3, respectively in all patients with appendicitis versus normal appendix; 9.400×10^3 and 8.080×10^3, respectively in patients with inflamed versus normal appendix and 11.100×10^3 and 7.540×10^3, respectively in patients with complicated versus normal appendix. At these cutoff points, sensitivity, specificity, PPV, NPV, LR (+) and LR (−) for WBCs and neutrophils were for normal versus all abnormal appendix for WBCs: 76.81, 65.52%, 97.0%, 16.1%, 2.23%, 0.35%; for neutrophils: 70.96%, 65.52%, 96.8%, 13.3%. 2.06%. 0.44%; for normal versus inflamed appendix for WBCs: 75.43%, 65.52%, 96.4%, 18.1%, 2.19%, 0.38%; for neutrophils: 65.43%, 68.97%, 96.2%. 14.2%, 2.11, 0.50%; for normal versus complicated appendix for WBCs: 76.62%, 72.41%, 88.10%, 53.80%, 2.78%, 0.32%; for neutrophils: 81.82%, 65.52%, 86.30%. 57.60%, 2.37, 0.28% (Table 3; Figures 1, 2 and 3).

Discussion

Although the incidence of AA appears to have been waning slightly over the past few decades, it remains a frequent cause of acute abdominal pain and urgent operative intervention. The analysis of a patient with possible appendicitis can be divided into 3 parts: history, physical examination, and routine laboratory and radiological tests. The pain was reported in 456 (100%) of our cases which was mostly localized than generalized and mostly more than 12 hours. In this respect, Mughal and Soomro [12] have noted pain in 66.7% of patients while, Soomro [13] reported abdominal pain in 98.27% of appendicitis patients. Pain involves whole abdomen when there is perforation leading to peritonitis [14]. This was also true in this series as in complicated appendicitis; generalized pain was more than in normal or inflamed appendicitis. In our cases, second most common presenting symptom was vomiting 76.8% followed by anorexia72.9%, nausea 55.0%, fever 49.1%, diarrhea 4.8% then dysuea 3.1%. Salari and Binesh [15] reported anorexia in 84.48% of patients in pediatric age group while, Soomro [13] reported anorexia in 86.20% of patients. At

Table 3 Performance characteristics estimate of normal versus different groups

Parameters	Cutoff point	Sensitivity	Specificity	PPV	NPV	LR(+)	LR(−)
			normal versus all abnormal appendix (*n* = 456)				
WBCs count 95% CIs	9.400 X10^3	76.81 (72.5 - 80.7)	65.52 (45.7 - 82.1)	97.0 (4.6 - 98.6)	16.1 (10.0 - 24.0)	2.23 (1.7- 2.9)	0.35 (0.2 - 0.6)
Neutrophil count 95% CIs	7.540X10^3	70.96 (66.4 - 75.2)	65.52 (45.7 - 82.1)	96.8 (94.2 - 98.5)	13.3 (8.2 - 20.0)	2.06 (1.6 - 2.7)	0.44 (0.3 - 0.7)
			normal versus inflamed appendix (*n* = 379)				
WBCs count 95% CIs	9.400 X10^3	75.43 (70.6 - 79.8)	65.52 (45.7 - 82.1)	96.4 (93.4 - 98.2)	18.1 (11.2 - 26.9)	2.19 (1.7 - 2.9)	0.38 (0.2 - 0.6)
Neutrophil count 95% CIs	8.080X10^3	65.43 (60.2 - 70.4)	68.97 (49.2 - 84.7)	96.2 (92.9 - 98.3)	14.2 (8.9 - 21.1)	2.11 (1.6 - 2.7)	0.50 (0.3 - 0.9)
			normal versus complicated appendix (*n* = 106)				
WBCs count 95% CIs	11.100 X10^3	76.62 (65.6 - 85.5)	72.41 (52.8 - 87.3)	88.10 (77.8 - 94.7)	53.80 (37.2 - 69.9)	2.78 (2.1 - 3.6)	0.32 (0.2 - 0.7)
Neutrophil count 95% CIs	7.540X10^3	81.82 (71.4 - 89.7)	65.52 (45.7 - 82.1)	86.30 (76.2 - 93.2)	57.60 (38.9 - 74.8)	2.37 (1.8 - 3.2)	0.28 (0.1 - 0.6)

WBCs white blood cells, *95% CIs* 95% confidence intervals, *NPV* negative predictive value, *PPV* positive predictive value, *LR* likelihood ratio.

operation, we found 29 (6.4%) patients with normal appendix, 350 (76.8%) with inflamed appendix, 77 (16.9%) with complicated appendix. Soomro [13] reported that at operation 31 (53.44%) patients with simple appendicitis and 26 (44.82%) patients with complicated appendicitis. In literature the rate of perforated and gangrenous appendicitis has been quoted as 16-57% [14,16].

Acute appendicitis remains a challenging diagnosis. Almost one-third of patients have atypical clinical features. The wide use of ultra sonography and computer tomography scan has not effectively decreased the rate of perforated appendicitis or number of negative appendectomies in large population studies [3] despite the hopeful results of some case series in tertiary care academic hospitals [1,17]. Some authors have assessed the diagnostic value of inflammatory markers with varied designs and results [7,18-20]. Variety of designs explains the lack of evidence in the two meta-analysis published to date about inflammatory markers diagnostic utility [9,21]. Although, over the last few decades, several inflammation markers have been proposed to increase diagnostic accuracy in AA including phospholipase A2, [4] amyloid A, [22] leukocyte elastase, [23] neutrophil count, [9] several interleukins and cytokines, [24] WBCs and neutrophil counts are certainly the most widely used.

In this study, WBCs and neutrophil counts were significantly higher in patients with inflamed and complicated than normal appendix and in complicated than inflamed appendix. Several reports suggest that an elevated leukocyte count is usually the earliest laboratory test to indicate appendiceal inflammation, and most of the patients with acute appendicitis present with leukocytosis [25] despite several studies that acknowledge the limitations of

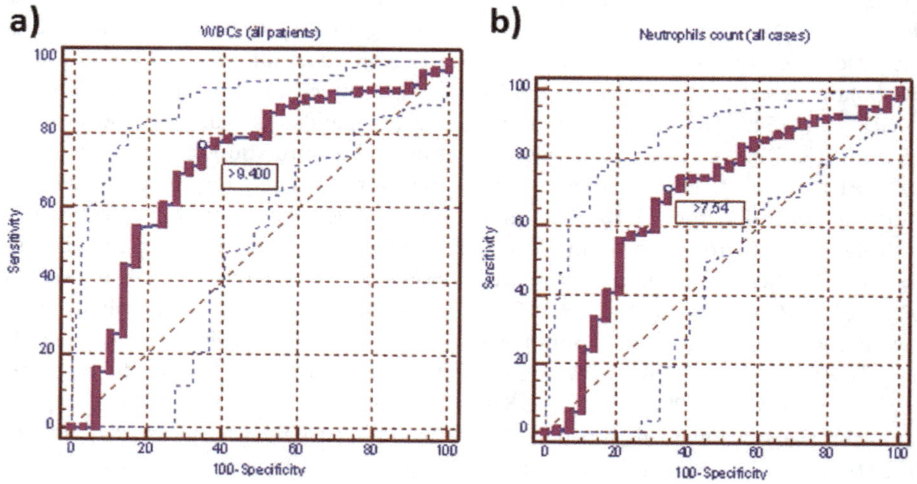

Figure 1 Receiver-operating characteristic curve (ROC) for white blood cells and neutrophil counts in all appendectomy patients. a) ROC for white blood cells in all appendectomy patients. ROC for white blood cell count of all appendectomy patients. Area under the curve (AUC) was 0.701 (standard error, 0.055; 95% CI =0.671-0.755). Ideal white blood cell count cutoff value was 9,400 cells/mm^3, this yields sensitivity of 76.8% and specificity of 65.5%. **b)** ROC for neutrophils count of all appendectomy patients. AUC is 0.680 (standard error, 0.056; 95% CI = 0.635-0.722). Neutrophils count ideal cutoff value was 7.540 ×10^3 cells/mm^3, this yields sensitivity of 71.0% and specificity of 65.5%.

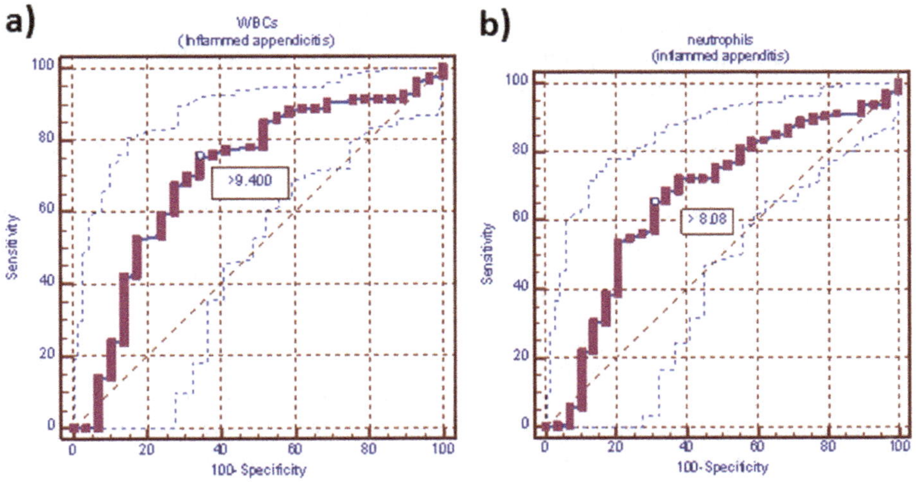

Figure 2 Receiver-operating characteristic curve (ROC) for white blood cells and neutrophil counts in inflamed appendicitis patients. a) ROC for white blood cells in inflamed appendicitis patients. Area under curve (AUC) is 0.704 (standard error, 0.055; 95% CI =0.655-0.749). White blood cell count ideal cutoff value was 9,400 $\times 10^3$ cells/mm^3; this yields sensitivity of 75.4% and specificity of 65.5%. **b)** ROC for neutrophils count in inflamed appendicitis patients. AUC was 0.664 (standard error, 0.056; 95% CI = 0.614-0.712). Neutrophils count ideal cutoff value was 8.080 $\times 10^3$ cells/mm^3, this cutoff value yields sensitivity of 65.4% and specificity of 69.0%.

this test [26,27]. Sack et al. [28].found that WBCs count was clearly elevated in children with phlegmonous and perforated appendicitis. Mughal and Soomro [12] found total leucocytes and neutrophil counts elevated in all their patients. Soomro [13] reported elevation of total leucocytes and neutrophils counts in 53.33% of their patients. Meanwhile, Yokoyama et al. [29] reported that WBCs counts and neutrophil percentage are not useful for surgical indication.

Previous studies assessing the relationship between WBCs count and appendicitis have their findings reported in a variety of ways, including comparing mean values for total WBCs count in patients with and without appendicitis, and variously using *P*-values, sensitivity, specificity, PPV and NPV [23,30]. These studies can be difficult to interpret, because both PPV and NPV depend on disease prevalence. Moreover, sensitivity and specificity alone do not allow clinicians to directly apply

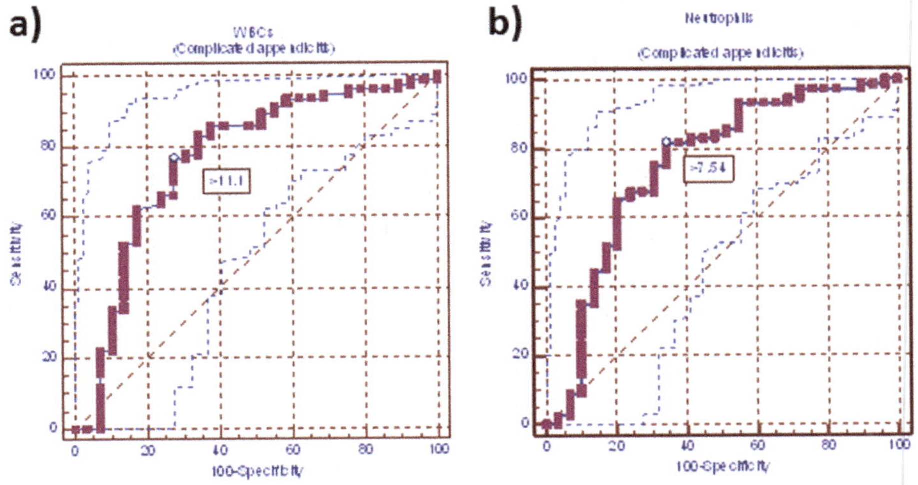

Figure 3 Receiver-operating characteristic curve (ROC) for white blood cells and neutrophil counts in complicated appendicitis patients. a) ROC curve for white blood cell count in complicated appendicitis patients. Area under curve (AUC) was 0.763 (standard error, 0.058; 95% CI = 0.670-0.840). White blood cell count ideal cutoff value was 11.100 $\times 10^3$ cells/mm^3, this cutoff value yields sensitivity of 75.4% and specificity of 65.5%. **b)** ROC curve for neutrophils count in complicated appendicitis patients. AUC was 0.749 (standard error, 0.060; 95% CI = 0.656-0.828). Neutrophils count ideal cutoff value was 7.540 $\times 10^3$ cells/mm^3, this cutoff value yields sensitivity of 81.8% and specificity of 65.5%.

diagnostic tests results to individual patients. Grönroos et al. [4] were the first to report that an increased leukocyte count was a very early marker of appendiceal inflammation in adult patients, according to ROC analysis. Contrary to descriptive and comparing statistical methods, analysis of ROC curves allows the estimation and verification of diagnostic suitability of diagnostic parameters. LR(+) is defined as the true-positive rate over the false-positive rate. It allows the clinician to assess the likelihood that a patient with a given test result (i.e., elevated WBCs count) has that disease. Additionally, LR is independent of disease prevalence. Generally, a clinically useful diagnostic test has an LR >10 or <0.1.

In this study, cut-off values, at which greatest sum of sensitivity and specificity was obtained, in WBCs and neutrophils counts were (9.400×10^3 and 7.540×10^3, respectively) in all patients with appendicitis versus normal appendix. At these cutoff points, AUC (95% CI) for WBCs and neutrophils were 0.701 (standard error, 0.055; 95% CI = 0.671-0.755) and 0.680 (standard error, 0.055; 95% CI = 0.635-0.722). WBCs and neutrophils sensitivity were 76.81%, 70.96%, specificity 65.52%, 65.52%, PPV 97.0%, 96.8%, NPV 16.1%, 13.3%, LR(+) 2.23, 2.06 and LR(–) 0.35, 0.44. Meanwhile, when we took only cases with inflamed appendicitis versus normal appendix, cut-off values in WBCs and neutrophils counts were 9.400×10^3 and 8.080×10^3, respectively. At these cutoff points, AUC (95% CI) for WBCs and neutrophils were 0.704 (standard error, 0.055; 95% CI = 0.655-0.749) and 0.664 (standard error, 0.056 95% CI = 0.614-0.712). WBCs and neutrophils sensitivity were 75.43%, 65.43%, specificity 65.52%, 68.97%, PPV 96.4%, 96.2%, NPV 18.1%, 14.2%, LR (+) 2.19, 2.11 and LR(–) 0.38, 0.50. While, when we took only cases with complicated appendicitis versus normal appendix, cut-off values in WBCs and neutrophils counts were 11.100×10^3 and 7.540×10^3, respectively. At these cutoff points, AUC (95% CI) for WBCs and neutrophils were 0.763 (standard error, 0.058; 95% CI = 0.670 - 0.840) and 0.749 (standard error, 0.060; 95% CI = 0.656 - 0.828). WBCs and neutrophils sensitivity were 76.62%, 81.82%, specificity 72.41%, 65.52%, PPV 88.10%, 86.30%, NPV 53.80%, 57.60%, LR(+) 2.78, 2.37 and LR(–) 0.32, 0.28. ROC curve analysis of our data suggests that there is no value of WBCs or neutrophils counts that is sensitive and specific enough to be clinically useful. An ideal test has an AUC of 1, while a perfectly random test has an AUC of 0.5. Generally, a "good" test has an AUC >0.8 and an "excellent" test has an AUC >0.9. In this respect, it had been reported that inflammatory markers such as WBCs is poorly reliable in confirming the presence of AA because of their low specificity in adults and children [2,7,31]. Sensitivity and specificity for WBCs count determined in this study is comparable with various national [32,33] and international [6,33-35] studies in which sensitivity ranges from 80.0–88.7%, while specificity ranges from 61.5-87.0%. So, leukocyte count by itself is not completely preventive against negative appendectomy, a finding consistent with our results.

Other investigators have constructed ROC curves for WBCs count and appendicitis with similar results. Körner et al. [36] found AUC of 0.69 (95% CI = 0.65-0.73), statistically no different from our results. Grönroos et al. [4] found a AUC of 0.730 (standard error = 0.041). Rodriguez- Sanjuan et al. [37] found an AUC of 0.67 (standard error = 0.08) for WBCs count and appendicitis in children. Paajanen et al. [18] found an AUC of 0.76. Andersson et al. [38] found an AUC of 0.80 (standard error = 0.02) for patients admitted to hospital for suspected appendicitis. An elevated total WBCs count might erroneously lead a surgeon to operate when other features of clinical scenario do not warrant or alternatively delay intervention as a result of a normal WBCs count. In support, of Guss and Richards [39] showed an association between delay in operative intervention and higher rate of perforated appendix in patients presenting to emergency with eventual diagnosis of appendicitis and normal WBCs count.

Limitations

The main limitation of this study that it is retrospective so there is biases in inclusion criteria of the patients which included all patients who underwent appendectomy, another prospective study containing all patients with abdominal pain with suspension of appendicitis must be made.

Conclusion

Leukocyte and neutrophils counts should not be used as diagnostic criteria for acute appendicitis because of its low sensitivity and specificity and must depend on clinical data as they are superior in decision-making appendectomy. WBCs and neutrophils counts do not indicate disease severity. WBCs and neutrophils counts in appendicitis evaluation does not enhance clinical decision making. The sensitivity of these tests is insufficient to achieve reliable rule-out.

Abbreviations

AA: Acute appendicitis; AUC: Area under curve; LR: Likelihood ratios; NPV: Negative predictive value; PPV: Positive predictive value; ROC: Receiver operating characteristic curves; WBCs: White blood cells.

Competing interests

The authors declare that they have no competing interests.

Authors' contributions

ZA carried out the design the study, collection and analysis of data, drafting and approved the final manuscript for publication.

References

1. Cardall T, Glasser J, Guss DA: **Clinical value of the total white blood cell count and temperature in the evaluation of patients with suspected appendicitis.** *Acad Emerg Med* 2004, **11**(10):1021–1027.
2. Yang HR, Wang YC, Chung PK, Chen WK, Jeng LB, Chen RJ: **Laboratory tests in patients with acute appendicitis.** *ANZ J Surg* 2006, **76**(1–2):71–74.
3. Flum DR, McClure TD, Morris A, Koepsell T: **Misdiagnosis of appendicitis and the use of diagnostic imaging.** *J Am Coll Surg* 2005, **201**(6):933–939.
4. Grönroos JM, Forsström JJ, Irjala K, Nevalainen TJ: **Phospholipase A2, C-reactive protein, and white blood cell count in the diagnosis of acute appendicitis.** *Clin Chem* 1994, **40**(9):1757–1760.
5. Cağlayan F, Cakmak M, Cağlayan O, Cavuşoglu T: **Plasma D-lactate levels in diagnosis of appendicitis.** *J Invest Surg* 2003, **16**(4):233–237.
6. Yang HR, Wang YC, Chung PK, Chen WK, Jeng LB, Chen RJ: **Role of leukocyte count, neutrophil percentage, and C-reactive protein in the diagnosis of acute appendicitis in the elderly.** *Am Surg* 2005, **71**(4):344–347.
7. Grönroos JM, Grönroos P: **Leucocyte count and C reactive protein in the diagnosis of acute appendicitis.** *Br J Surg* 1999, **86**(4):501–504.
8. Ng KC, Lai SW: **Clinical analysis of the related factors in acute appendicitis.** *Yale J Biol Med* 2002, **75**(1):41–45.
9. Andersson RE: **Meta-analysis of the clinical and laboratory diagnosis of appendicitis.** *Br J Surg* 2004, **91**(1):28–37.
10. Kharbanda AB, Taylor GA, Fishman SJ, Bachur RG: **A clinical decision rule to identify children at low risk for appendicitis.** *Pediatrics* 2005, **116**(3):709–716.
11. Zweig MH, Campbell G: **Receiver-operating characteristic (ROC) plots: a fundamental evaluation tool in clinical medicine.** *Clin Chem Clin Chem* 1993, **39**(4):561–577.
12. Mughal SA, Soomro S: **Acute appendicitis in children.** *J Surg Pakistan* 2007, **12**:123–125.
13. Soomro BA: **Acute appendicitis in children.** *J Surg Pak (Int)* 2008, **13**(4):151–154.
14. Lee SL, Ho HS: **Acute appendicitis: is there a difference between children and adults?** *Am Surg* 2006, **72**(5):409–413.
15. Salari AK, Binesh F: **Diagnostic value of anorexia in acute appendicitis.** *Pak J Med Sci* 2007, **23**:68–70.
16. Kirshan S: **Small bowel and appendix**. In *General surgery – Board review series*. Edited by Crabtree TD. London: Lippencott-Williams and Wilkins; 2000:195–196.
17. Balthazar EJ, Rofsky NM, Zucker R: **Appendicitis: the impact of computed tomography imaging on negative appendectomy and perforation rates.** *Am J Gastroenterol* 1998, **93**(5):768–771.
18. Paajanen H, Mansikka A, Laato M, Ristamäki R, Pulkki K, Kostiainen S: **Novel serum inflammatory markers in acute appendicitis.** *Scand J Clin Lab Invest* 2002, **62**(8):579–584.
19. Kessler N, Cyteval C, Gallix B, Lesnik A, Blayac PM, Pujol J, Bruel JM, Taourel P: **Appendicitis: evaluation of sensitivity, specificity, and predictive values of US, Doppler US, and laboratory findings.** *Radiology* 2004, **230**(2):472–478.
20. Wu HP, Huang CY, Chang YJ, Chou CC, Lin CY: **Use of changes over time in serum inflammatory parameters in patients with equivocal appendicitis.** *Surgery* 2006, **139**(6):789–796.
21. Hallan S, Asberg A: **The accuracy of C-reactive protein in diagnosing acute appendicitis - a meta-analysis.** *Scand J Clin Lab Invest* 1997, **57**(5):373–380.
22. Lycopoulou L, Mamoulakis C, Hantzi E, Demetriadis D, Antypas S, Giannaki M, Bakoula C, Chrousos G, Papassotiriou I: **Serum amyloid A protein levels as a possible aid in the diagnosis of acute appendicitis in children.** *Clin Chem Lab Med* 2005, **43**(1):49–53.
23. Eriksson S, Granström L, Olander B, Pira U: **Leukocyte elastase as a marker in the diagnosis of acute appendicitis.** *Eur J Surg* 1995, **161**(12):901–905.
24. Dalal I, Somekh E, Bilker-Reich A, Boaz M, Gorenstein A, Serour F: **Serum and peritoneal inflammatory mediators in children with suspected acute appendicitis.** *Arch Surg* 2005, **140**(2):169–173.
25. Hallan S, Asberg A, Edna TH: **Additional value of biochemical tests in suspected acute appendicitis.** *Eur J Surg* 1997, **163**(7):533–538.
26. Sarosi GA, Turnage RH: **Appendicitis**. In *Sleisenger and Fortran's Gastrointestinal and Liver Disease*. 7th edition. Edited by Feldman M, Friedman LS, Sleisenger MH. Philadelphia, PA: Elsevier; 2002. 2092.
27. Wolfe JM, Henneman PL: **Acute appendicitis**. In *Rosen's Emergency Medicine: Concepts and Clinical Practice*. 3rd edition. Edited by Marx JA, Hockberger RS, Walls RM. St. Louis, MO: Mosby; 2002:1293–1294.
28. Sack U, Biereder B, Elouahidi T, Bauer K, Keller T, Tröbs RB: **Diagnostic value of blood inflammatory markers for detection of acute appendicitis in children.** *BMC Surg* 2006, **28**:6–15.
29. Yokoyama S, Takifuji K, Hotta T, Matsuda K, Nasu T, Nakamori M, Hirabayashi N, Kinoshita H, Yamaue H: **C-Reactive protein is an independent surgical indication marker for appendicitis: a retrospective study.** *World J Emerg Surg* 2009, **4**:36.
30. Lee SL, Walsh AJ, Ho HS: **Computed tomography and ultrasonography do not improve and may delay the diagnosis and treatment of acute appendicitis.** *Arch Surg* 2001, **136**(5):556–562.
31. Gronroos JM: **Do normal leucocyte count and C-reactive protein value exclude acute appendicitis in children?** *Acta Paediatr* 2001, **90**(6):649–651.
32. Khan MN, Davie E, Irshad K: **The role of white cell count and C-reactive protein in the diagnosis of acute appendicitis.** *J Ayub Med Coll Abbottabad* 2004, **16**(3):17–19.
33. Gulzar S, Umar S, Dar GM, Rasheed R: **Acute appendicitisrole of clinical examination in making a confident diagnosis.** *Pak J Med Sci* 2005, **21**(2):125–132.
34. Bener A, Suwaid MH, Ghazawi IE: **Diagnosis of appendicitis.** *Can J Rural Med* 2002, **7**:26–29.
35. de Carvalho BR, Diogo-Filho A, Fernandes C, Barra CB: **Leukocyte count, C-reactive protein, alpha-1 acid glycoprotein and erythrocytes sedimentation rate in acute appendicitis.** *Arq Gastroenterol* 2003, **40**(1):25–30.
36. Körner H, Söreide JA, Söndenaa K: **Diagnostic accuracy of inflammatory markers in patients operated on for suspected acute appendicitis: a receiver operating characteristic curve analysis.** *Eur J Surg* 1999, **165**(7):679–685.
37. Rodríguez-Sanjuán JC, Martín-Parra JI, Seco I, García-Castrillo L, Naranjo A: **C-reactive protein and leukocyte count in the diagnosis of acute appendicitis in children.** *Dis Colon Rectum* 1999, **42**(10):1325–1329.
38. Andersson RE, Hugander AP, Ghazi SH, Ravn H, Offenbartl SK, Nyström PO, Olaison GP: **Diagnostic value of disease history, clinical parameters, and inflammatory parameters of appendicitis.** *World J Surg* 1999, **23**(2):133–140.
39. Guss DA, Richards C: **Normal total WBC and operative delay in appendicitis.** *Cal J Emerg Med* 2000, **1**(2):7–8.

Ex-vivo and live animal models are equally effective training for the management of a penetrating cardiac injury

Yoshimitsu Izawa[1,2*], Shuji Hishikawa[1,2,3], Tomohiro Muronoi[2], Keisuke Yamashita[2], Hiroyuki Maruyama[3], Masayuki Suzukawa[2] and Alan Kawarai Lefor[1,3]

Abstract

Background: Live tissue models are considered the most useful simulation for training in the management for hemostasis of penetrating injuries. However, these models are expensive, with limited opportunities for repetitive training. Ex-vivo models using tissue and a fluid pump are less expensive, allow repetitive training and respect ethical principles in animal research. The purpose of this study is to objectively evaluate the effectiveness of ex-vivo training with a pump, compared to live animal model training. Staff surgeons and residents were divided into live tissue training and ex-vivo training groups. Training in the management of a penetrating cardiac injury was conducted for each group, separately. One week later, all participants were formally evaluated in the management of a penetrating cardiac injury in a live animal.

Results: There are no differences between the two groups regarding average years of experience or previous trauma surgery experience. All participants achieved hemostasis, with no difference between the two groups in the Global Rating Scale score (ex-vivo: 25.2 ± 6.3, live: 24.7 ± 6.3, $p = 0.646$), blood loss (1.6 ± 0.7, 2.0 ± 0.6, $p = 0.051$), checklist score (3.7 ± 0.6, 3.6 ± 0.9, $p = 0.189$), or time required for repair (101 s ± 31, 107 s ± 15, $p = 0.163$), except overall evaluation (3.8 ± 0.9, 3.4 ± 0.9, $p = 0.037$). The internal consistency reliability and inter-rater reliability in the Global Rating Scale were excellent (0.966 and 0.953 / 0.719 and 0.784, respectively), and for the checklist were moderate (0.570 and 0.636 / 0.651 and 0.607, respectively). The validity is rated good for both the Global Rating Scale (Residents: 21.7 ± 5.6, Staff: 28.9 ± 4.7, $p = 0.000$) and checklist (Residents: 3.4 ± 0.9, Staff Surgeons: 3.9 ± 0.3, $p = 0.003$). The results of self-assessment questionnaires were similarly high (4.2–4.9) with scores in self-efficacy increased after training (pre: 1.7 ± 0.8, post: 3.2 ± 1.0, $p = 0.000$ in ex-vivo, pre: 1.9 ± 1.0, post: 3.7 ± 0.7, $p = 0.000$ in live). Scores comparing pre-training and post-evaluation (pre: 1.7 ± 0.8, post: 3.7 ± 0.9, $p = 0.000$ in ex-vivo, pre: 1.9 ± 1.0, post: 3.8 ± 0.7, $p = 0.000$ in live) were increased.

Conclusion: Training with an ex-vivo model and live tissue training are similar for the management of a penetrating cardiac injury, with increased self-efficacy of participants in both groups. The ex-vivo model is useful to learn hemostatic skills in trauma surgery.

Keywords: Trauma surgery, Ex-vivo training, Surgical education, Simulation, Objective Structured Assessment of Technical Skills, Self-efficacy

* Correspondence: damagecontrolresuscitation@gmail.com
[1]Center of Development for Advanced Medical Technology, Jichi Medical University, 3311-1 Yakushiji, Shimotsukeshi, Tochigiken 329-0498, Japan
[2]Department of Emergency and Critical Care Medicine, Jichi Medical University, 3311-1 Yakushiji, Shimotsukeshi, Tochigiken 329-0498, Japan
Full list of author information is available at the end of the article

Background

Simulation training is essential for learning a variety of skills in medical training. Concerns for patient safety and super-specialization have increased the need for simulation-based training. Simulation training for hemostasis in trauma surgery is especially desired because hemostasis is critical to save severely injured patients and there are limited opportunities for surgeons to learn the skills needed to treat traumatically injured patients in clinical practice [1, 2]. The number of surgical procedures performed by trainees has been decreasing with advancements in non-operative management [1]. Various simulation courses are conducted around the world in part to make up for limited real-life experience [3–5].

Live tissue training is considered by some to be the most useful simulation for training in the hemostasis of traumatic injuries [6, 7]. However, these programs are expensive, repetitive training is impractical, and ethical issues regarding the use of live animals have gained intense focus [7]. These factors limit the conduct of live tissue training programs. Other methods, such as cadaver training, virtual reality and bench model training, are less suitable for training in hemostatic skills because of decreased reality or a total lack of bleeding [6, 7].

Ex-vivo tissue can be used for simulation training for technical skills [8, 9]. It is generally considered to have mid-level fidelity, is financially reasonable and conducive to repetitive training. We previously conducted a pilot study in the use of a circulation pump for ex-vivo training in trauma surgery, with subjective evaluation [8]. The pump mimics circulation, and appears similar to live tissue. However, objective assessment of this method has not been conducted.

The purpose of this study is to objectively evaluate the effectiveness of ex-vivo training with a pump, compared to live tissue training, for the management of a penetrating cardiac injury.

Methods

Institutional Animal Experiment Committee approval was obtained before beginning this study. This study was conducted in the Center for Development of Advanced Medical Technology (CDAMtec) at Jichi Medical University.

Participants

Staff surgeons and residents at Jichi Medical University Hospital took part in this study. This program was the first time any of the participants managed a penetrating cardiac injury. Participants were surveyed regarding their level of training, years of experience and details of their previous trauma surgery experience.

Study design

This is a comparative study comparing ex-vivo training and live tissue training (Fig. 1). Participants were divided into two groups, an ex-vivo training group and a live tissue training group. Participants were randomly assigned based on their last name. However, there were a few changes because of emergency clinical responsibilities on the day of the training. After completing a pre-training questionnaire (Fig. 2) and obtaining informed consent about participation in the study, participants were trained by experienced trauma surgeons to achieve hemostasis of a penetrating cardiac wound and then repair the wound with explanations and demonstrations. Participants then practiced achieving hemostasis of a one centimeter cardiac injury with help from the instructor. The ex-vivo group did this using an ex-vivo tissue model, and the live group performed this on a live, anesthetized pig. After the training, a post-training questionnaire was completed (Fig. 3).

One week after the training session, all participants managed a standard one centimeter penetrating cardiac wound in a live animal using the skills acquired during the previous training session. Each participant managed the wound individually, and was assessed with an Objective Structured Assessment of Technical Skills (OSATS) instrument. After the evaluation, a post-evaluation survey form was completed by the participants (Fig. 3).

Ex-vivo training session (Fig. 4)

Ex-vivo training was performed using porcine hearts from animals used in other experiments or training. The ex-vivo hearts were harvested and frozen, the frozen organs thawed and connected to a circulation pump before the training session. During the training, a one centimeter penetrating wound was made in the right ventricle. Participants learned how to stop bleeding initially with digital pressure, and then repair the injury with direct suture, under the guidance of an instructor.

Live tissue training session (Fig. 5)

Live tissue training was performed with pigs (Crossbred KCG or Mexican hairless miniature pig, approximately 30–40 kg under general anesthesia (Sevoflurane 2–5 %). After performing a median sternotomy and incising the pericardium, a penetrating injury about one centimeter long was made in the right ventricle by the instructor. Participants achieved hemostasis using digital pressure and then repaired the injury with direct suture.

Evaluation session

Participants were evaluated by direct observation in their management of a cardiac injury in the live animal model conducted one week after the training session. The

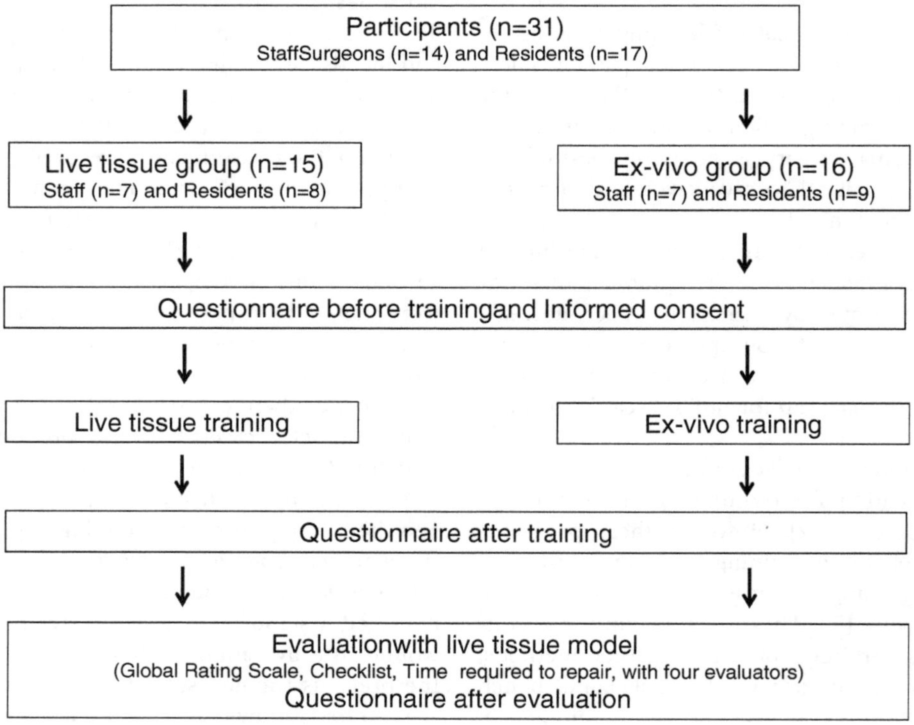

Fig. 1 Study flowchart

animals were the same type and size used in the training session. The evaluation session was conducted similarly for all participants. Four evaluators assessed each participant, and completed an evaluation form using the OSATS instrument. The time required to repair the injury by each of the participants was recorded. The evaluators were blinded to whether participants had undergone training with live tissue or an ex-vivo model.

There were six evaluators in total, and four of the six assessed the performance of each participant using the OSATS. Two of the six were experienced surgeons with more than 25y experience in acute care surgery. Two were board certified surgeons and others included an experienced veterinarian, and an experienced veterinary technician with more than 30 years of experience in veterinary care and surgery.

OSATS is widely accepted as a reliable and valid evaluative tool for simulation [10, 11]. This OSATS instrument included a Global Rating Scale and checklist. The Global Rating Scale includes nine items (Fig. 6). Item 1–7 are standard, and we added two items including, "amount of hemorrhage" and "overall evaluation". In eight of the nine items, a five-point Likert scale (1 = poor ~ 5 = excellent) was used. One item, "amount of hemorrhage", was a three-point qualitative scale (1 = little, 2 = intermediate and 3 = a lot). The checklist included four Yes/No questions (Fig. 7). The questions on the checklist are task-specific and more concrete, different from the global rating scale.

Reliability and validity of the OSATS were evaluated in this study. The internal consistency reliability was analyzed by Cronbach's α. The inter-rater reliability was analyzed by inter-class correlation. The validity was evaluated by comparing the outcome of the Global Rating Scale (as the sum of the seven component scores, each score range 1–5, overall range 7–35) and checklist score (4 items scored 0 or 1, overall range 0–4) of staff surgeons and residents, using a sum of the scores.

Participants completed questionnaires at three separate time points: pre-training post-training and post-evaluation. The questionnaires utilized a five point Likert scale (1 = poor ~ 5 = excellent) and included an assessment of self-efficacy (self-confidence) (Figs. 2 and 3).

Statistical analysis

Data were analyzed with SPSS (IBM, Armonk NY) version 22.0. Continuous variables are presented as means with standard deviations. Mann Whitney's *U* test is used for continuous variables because most data were non-normal distributions. Wilcoxon signed-rank test is used for paired continuous variables. Inter-class correlation is

Questionnaire before training

Date: ______________________

Name: ______________________

Years after medical school graduation: (   ) years

Group:(live · ex-vivo)

How many times have you ever participated in chest or abdominal trauma operation?
(   ) times

I am looking forward to this training.
(5 4 3 2 1)
(I strongly agree ← → I strongly disagree)

I am interested in trauma surgery.
(5 4 3 2 1)
(I strongly agree ← → I strongly disagree)

I am confident in performing hemostasis procedures for a cardiac injury.
(5 4 3 2 1)
(I strongly agree ← → I strongly disagree)

Fig. 2 Pre-training questionnaire

used for the assessment of inter-rater reliability. Statistical significance was set at a *P*-value less than .05.

Results

Study participants

There are no statistical differences between the two study groups, although the number of years after medical school graduation and trauma surgery experience in the ex-vivo training group was slightly higher than in the live tissue group (Table 1).

Evaluation of management of a penetrating cardiac injury

All participants were able to achieve hemostasis. Table 2 shows the results of the Global Rating Scale, amount of hemorrhage, overall evaluation, checklist and time required to repair. There was a significant difference in the overall evaluation between the two study groups, with the ex-vivo group being significantly higher. The amount of hemorrhage before achieving hemostasis was higher in the live tissue trained group, but this difference did not quite reach statistical significance.

Table 3 shows the internal consistency reliability and inter-rater reliability for both the Global Rating Scale and checklist. The internal consistency reliability scores were better in both groups than the inter-rater reliability, but the results were reasonable for all four evaluations. Although two instructors could not participate in all evaluations, two different instructors served as substitutes, and the inter-rater reliability scores remained excellent.

Table 4 shows the validity by comparing the Global Rating Scale and checklist scores between residents and staff surgeons. There is a significant difference between residents and staff surgeons, with the validity for both rating scales significantly greater for staff surgeons than for residents.

Tables 5 and 6 show the results of pre-training, post-training and post-evaluation questionnaires. Table 5

Questionnaire post training / post evaluation

Date : ______________________________

Name : ______________________________

Group : (live ・ ex-vivo)

I am satisfied with this training.
(5 4 3 2 1)
(I strongly agree ← → I strongly disagree)

My interest in trauma care has increased.
(5 4 3 2 1)
(I strongly agree ← → I strongly disagree)

I am confident to perform hemostatic procedures for a cardiac injury.
(5 4 3 2 1)
(I strongly agree ← → I strongly disagree)

I would recommend this training to my colleagues.
(5 4 3 2 1)
(I strongly agree ← → I strongly disagree)

I obtained new knowledge and skills to achieve hemostasis of a cardiac injury.
(5 4 3 2 1)
(I strongly agree ← → I strongly disagree)

I would like to repeat this training.
(5 4 3 2 1)
(I strongly agree ← → I strongly disagree)

Fig. 3 Post-training and post-evaluation questionnaire

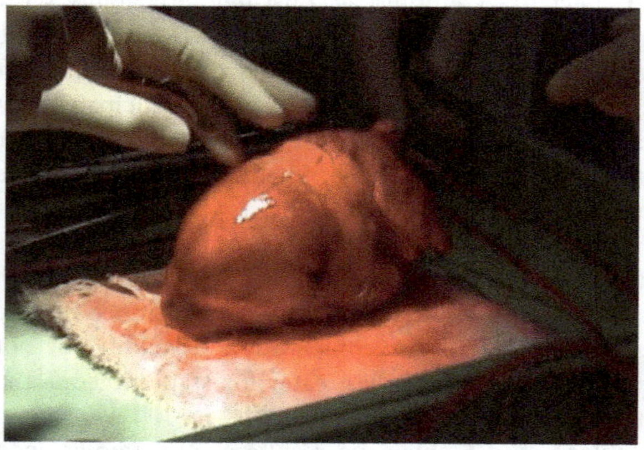

Fig. 4 Ex-vivo tissue: cardiac injury

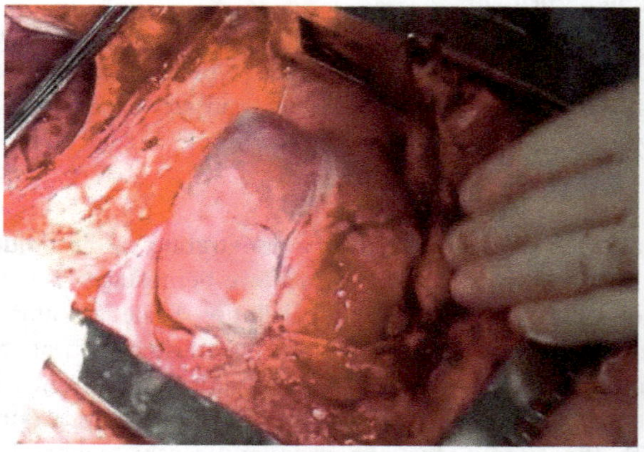

Fig. 5 Live tissue training: cardiac injury

Global Rating Scale

Date: ( )
Participant Name: ( )
Evaluator Name: ( )

1. Respect for Tissue
   5 4 3 2 1
   Excellent ←—→ Poor

2. Time and Motion
   5 4 3 2 1
   Excellent ←—→ Poor

3. Instrument handling
   5 4 3 2 1
   Excellent ←—→ Poor

4. Knowledge of instrument
   5 4 3 2 1
   Excellent ←—→ Poor

5. Use of assistant
   5 4 3 2 1
   Excellent ←—→ Poor

6. Flow of operation and forward planning
   5 4 3 2 1
   Excellent ←—→ Poor

7. Knowledge of specific procedure
   5 4 3 2 1
   Excellent ←—→ Poor

8. Amount of hemorrhage
   3 2 1
   Large ← → Small

9. Overall evaluation
   5 4 3 2 1
   Excellent ←—→ Poor

Fig. 6 Global Rating Scale score sheet, including evaluations of amount of hemorrhage and overall evaluation

Checklist

Date: ( )
Participant Name: ( )
Evaluator Name: ( )

1. Applied pressure to stop bleeding first
   done correctly / not done or done incorrectly

2. Applied appropriate pressure
   done correctly / not done or done incorrectly

3. Appropriate suture
   done correctly / not done or done incorrectly

4. Tied appropriately
   done correctly / not done or done incorrectly

Fig. 7 Evaluation checklist

shows that the two study groups had no differences in their subjective self-assessment before the training. Table 6 shows no differences in subjective evaluations comparing the two study groups after training and after the evaluation session. There was a small, but not statistically significant difference in the satisfaction scores after the training session, but this difference did not appear after the evaluation session.

Table 7 shows the assessment of self-confidence comparing the results at all three time points, pre-training, post-training and post evaluation. Confidence levels are similar in the two study groups at the pre-training time point, with both groups showing significantly more confidence both post-training and post-evaluation. Comparing post-evaluation to post-training shows that the two study groups had similar confidence levels after the evaluation session, but that the live tissue group felt more confident at post-training.

Interestingly, after the training session, the live tissue group had significantly more self-confidence (score 3.7) than the ex-vivo (score 3.2, $p < .05$) trained group. However, after the evaluation session, while the self-confidence of both groups was significantly greater compared to pre-training, there was no longer a difference in the self-confidence level of the two groups.

Discussion

We conducted training using an ex-vivo model with a pump, and compared it with use of a live animal model

Table 1 Characteristics of study participants: years after medical school graduation and previous experience in trauma surgery

Study group (*n* = number of participants)	Ex-vivo (*n* = 16; residents 9, Staff Surgeons 7)	Live tissue (*n* = 15; residents 8, Staff Surgeons 7)	*P*-value
Years after medical school graduation (mean years (Standard Deviation))	4.6 (4.9)	3.5 (2.4)	0.654
Prior experience in chest and abdominal trauma surgery (mean number of procedures (Standard Deviation))	4.5 (7.0)	2.2 (3.1)	0.861

to teach the management of penetrating cardiac injuries. After training, all participants were objectively evaluated in their management of a penetrating cardiac injury. All participants were able to achieve hemostasis at the injury site on the surface of the right ventricle. Objective assessment revealed that ex-vivo training was as effective as live tissue training, based on the evaluation conducted. The reliability and validity of the OSATS instrument were good. Participant responses to subjective questionnaires were positive and the level of self-efficacy increased.

Live tissue training is considered by some to be the most effective way to learn hemostatic skills for trauma surgery [6, 7]. Other training models, such as cadaver training, bench model training, or virtual reality training, do not have active blood circulation to mimic live tissue training. However, the ex-vivo system used in this study simulates active bleeding with an external pump which facilitates learning hemostatic procedures in a more realistic environment without a live animal [8].

Ethical issues regarding the use of experimental animals are also important [7] and ex-vivo training models are a good response to these ethical issues. Burch and Russel proposed the 3R's for animal ethics [12], including Reduction, Replacement and Refinement. Although cadaver training and virtual reality training are beneficial from an ethical standpoint, these models may not be suitable for learning hemostatic skills. There are few studies comparing the effectiveness of training using these modalities with training using a live animal model [7]. The ex-vivo model described here using a pump provides the opportunity to learn hemostatic skills in trauma surgery with objective results similar to training with a live animal and respects the principles represented by the 3R's.

Although we did not calculate exact costs in this study, estimates can be made, based on average charges at our institution. The direct cost of the ex-vivo training is the facility fee and the price of the sutures. The facility fee is equivalent to the electrical charges of the circulation pump and the refrigerator for preservation of the harvested organs, which we estimate to about US$20 for one session. The sutures cost about US$50 per session, for a total cost of about US$70. Live tissue training requires the cost of the pig, the fee for general anesthesia, and the sutures. The pig costs about US$1800, and the cost of anesthesia and the facility fee is about US$300 for a total cost of about US$2150, with the sutures. While these are only estimates, the cost of live tissue training is far greater than ex-vivo training.

One factor which influences the results of the objective evaluation is the size of the penetrating cardiac injury. The amount of hemorrhage was not excessive because the stab wound was just one centimeter long. It was relatively easy to stop the bleeding. If the injury were larger, hemostasis would be more difficult and a greater difference in results may have been observed. Another important factor is the location of the wound in the heart, which directly affects the ease of achieving hemostasis. If the injury was created in the left atrium, the results may have been different. Manipulation of an ex-vivo heart during the procedure

Table 2 Global Rating Scale score, amount of hemorrhage, overall evaluation, checklist and time required to repair comparing ex-vivo and live tissue groups

Study group (*n* = number of evaluation forms)	Ex-vivo (*n* = 64)	Live tissue (*n* = 60)	*P* value
Global Rating Scale (sum of scores for seven items, Range 7–35)	25.2 (6.3)	24.7 (6.3)	0.646
Amount of hemorrhage (Range 1–3)	1.6 (0.7)	2.0 (0.6)	0.051
Overall evaluation	3.8 (0.9)	3.4 (0.9)	0.037
Checklist	3.7 (0.6)	3.6 (0.9)	0.189
Time required (seconds)[a]	101 (31), n=16	107 (15), n=15	0.163

Scores shown are mean (Standard Deviation), using a 5-point Likert scale (range 1–5), except hemorrhage which is rated on a 3-point scale (1 = little, 2 = intermediate, 3 = a lot). Checklist scores are range 0–4. Scores shown are the mean of the four evaluations for all participants

[a]values of n shown for time are number of participants

Table 3 Internal consistency reliability and inter-rater reliability of Global Rating Scale and checklist scores

Study group		Ex-vivo	Live tissue
Internal consistency reliability, Cronbach's α (Seven items)	Global Rating Scale	0.966	0.953
	Checklist	0.570	0.636
Inter-rater reliability, inter-class correlation score (Four evaluators)	Global Rating Scale	0.719	0.784
	Checklist	0.651	0.607

Table 4 Validity of Global Rating Scale and checklist scores: Residents and staff surgeons, four evaluations for each participant (Mann–Whitney *U* test)

Group (*n* = number of evaluation forms)	Residents (*n* = 68)	Staff surgeons (*n* = 56)	*P* value
Global Rating Scale (mean and standard deviation, sum of seven scores each score range 1–5, with overall range 7–35)	21.7 (5.6)	28.9 (4.7)	0.000
Checklist score (range 0–4)	3.4 (0.9)	3.9 (0.3)	0.003

does not have a physiologic effect, limiting the reality of the simulation.

The overall evaluation of the ex-vivo group was statistically significantly higher than that of the live tissue group. Among other evaluation items, such as amount of hemorrhage and time required to repair, there was no significant difference between the two groups, but the mean scores of the ex-vivo group are higher than those of the live tissue group, though the characteristics of participants are similar in both groups. The pressure of the bleeding with the ex-vivo model, seemed higher than that in the live tissue model according to some participants [8], and might influence the difference in scores. The impression of higher pressure bleeding with the ex-vivo model might give participants the impression that repair of the injury in the live tissue model is easier than during the training session.

The OSATS instrument had good reliability and validity and was useful as an evaluation tool. OSATS is widely used for the evaluation of technical skills in simulation [10, 11, 13–16]. The internal consistency reliability and inter-rater reliability analysis of the Global Rating Scale were high and those for the checklist were moderate. The validity was evaluated by comparing the results of residents and staff surgeons, and a significant difference was observed, which means that the OSATS used in this study can identify differences between the study groups. Overall, the evaluation tools demonstrated that training with this ex-vivo model is as useful as live tissue training for the management of a penetrating cardiac injury in a porcine model simple.

Table 5 Pre-training questionnaire

Study group (*n* = number of participants)	Ex-vivo (*n* = 16)	Live tissue (*n* = 15)	*P* value
I am looking forward to this training.	4.4 (0.7)	4.4 (0.8)	0.984
I am interested in trauma surgery.	4.2 (0.9)	4.2 (0.9)	0.984
I am confident in performing hemostatic procedures for a cardiac injury.	1.7 (0.8)	1.9 (1.0)	0.545

Scores shown are mean (Standard Deviation), using a 5-point Likert scale (range 1–5)

The subjective evaluations also revealed the usefulness of training with this ex-vivo model. All responses to items in the questionnaires showed that the training was perceived well by the participants. Self-confidence in both groups significantly increased after the training. Self-confidence carries the same meaning as self-efficacy, which was advocated by Bandura in 1977 [17]. Bandura described that self-efficacy means"people's judgments of their capabilities to organize and execute courses of action required to attain designated types of performances [18]." In other words, it is a belief that one can accomplish a specific task. Self-efficacy is a very important characteristic for physicians and surgeons who perform procedures [19], particularly in emergency situations [20, 21]. Training with the ex-vivo model significantly increased the self-efficacy of participants for the repair of a penetrating cardiac injury. It was of interest that the increased self-efficacy in the live tissue trained group compared to the ex-vivo group was not sustained. Self-efficacy of the two groups was equal after the evaluation session.

This training is suitable for resident training as it facilitates repetitive practice. Aboud et al. reported that cadaver training for placement of an Intra-Aortic Balloon can be performed with a fluid pump to mimic circulation [22], but based on the description of the procedure, is far more complex than the system employed in this training program. This ex-vivo model is reasonable and needs less work to perform the training.

There are some limitations to this study. First, hemostasis is just one factor in the care of trauma patients. There are other technical skills required to save patients with penetrating cardiac injuries, such as performing a thoracotomy or median sternotomy to gain access to the injury site. Decision making and team dynamics for trauma are extremely important in emergency care. This ex-vivo training does not provide training for all of the requisite skills. Actual patient care experience in clinical practice is essential. There are a number of formal training programs to teach skills needed in the care of trauma patients. Second, the physical features of live tissue cannot be reproduced completely with this ex-vivo model, such as coagulation and motion of the heart. Third, a complex injury cannot be simulated using this ex-vivo model. Management of a single type of injury is a limitation using this model and this level of fidelity is suitable for learning basic procedures in trauma surgery. Fourth, the sample size is somewhat small. As Table 1 shows, there are differences between the two groups for time since graduation and prior experience (number of procedures) in chest and abdominal

Table 6 Post training and post evaluation questionnaires

Study group (*n* = number of participants)	Questionnaire	Ex-vivo (*n* = 16)	Live tissue (*n* = 15)	*P* value
I am satisfied with this training.	Post-training	4.5 (0.6)	4.9 (0.3)	0.078
	Post-evaluation	4.8 (0.4)	4.9 (0.4)	0.599
My interest in trauma care has increased.	Post-training	4.4 (0.9)	4.6 (0.8)	0.423
	Post-evaluation	4.6 (0.6)	4.6 (0.5)	1.000
I am confident to perform hemostatic procedures for a cardiac injury.	Post-training	3.2 (1.0)	3.7 (0.7)	0.140
	Post-evaluation	3.7 (0.9)	3.8 (0.7)	0.770
I would recommend this training to my colleagues.	Post-training	4.3 (0.7)	4.6 (0.5)	0.318
	Post-evaluation	4.6 (0.6)	4.7 (0.5)	1.000
I obtained new knowledge and skills to achieve hemostasis of a cardiac injury.	Post-training	4.6 (0.6)	4.9 (0.4)	0.247
	Post-evaluation	4.6 (0.5)	4.8 (0.6)	0.202
I would like to repeat this training.	Post-training	4.3 (0.8)	4.5 (0.6)	0.495
	Post-evaluation	4.8 (0.4)	4.6 (0.5)	0.495

Scores shown are mean (Standard Deviation), using a 5-point Likert scale (range 1–5). *P*-values shown are comparing the two study groups, ex-vivo and live tissue

trauma surgery. While the differences are not significant, a significant difference may be identified with a larger sample size. Power analysis shows that the sample size required is 186 ($\alpha = 0.05$, $1\text{-}\beta = 0.8$), supporting the need for further study of the ex-vivo model.

Although this ex-vivo model has some limitations, simulation is an important modality in training for the care of injured patients. Utilizing this ex-vivo model is intended to bolster the competence of surgeons, and will hopefully lead to the increased survival of severely injured patients.

Conclusions

Ex-vivo training with a pump was as useful as live tissue training to learn hemostatic techniques for a penetrating cardiac injury. This training increased the self-efficacy of participants, and objective scores of results showed no differences for training with an ex-vivo model or live tissue. This study supports the use of ex-vivo models for training in hemostasis, at lower cost and respecting the principle of 3R's for animal research.

Table 7 Confidence level comparing pre-training, post-training and post-evaluation

Study group (*n* = number of participants)	Pre-training (*n* = 31)	Post-training (*n* = 31)	Post-evaluation (*n* = 31)
Ex-vivo	1.7 (0.8)	3.2 (1.0), $p = 0.00$	3.7 (0.9), $p = 0.00$
Live tissue	1.9 (1.0)	3.7 (0.7), $p = 0.00$, $p^{**} < .05$	3.8 (0.7), $p = 0.00$

Scores shown are mean (Standard Deviation), using a 5-point Likert scale (range 1–5). *P*-values shown are comparison with the pre-training questionnaire for each of the two study groups, while p^{**} compares the live tissue and ex-vivo group for the post-training evaluation (Wilcoxon signed-rank test)

Acknowledgements
Some part of this study was presented in the 10th Annual Congress of Korean Society of Acute Care Surgery, 4th Joint Scientific Congress of KSACS and JSACS in Busan, Republic of Korea on April 9th, 2016.

Funding
This study was supported by the Ministry of Education, Culture, Sports, Science and Technology (MEXT)-Supported Program for the Strategic Research Foundation at Private Universities.

Authors' contributions
YI: Conceived the trial, conducted the training, collected and analyzed data, prepared the manuscript. SH: Conducted the training, collected data. TM: Collected the data. KY: Collected the data. HM: Collected data. MS: Conceived the trial. AKL: Conceived the trial, analyzed the data, preparation of manuscript. All authors read and approved the final manuscript.

Competing interests
The authors declare that they have no competing interests.

Author details
[1]Center of Development for Advanced Medical Technology, Jichi Medical University, 3311-1 Yakushiji, Shimotsukeshi, Tochigiken 329-0498, Japan. [2]Department of Emergency and Critical Care Medicine, Jichi Medical University, 3311-1 Yakushiji, Shimotsukeshi, Tochigiken 329-0498, Japan. [3]Department of Digestive Surgery, Jichi Medical University, 3311-1 Yakushiji, Shimotsukeshi, Tochigiken 329-0498, Japan.

References

1. Spain DA, Miller FB. Education and training of the future trauma surgeon in acute care surgery: trauma, critical care, and emergency surgery. Am J Surg. 2005;190:212–7.
2. Fakhry SM, Watts DD, Michetti C, Hunt JP, EAST Multi-Institutional Blunt Hollow Viscous Injury Research Group. The resident experience on trauma: declining surgical opportunities and career incentives? Analysis of data from a large multi-institutional study. J Trauma. 2003;54:1–7.
3. Jacobs LM, Burns KJ, Luk SS, Marshall 3rd WT. Follow-up survey of participants attending the Advanced Trauma Operative Management (ATOM) Course. J Trauma. 2005;58:1140–3.
4. Jacobs L, Burns K, Luk S, Hull S. Advanced trauma operative management course: participant survey. World J Surg. 2010;34:164–8. doi:10.1007/s00268-009-0276-z.
5. Kuhls DA, Risucci DA, Bowyer MW, Luchette FA. Advanced surgical skills for exposure in trauma: a new surgical skills cadaver course for surgery residents and fellows. J Trauma Acute Care Surg. 2013;74:664–70. doi:10.1097/TA.0b013e31827d5e20.

6. Reznick RK, MacRae H. Teaching surgical skills – change in the wind. N Engl J Med. 2006;355:2664–9.
7. Stefanidis D, Yonce TC, Green JM, Coker AP. Cadavers versus pigs: which are better for procedural training of surgery residents outside the OR? Surgery. 2013;154:34–7. doi:10.1016/j.surg.2013.05.001.
8. Izawa Y, Hishikawa S, Muronoi T, Yamashita K, Suzukawa M, Lefor AT. Ex-vivo porcine organs with a circulation pump are effective for teaching hemostatic skills. World J Emerg Surg. 2012;7:5. doi:10.1186/1749-7922-7-5.
9. Thomas MB, Dandolu V, Caputo P, Milner R, Hernandez E. Resident education in principles and technique of bowel surgery using an ex-vivo porcine model. Obstet Gynecol Int. 2010;2010:852647. doi:10.1155/2010/852647.
10. Steigerwald SN, Park J, Hardy KM, Gillman L, Vergis AS. Establishing the concurrent validity of general and technique-specific skills assessments in surgical education. Am J Surg. 2016;211:268–73. doi:10.1016/j.amjsurg.2015.04.024.
11. van Hove PD, Tuijthof GJ, Verdaasdonk EG, Stassen LP, Dankelman J. Objective assessment of technical surgical skills. Br J Surg. 2010;97:972–87. doi:10.1002/bjs.7115.
12. Russell WMS, Burch RL. The Principles of Humane Experimental Technique. London: Methuen and Co. Ltd.; 1959.
13. Martin JA, Regehr G, Reznick R, MacRae H, Murnaghan J, Hutchison C, Brown M. Objective structured assessment of technical skill (OSATS) for surgical residents. Br J Surg. 1997;84:273–8.
14. Faulkner H, Regehr G, Martin J, Reznick R. Validation of an objective structured assessment of technical skill for surgical residents. Acad Med. 1996;71:1363–5.
15. Reznick R, Regehr G, MacRae H, Martin J, McCulloch W. Testing technical skill via an innovative 'bench station' examination. Am J Surg. 1997;173:226–30.
16. Ault G, Reznick R, MacRae H, Leadbetter W, DaRosa D, Joehl R, et al. Exporting a technical skills evaluation technology to other sites. Am J Surg. 2001;182:254–6.
17. Bandura A. Self-efficacy: toward a unifying theory of behavioral change. Psychol Rev. 1977;84:191–215.
18. Bandura A. Social foundations of thought and action: a social cognitive theory. Englewood Cliffs: Prentice Hall; 1986.
19. Artino Jr AR. Academic self-efficacy: from educational theory to instructional practice. Perspect Med Educ. 2012;1:76–85. doi:10.1007/s40037-012-0012-5.
20. Hall AB, Riojas R, Sharon D. Comparison of self-efficacy and its improvement after artificial simulator or live animal model emergency procedure training. Mil Med. 2014;179:320–3. doi:10.7205/MILMED-D-12-00446.
21. Martinic G. The use of animals in live-tissue trauma training and military medical research. Lab Anim (NY). 2011;40:319–22. doi:10.1038/laban1011-319.
22. Aboud ET, Krisht AF, O'Keeffe T, Nader R, Hassan M, Stevens CM, Ali F, Luchette FA. Novel simulation for training trauma surgeons. J Trauma. 2011;71:1484–90. doi:10.1097/TA.0b013e3182396337.

18

ICEAGE (Incidence of Complications following Emergency Abdominal surgery: Get Exercising): study protocol of a pragmatic, multicentre, randomised controlled trial testing physiotherapy for the prevention of complications and improved physical recovery after emergency abdominal surgery

Ianthe Boden[1,2*], Kate Sullivan[1,3], Claire Hackett[4], Brooke Winzer[5], Rebecca Lane[6], Melissa McKinnon[4] and Iain Robertson[7,8]

Abstract

Background: Postoperative complications and delayed physical recovery are significant problems following emergency abdominal surgery. Physiotherapy aims to aid recovery and prevent complications in the acute phase after surgery and is commonplace in most first-world hospitals. Despite ubiquitous service provision, no well-designed, adequately powered, parallel-group, randomised controlled trial has investigated the effect of physiotherapy on the incidence of respiratory complications, paralytic ileus, rate of physical recovery, ongoing need for formal sub-acute rehabilitation, hospital length of stay, health-related quality of life, and mortality following emergency abdominal surgery. We hypothesise that an enhanced physiotherapy care package of additional education, breathing exercises, and early rehabilitation prevents postoperative complications and improves physical recovery following emergency abdominal surgery compared to standard care alone.

(Continued on next page)

* Correspondence: ianthe.boden@ths.tas.gov.au
[1]Physiotherapy Department, Launceston General Hospital, Charles St, Launceston, Tasmania 7250, Australia
[2]Department of Physiotherapy, The University of Melbourne, Melbourne, Victoria 3052, Australia
Full list of author information is available at the end of the article

(Continued from previous page)
Methods: The Incidence of Complications following Emergency Abdominal surgery: Get Exercising (ICEAGE) trial is a pragmatic, investigator-initiated, multicentre, patient- and assessor-blinded, parallel-group, active-placebo controlled randomised trial, powered for superiority. ICEAGE will compare standard care physiotherapy to an enhanced physiotherapy care package in 288 participants admitted for emergency abdominal surgery at three Australian hospitals. Participants will be randomised using concealed allocation to receive either standard care physiotherapy (education, single session of coached breathing exercises, and daily early ambulation for 15 min) or an enhanced physiotherapy care package (education, twice daily coached breathing exercises for a minimum 2 days, and 30 min of daily supervised early rehabilitation for minimum five postoperative days). The primary outcome is a respiratory complication within the first 14 postoperative hospital days assessed daily with standardised diagnostic criteria. Secondary outcomes include referral for sub-acute rehabilitation services, discharge destination, paralytic ileus, hospital length of stay and costs, intensive care unit utilisation, 90-day patient-reported complications and health-related quality of life and physical capacity, and mortality at 30 days and at 1 year following surgery.

Discussion: The morbidity, mortality, and fiscal burdens following emergency abdominal surgery are some of the worst within surgery. Physiotherapy may be an effective, low-cost, minimal harm intervention to improve outcomes and reduce hospital utilisation following this surgery type. ICEAGE will test the benefits of this commonly provided intervention within a methodologically robust, multicentre, double-blinded, active-placebo controlled randomised trial.

Keywords: Emergency surgery, Abdominal surgery, Complications, Physiotherapy, Breathing exercises, Postoperative pulmonary complication, Pneumonia, Ileus, Rehabilitation, Patient education

Background

Globally, millions of people every year require urgent time-critical emergency abdominal surgery to resolve potentially catastrophic small bowel obstructions, gastro-intestinal tract perforations, haemorrhage, invasive cancerous tumours, blunt force/penetrative trauma injuries, and peritonitis [1]. Emergency surgery accounts for approximately 11% of total surgical cases in the USA yet disproportionately can contribute to half of all surgical deaths and a third of all complications [2]. Postoperative outcomes following emergency abdominal surgery are generally poorer when compared to elective surgery. The most common serious complication after emergency abdominal surgery is a postoperative pulmonary complication (PPC) with an incidence rate of 20–50% [3–5]. Emergency surgery is the single greatest risk factor for a PPC, much greater than the risk attributed to other types of surgery and existing patient comorbidities [5]. The consequences of developing a PPC are serious with doubled health costs [6], longer hospital stay [5, 7], and higher mortality [5, 7, 8]. Understandably, efforts to improve postoperative outcomes following emergency abdominal surgery are strongly advocated [9].

Promising findings of reduced morbidity and mortality following the introduction of multidisciplinary perioperative care bundles, including increased physiotherapy [10, 11], are yet to be confirmed in randomised controlled trials. The size of the contribution of each individual treatment component within a care bundle also limits interpretation of findings. It is unknown whether physiotherapy can independently improve outcomes after emergency abdominal surgery.

Although the provision of physiotherapy to emergency abdominal surgery patients is ubiquitous in high-income countries [12], no clinical trials exist that have investigated the effect of physiotherapy on PPCs and overall recovery in this high-risk, high-care burden cohort over and above standard care [13].

Methods/design

Trial objectives

The primary objective of the Incidence of Complications following Emergency Abdominal surgery: Get Exercising (ICEAGE) trial is to estimate the effectiveness of physiotherapy on the incidence of PPC, including pneumonia, in patients following emergency open abdominal surgery.

Secondary objectives are to estimate the possible effect physiotherapy may have on prolonged postoperative ileus incidence, rates of referrals for formal sub-acute rehabilitation services, discharge destination, hospital length of stay (LOS) and costs, readiness to discharge from hospital, intensive care unit (ICU) LOS and readmissions, and rate of change to physical function and quality of life (QOL) whilst in hospital and at 90 days, and 1-year mortality.

Trial design

ICEAGE is a pragmatic, multicentre, parallel-group, randomised controlled trial. It is patient and assessor blinded, and powered for superiority. Eligible patients will be randomly assigned via concealed allocation into one of two physiotherapy treatment arms (Table 1). The control group will receive standard care physiotherapy from the first postoperative day consisting of education on prevention of complications with upright positioning, ambulation, and breathing exercises; a single deep breathing and coughing (DB&C) coaching session; and no more than 15 min of supervised ambulation once daily until a threshold score is met to discharge from this service. The intervention group will receive an enhanced physiotherapy care package from the first postoperative day consisting of (i) education on prevention of complications with upright positioning, ambulation, and breathing exercises; (ii) at least twice daily coached DB&C for the first two postoperative days; and (iii) at least 30 min of supervised early rehabilitation daily for the first five postoperative days. The mode of ambulation and respiratory physiotherapy will be standardised for both groups. The difference between groups will be (1) additional reminders and education as necessary for performance of independent exercises, (2) longer duration of ambulation and/or provision of individualised rehabilitation exercises, and (3) increased number of coached DB&C sessions (see Fig. 1 for the ICEAGE trial CONSORT diagram).

Trial setting

The three participating centres represent a range of hospital types in Australia. The Launceston General Hospital (Launceston, Tasmania, Australia) is a regional primary referral hospital; the Princess Alexandra Hospital (Brisbane, Queensland, Australia), a metropolitan primary referral hospital; and Northeast Health Wangaratta (Wangaratta, Victoria, Australia), a sub-regional secondary referral hospital, are all government-funded, university-affiliated, teaching hospitals.

Eligibility and exclusion criteria

Local investigators will screen daily surgery lists and recruit eligible patients from the ICU and wards at participating hospitals. Eligible patients will be adults over 18 years having open emergency abdominal surgery. This is defined as time-critical surgery (within 48 h of decision to operate) for a condition that is an immediate or intermediate threat to life or organ survival, involving at least one incision greater than, or equal to, 5 cm anywhere in the abdomen and through the fascia, for an existing hospital patient or a person admitted through the emergency department and requiring at least an overnight stay. Exclusion criteria are as follows: procedures solely involving inguinal hernia repairs, appendectomies, organ transplantation, thoracic, or gynaecological surgery; a PPC diagnosis anytime in the 24 h prior to eligibility screening; a pre-existing condition where the patient is unable to stand upright and ambulate for 1 min without a seated rest; severe cognitive impairment; unable to understand spoken English without the assistance of an interpreter (as determined by the research assistant, site investigator or ward physiotherapist performing eligibility screening); within 7 days of elective abdominal surgery; planned repeat surgery within 5 days of emergency procedure; approaching imminent death or withdrawal of medical treatment within 48 h of their surgical procedure; medical orders not to participate in early active rehabilitation; patients unable to be randomised by the research team within 48 h of surgery; enrolment in another clinical trial with similar endpoints; and previous enrolment in ICEAGE.

Randomisation and allocation

An administrative assistant independent of the trial will prepare 288 consecutively numbered (1 to 288) opaque envelopes each containing an allocation card wrapped in extra paper or aluminium foil [14]. Allocation sequence is determined by a computer-generated (http://www.randomizer.org/) blocked random number table (6 blocks of 48) with large blocks to minimise guessing of allocation sequence. The randomisation table will be sealed in an opaque envelope, locked within the primary centres' research institute, and made unavailable to trial personnel until trial completion. The number of consecutively numbered envelopes provided to each site will be dependent on funding agreements (i.e. funded to recruit one block of 48 participants, or, on a per patient recruit basis till the end of the trial).

Once a patient has been deemed eligible, the treating ward physiotherapist receives the group allocation by first writing patient details on the next consecutively numbered sealed opaque envelope and then opening it. If numerous new patients are eligible on the same day at a site, envelopes will be allocated in alphabetical order of surname. If an envelope is not available at the time of randomisation, a coin can be tossed by the treating physiotherapist and the result written on a card and countersigned by an independent observer. This card will be placed within the envelope that should have been allocated for that patient. If an envelope is erroneously opened out of sequence, the reason for doing so will be documented on it and the patient will be treated as per allocation card. Any aberrations to sequential allocation will be recorded. Envelopes will be kept securely by the ward physiotherapist or site investigator until hospital discharge and then integrated with the consent form and filed securely by the site investigator. Potential selection bias will be studied by extracting basic demographic data and planned surgical procedure from the medical records of all included and excluded patients.

Trial withdrawal

A patient is withdrawn if they withdraw their consent or do not provide consent following randomisation.

Table 1 TIDieR descriptions of ICEAGE interventions

TIDieR criterion	Control	Intervention
Item 1. Brief name: provide the name or a phrase that describes the intervention	Standard care: 'talk, walk, breathe'	Enhanced physiotherapy care: 'talk more, exercise more, breathe more'
Item 2 a) Describe any rationale, theory essential to the intervention	After emergency abdominal surgery the most common cause of morbidity and mortality is a postoperative pulmonary complication (PPC). Postoperative physiotherapy is routinely provided in intensive care units and surgical wards across Australia in an effort to prevent respiratory complications and enhance physical recovery after this major surgery type. Despite ubiquitous provision of this service, the effectiveness of postoperative physiotherapy is unknown.	Treatment components: 'Talk more': Repeated education sessions and reminders are allowed to be provided at the discretion of the physiotherapist. It is possible that more education will lead to greater motivation and increased independent performance of breathing and walking exercises.
Item 2 b) Describe goal of the elements essential to the intervention	Treatment components: 'Talk': The patient is informed of their risk of postoperative complications due to surgery and prolonged bed rest impairing their lungs and muscles. Education aims to inform, motivate, encourage, and inspire participation in exercises as prescribed. A booklet provides a written record of what was verbally taught. 'Walk': Early ambulation away from the bedside after surgery may prevent complications and physical decline after surgery. 'Breathe': Breathing and coughing exercises increase lung volumes, prevent postoperative atelectasis, improve gas exchange, clear stagnant secretions, and prevent postoperative pulmonary complications.	'Exercise more': The goal is to provide at least double the amount of physical activity daily. Daily physical activity will comprise of both ambulation and functional bed/chair/standing exercises. It is possible that there is a dose-dependent relationship with physical activity after surgery. Additional supervised physical activity early following surgery may hasten physical recovery and prevent complications more effectively. 'Breathe more': The goal is to provide at least four times the amount of coached breathing exercises in the first 2 days after surgery. It is possible that more breathing exercises performed early after surgery results in a greater risk reduction in the incidence of PPC.
Item 3. What (materials): describe any physical or informational materials used in the intervention, including those provided to participants or used in intervention delivery or in training of intervention providers.	Participant information materials: A booklet containing written and pictorial information regarding PPC and their potential prevention with early ambulation and breathing exercises to consolidate the learnt knowledge from verbal education and training. Intervention providers: Familiarisation with protocol prior to treating intervention participants. Badge cards containing the treatment protocol Template for documentation of treatment delivery Data entry sheets with further details of protocol	Participant information materials: As per control Intervention providers: As per control
Item 4. What (procedures): describe each of the procedures, activities, and/or processes used in the intervention, including any enabling or support activities	'Talk': once off Patients will have a single face-to-face education session following surgery with their physiotherapist. Patients will be educated on the benefit of walking and breathing exercises to prevent complications and improve recovery after surgery. Participants will be educated on the effect of surgery and bedrest to their lungs and muscles, and the benefit of walking and breathing exercises to prevent complications and improve recovery after surgery. Participants will be encouraged to perform the taught breathing exercises independently every hour during the day until they are walking at least 5 min, four times a day. Participants will also be strongly en couraged by their treating physiotherapist to sit upright, sit out of bed, walk away from their bed side (if safe to do so), or march on the spot be side their bed, as many times as they can during	'Talk more': at least once, then as often as required As per the control group. In addition, intervention group participants will receive extra reminders and prompts during the first five postoperative days to perform the prescribed rehabilitation and breathing exercises independently. Pragmatically, the number of additional education sessions and the use of exercise diaries and instruction sheets will be at the discretion of each treating physiotherapist based on their clinical experience and the individual needs of the intervention group participant.

Table 1 TIDieR descriptions of ICEAGE interventions *(Continued)*

TIDieR criterion	Control	Intervention
	the following days to aid in the prevention of PPCs Participants will be provided with an education booklet. This booklet contains written and pictorial information about abdominal surgery, expected types of pain management, medical lines and drains, postoperative recovery process, and how to prevent postoperative respiratory complications with early ambulation and self-directed breathing exercises. The breathing exercises are prescribed within with the recommended prescription of reps and sets.	
	'Walk': once daily ambulation only, < 15 min Initiation—as soon as practical after surgery Duration—no more than 15 min of total work time Frequency—once daily until a threshold score is met Intensity—rating of perceived exertion > 3/10, breathing deeper than at rest. Type—continuous activity for a minimum 1 min aiming for up to 15 min continuous as patient can tolerate. Allowable to train in intervals with work/rest ratio of 1:1 Mode—ambulation only. At every session the participant will be progressed sequentially through the protocol stages aiming to achieve a walking time of at least 10-min, but no more than 15-min. Successful ambulation is defined as continuously marching on the spot beside the bed or walking away from the bedside for more than 1 min. If a participant is unable to participate in upright ambulation, then no other non-ambulation exercises will be provided that day.	'Exercise more': once daily, ambulation and exercises, > 30 min Initiation—as soon as practical after surgery Duration—at least 30 min of total work time Frequency—once daily for at least the first 5 postoperative days and then until a threshold score is met Intensity—rating of perceived exertion > 3/10, breathing deeper than at rest. Type—continuous activity for a minimum 1 min aiming for as long as patient can tolerate. Allowable to train in intervals with work/rest ratio of 1:1 Mode—functional exercise programme starting with ambulation as per the control group protocol aiming for at least 15 min and if possible to at least 30 min of walking. If walking time is less than 30 min, non-ambulatory physical activity is continued to be provided until the minimum 30 min of activity time is achieved (not including rest periods). Physical activity is provided in a sequential step-down process starting with the highest activity possible and moving to less intense. These exercises consist of chair- or bed-based progressive low resistance, high repetition, lower and upper limb exercises of three–four sets as prescribed by the treating physiotherapist based on the individual patient's requirements and functional ability. If a participant is unconscious or acutely unwell, functional electrical stimulation of muscles and/or passive movements of limbs can be used as a physical activity.
	'Breathe': once off coached session Participants will receive a single physiotherapy coached deep breathing and coughing (DB&C) session within the first 2 days following surgery, or once the ward physiotherapist considers a patient conscious enough to understand and participate in this session. Physiotherapists will treat patients in upright sitting either in a bed or in a chair. The coached DB&C exercises will consist of two sets of 10 slow-flow breaths to maximum inspiratory capacity with two to three inspiratory sniff breath-stacking manoeuvres at the end of each deep breath followed by a 3- to 5-s breath hold. Each set of 10 breaths are followed by three coughs, or a forced expiratory technique with an open glottis called a 'huff', with a small firm pillow, or suitable substitute, pressed over on the abdominal	'Breathe more': at least four coached sessions in the first 2 days: As per the control group. Additionally, intervention group participants will receive at least three additional physiotherapist-coached DB&C sessions in the first two postoperative days. At least four sessions will be provided in total. Beyond the second day additional, coached DB&C can be provided at the discretion of the treating physiotherapist if they consider the patient incapable of performing exercises unsupervised or they consider the patient requires additional respiratory exercises to prevent a PPC.

Table 1 TIDieR descriptions of ICEAGE interventions *(Continued)*

TIDieR criterion	Control	Intervention
	incision to support the wound and to encourage greater expiratory force. The treating physiotherapist will have the discretion to place hands on the patient's chest wall during the coaching sessions to provide tactile feedback of performance. Total prescribed dosage of DB&C exercises is 20 breaths and six forced expiratory efforts every hour. The participants were encouraged to perform these every hour during the day until they were ambulant out of bed at least four times a day, for a minimum of 5 min at a time. No other prophylactic respiratory physiotherapy interventions or reminders to perform the taught DB&C exercises will be provided by the physiotherapist, this includes, but is not limited to, the following: manual or ventilator hyperinflation or recruitment manoeuvres in ventilated patients, manual techniques, positive expiratory pressure devices, incentive spirometers, or non-invasive ventilation.	
Item 5. Who provided: for each category of intervention, provider (for example, psychologist, nursing assistant), describe their expertise, background, and any specific training given	Qualified physiotherapists of varying experience levels at three different hospitals: new graduates, senior physiotherapists, and consultant level physiotherapists. An allied health assistant can deliver the ambulation protocol once this is deemed safe to do so by the treating physiotherapist.	Qualified physiotherapists of varying experience levels at three different hospitals: new graduates, senior physiotherapists, and consultant level physiotherapists. All sessions will be conducted by a physiotherapist (not an allied health assistant) until at least the fifth postoperative day unless the supervising physiotherapist is confident that an assistant or participant will undertake the rehabilitation programme exactly as prescribed for the minimum 30 min.
Item 6. How: describe the modes of delivery (such as face to face or by some other mechanism, such as internet or telephone) of the intervention and whether it was provided individually or in a group	Face-to-face, individual sessions	Face-to-face, individual sessions
Item 7. Where: describe the type(s) of location(s) where the intervention occurred, including any necessary infrastructure or relevant features	Inpatient hospital wards, patient bedsides at three government-funded, university affiliated, teaching hospitals Hospitals include a sub-regional secondary referral hospital, a regional primary referral hospital, and a metropolitan primary referral hospital.	Inpatient hospital wards, patient bedsides at three government-funded, university-affiliated, teaching hospitals. Hospitals include a sub-regional secondary referral hospital, a regional primary referral hospital, and a metropolitan primary referral hospital.
Item 8. When and how much: describe the number of times the intervention was delivered and over what period of time including the number of sessions, their schedule, and their duration, intensity or dose	See item 4	See item 4
Item 9. Tailoring: if the intervention was planned to be personalised, titrated or adapted, then describe what, why, when, and how	No tailoring	'Talk'—Extra education sessions can be provided by physiotherapist as necessary based upon their clinical judgement and the requirements of the patient. 'Exercise more'—Physiotherapist can incorporate specific functional exercises to target identified individual physical impairments, within the exercise protocol as long as the exercises comply with the goal intensity, duration, and type. 'Breathe more'—Physiotherapist can provide more DB&C exercise sessions, in addition to the minimum of four coached sessions, in

Table 1 TIDieR descriptions of ICEAGE interventions *(Continued)*

TIDieR criterion	Control	Intervention
		response to clinical judgement of risk and respiratory vulnerability.
Item 10. Modifications: If the intervention was modified during the course of the study, describe the changes (what, why, when, how)	N/A	N/A
Item 11. How well (planned): if intervention adherence or fidelity was assessed, describe how and by whom, and if any strategies were used to maintain or improve fidelity, describe them	Planned interim analysis of provision of ambulation programme to ensure that in > 80% of patients ambulation duration is no more than 15 min and provided until discharge criteria is met	Planned interim analysis of provision of exercise programme to ensure that in 80% of patients exercise duration is at least 30 min and provided for a minimum of five postoperative days/sessions.
Item 12: How well (actual): if intervention adherence or fidelity was assessed, describe the extent to which the intervention was delivered as planned	The trial will be amended or ceased for futility if there are critical failures to recruitment rates, breaches to protocol, or minimal treatment separation between groups.	The trial will be amended or ceased for futility if there are critical failures to recruitment rates, breaches to protocol, or minimal treatment separation between groups.

Abbreviations: PPC postoperative pulmonary complications, *DB&C* deep breathing and coughing

Trial interventions

Standard care physiotherapy (control)

The control group will receive physiotherapy care that is typically delivered in Australian hospitals[12]. This comprises of education (talk), early supervised ambulation (walk) once daily from the first postoperative day, and a single session of coached DB&C exercises (breathe) (Table 1).

Patient education—'talk' Patients will be educated on their risk of a PPC and slow recovery after surgery. They will be educated on the benefit of walking and breathing exercises to prevent complications and improve recovery after surgery [15, 16]. Following the first successful ambulation session, all participants will be strongly encouraged by their treating physiotherapist to sit upright, sit out of bed, walk away from their bedside (if safe to do so), or march on the spot beside their bed, as many times as they can during the following days to aid in the prevention of PPCs. They will be encouraged to seek assistance from a nurse if necessary and to walk with their visitors, or independently, once they are able to walk away from the bedside safely. Patients will be encouraged to perform the coached DB&C exercises independently every hour during the day until they are walking at least 5 min, four times a day. Patients will be provided with an information booklet containing all the supplied verbal information in written and pictorial format.

Early supervised ambulation—'walk' The standardised ambulation protocol [16, 17] (Table 2) will be provided as soon as practical after surgery by a physiotherapist. Patients will receive one supervised ambulation session per day until a threshold score is met [18] (Additional file 1), or discharge from hospital, whichever occurs first. At every session, the participant will be progressed sequentially through the protocol stages aiming to achieve a walking time of at least 10 min, but no more than 15 min, at an intensity of at least three on the Borg 10-point visual analogue scale (VAS) of perceived exertion [19], and where breathing is deeper than at rest. The treating physiotherapist will use a stopwatch to ensure the treatment session does not exceed 15 min and can provide a walking aid if clinically indicated. If necessary, ambulation sessions can comprise of equal work/rest intervals. Shorter, but not longer, rest times are allowable. The final achieved ambulation stage corresponds to total time walked, including the marching on the spot time, and not including rest periods.

Successful ambulation is defined as continuously marching on the spot beside the bed or walking away from the bedside for more than 1 min. Time from surgery to time of first successful ambulation will be recorded. If participants are unavailable or unable to achieve ambulation for more than 1 min, the assisted ambulation session will be attempted once again on the same day. The reasons for participants being unable to ambulate or not achieving a minimum of 10 min will be recorded. If a participant is unable to participate in upright ambulation, then no other non-ambulatory exercises will be provided that day. All treating therapists will be provided with protocol badge cards and trained by the site investigator. An allied health assistant can deliver the ambulation protocol once this is deemed safe to do so by the treating physiotherapist. The professional qualification of the person assisting each ambulation session will be documented.

Coached respiratory exercises—'breathe' Participants will receive a single physiotherapy education and coached DB&C session within the first 2 days following surgery, or once the ward physiotherapist considers a patient cognitively capable of participation.

Physiotherapists will treat patients in upright sitting either in a bed or in a chair. The coached DB&C exercises will consist of two sets of 10 slow-flow breaths to maximum inspiratory capacity with two to three inspiratory sniff breath-stacking manoeuvres at the end of each deep

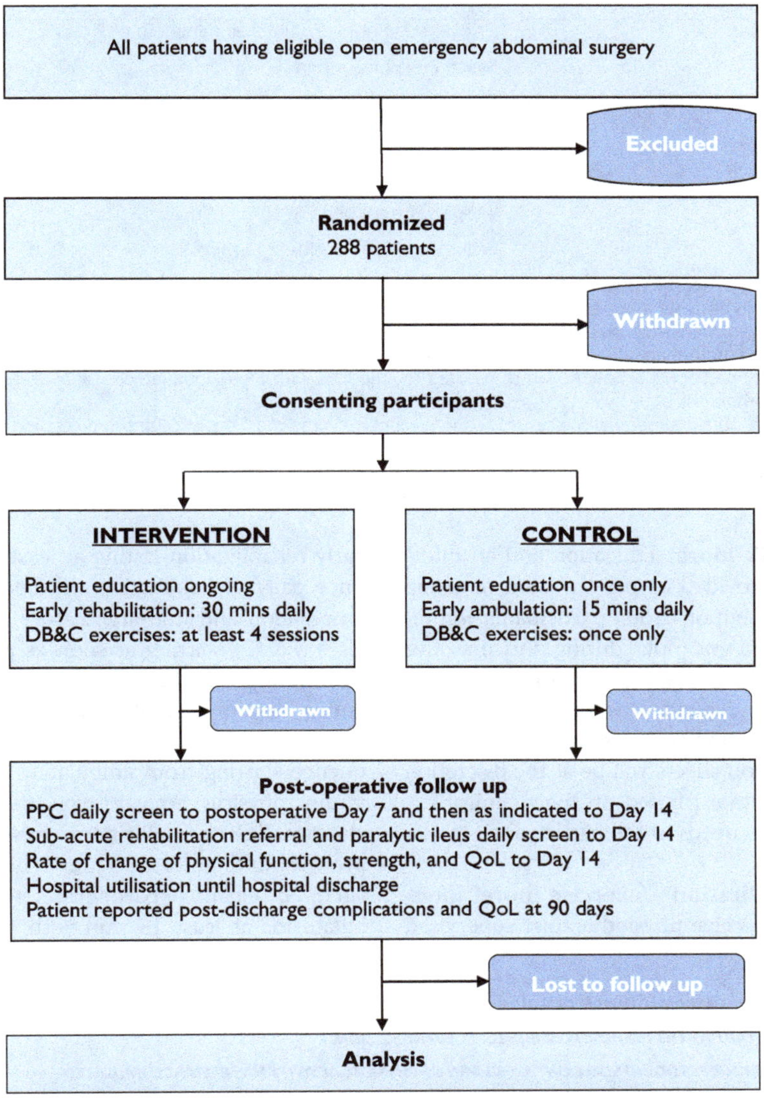

Fig. 1 CONSORT diagram of the ICEAGE trial. Abbreviations: DB&C deep breathing and coughing, PPC postoperative pulmonary complications, HRQOL health-related quality of life

breath followed by a 3- to 5-s breath hold [16, 17]. Each set of 10 breaths are followed by three coughs or forced expiratory technique with an open glottis called a 'huff,' with a small firm pillow, or suitable substitute, pressed over on the abdominal incision to support the wound and encourage greater expiratory force. The treating physiotherapist will have the discretion to place hands on the patient's chest wall during the coaching sessions to provide tactile feedback of performance. Total prescribed dosage of DB&C exercises is 20 breaths and six forced expiratory efforts every hour. No other prophylactic respiratory physiotherapy interventions or reminders to perform the taught DB&C exercises will be provided by the physiotherapist; this includes, but is not limited to, the following: manual or ventilator hyperinflation or recruitment manoeuvres in ventilated patients, manual techniques, positive expiratory pressure devices, or non-invasive ventilation.

Of note, all participants at Princess Alexandra Hospital and Northeast Health Wangaratta will be provided with an incentive spirometer by the nursing staff in the first 2 days after surgery as per routine nursing care at these hospitals. According to the pragmatic nature of this trial, this practice will continue and the incentive spirometer use will be recorded. Physiotherapists will not encourage incentive spirometer use in the control group.

Enhanced physiotherapy care (intervention)

The intervention group will receive the same care as the control group with the addition of the following (Table 1):

Table 2 ICEAGE ambulation protocol

Stage 1 (safety)	Sit over edge of bed/sit in chair minimum of 2 min
Stage 2 (safety)	March on spot 0–1 min
Stage 3 (ambulation)	March on spot/walk away from bedside 1–3 min
Stage 4 (ambulation)	March on spot/walk away from bedside 3–6 min
Stage 5 (ambulation)	Walk away from bedside 6–10 min
Stage 6 (ambulation)	Walk away from bedside 10–15 min
Stage 7 (ambulation)	Walk away from bedside > 15 min

Provide assisted early ambulation as soon as possible on the first postoperative day.
At each session, progress through each stage in sequence. Time achieved in the session is accumulative.
Aim to achieve rating of perceived exertion of greater than 3/10.
Aim to assist patient to ambulate more than 10 min (stage 6 or greater).
Once patient is able to ambulate past stage 3, patient can be assisted to ambulate with a physiotherapy assistant, as long as safe to do as determined by the ward physiotherapist.
Interval training is permissible to obtain target walking time. Each interval of rest time must not exceed the preceding work time. Total session time is the accumulative work time.
Provide assisted early ambulation once a day until discharged according to the discharge scoring tool.

Patient education—'talk more' Education and an information booklet will be provided as per the control group [15, 16]. In addition, intervention group participants will receive extra reminders and prompts during the first five postoperative days to perform the prescribed rehabilitation and breathing exercises independently. Pragmatically, the number of additional education sessions and the use of exercise diaries and instruction sheets will be at the discretion of each treating physiotherapist based on their clinical experience and the individual needs of the participant.

Supervised early rehabilitation—'exercise more' Intervention participants will receive physiotherapist supervised early rehabilitation lasting at least 30 min provided at least once daily. Rehabilitation will consist of a combination of ambulation and non-ambulatory chair- or bed-based exercises (Fig. 2) starting as soon as possible after surgery and continuing daily thereafter for at least the next five postoperative days or until at least five daily sessions are delivered. Exercises will be provided in a top-down hierarchical sequence starting from ambulation and aiming for the maximum physical activity type the participant is able to attempt. Exercise delivery progresses sequentially down the protocol until at least 30 min of activity have been accumulated. For example, participants will first be assisted to ambulate for at least 15 min with a goal to achieve at least

Early Rehabilitation Protocol

START AT THE HIGHEST POSSIBLE LEVEL EVERY SESSION.

PROGRESS DOWN SCALE UNTIL > 30-MIN OF PHYSICAL ACTIVITY HAS BEEN ACCUMULATED

1. Ambulation as per control protocol (Figure 2) although aim > 15mins
2. Lower limb closed-chain weight bearing exercises
   E.g. sit to stand. Start in raised bed progress to lower bed or ward chair as strength improves. Low resistance, 20 reps, 3-4 sets, 2 min rest between sets.
   Can include step ups, lunges in standing, mini-squats in standing
3. Upper limb or lower limb open-chain exercises in sitting
   Start against gravity progress to weight resisted as strength improves. Low resistance, 20 reps, 3-4 sets, 2 min rest between sets. Can include seated resisted foot pedals.
4. Dynamic sitting balance
   Sit over edge of bed or in chair. Patient to support themselves as much as able. Add in soft surface and/or reaching to targets as safety/patient status allows.
5. Active or active-assisted bed exercises
   Bridging in supine, hip flexion/extension/abduction, knee flexion/extension, ankle plantar/dorsiflexion. Start active-assisted and progress to active as soon as strength improves.
6. Deep breathing and coughing exercises
7. Passive mobilisation or passive muscle stimulation
   Passive cycling, functional electrical stimulation, passive limb movements

Fig. 2 ICEAGE exercise protocol. reps repetitions

30 min. If time ambulated is less than 30 min, the participant will attempt resistive lower limb exercises in standing for the remaining time or until fatigue limits the performance. If time still remains less than 30 min, participants will attempt upper limb/lower limb resistance exercises in sitting until fatigued. This process continues until a minimum total treatment time of 30 min has been reached. A treating physiotherapist is also permitted to prescribe a personalised training activity based on a detected functional deficit to be incorporated within the rehabilitation programme. These targeted and individualised sessions will be recorded.

This early rehabilitation protocol has been designed so that critically unwell ICU patients can participate [20, 21]. A conscious, intubated, and ventilated patient could be assisted out of bed to march on the spot once assessed as safe [20, 21], and an unconscious patient could participate in 30 min of passive limb movement [22, 23] and/or functional electrical stimulation of major muscles [24]. The initial starting exercise for each rehabilitation session will be made pragmatically at the discretion of the treating physiotherapist using their own past experience and knowledge base regarding the participant's current clinical and physiological status. No specific sedation score or assessment screening tool will be used to guide this decision.

Supervised activity in the intervention exercise protocol must aim to be continuous for more than 1 min, at an intensity of at least three on the Borg 10-point VAS of perceived exertion [18] and where breathing is deeper than at rest. The exception to this is for the passive limb exercises and functional electrical stimulation of muscles provided to unconscious or acutely unwell participants. Interval training is permitted; however, rest time cannot exceed the preceding active period. Once rest time becomes greater than the preceding work time, the exercise session is considered completed. The treating physiotherapist will use a stopwatch to ensure each rehabilitation session equals or exceeds 30 min. If a participant is unable to complete a 30-min session, the treating physiotherapist will document the reason. A further rehabilitation session later in the same day may be attempted to reach the 30-min threshold.

All sessions will be conducted by a physiotherapist until at least the fifth postoperative day unless the supervising physiotherapist is confident that a therapy assistant or the participant will undertake the rehabilitation programme exactly as prescribed for the minimum 30 min. After the fifth postoperative day, daily treatment with a physiotherapist or therapy assistant will continue until either a referral for sub-acute rehabilitation services is made (see endpoints), a participant is discharged from hospital, or once a threshold score is met [18] (Additional file 1), whichever occurs first. If the patient meets the discharge score prior to the fifth postoperative day, daily treatment will continue until the fifth postoperative day but cease thereafter.

Coached respiratory exercises—'breathe more' The mode, type, and timing of delivery of DB&C exercises will be provided as per the control group. Intervention group participants will receive at least three additional physiotherapist-coached DB&C sessions in the first two postoperative days. At least four sessions will be provided in total. The total number of sessions will be recorded. Beyond the second day, additional coached DB&C can be provided at the discretion of the treating physiotherapist if they consider the patient incapable of performing exercises unsupervised or requires additional respiratory exercises to prevent a PPC are indicated. Similar to the control group, no additional prophylactic respiratory interventions apart from the DB&C exercises will be provided.

Other components of postoperative care

Additional ambulation occasions or DB&C sessions conducted independently by the participant or assisted by other ward staff will not be measured nor controlled for as this would not be feasible or consistent with the pragmatic nature of this trial. All other aspects of patient care, including general anaesthesia, surgical techniques, intraoperative ventilation parameters, fluid delivery, prophylactic antibiotic prescription, pain management, use of lines and drains, general nursing care, and discharge planning, will be administered according to routine clinical practice at each participating centre.

The three participating sites have limited physiotherapy service on weekends and on public holidays. If protocol is unable to be delivered due to service limitations, this will be recorded.

Safety monitoring

Early rehabilitation of at least 30 min daily in ICU patents is safe when provided in consideration of the patient's immediate clinical status and haemodynamic stability [25]. The emergency abdominal surgery population, in comparison, will be generally less acute. No adverse events in this population have been reported in similar exercise treatment protocols [26]. The following events will be reported if they occur during a treatment session and only if it is standard procedure at each site to monitor these parameters during physiotherapy treatment: symptomatic blood pressure or heart rate change 20% from resting, new cardiac arrhythmia, or drop in oxygen saturation > 10% from baseline, which fails to recover within 2 min of ceasing activity; patient requires increased sedation or inotropic support; line detachment; fall; or severe nausea. Adverse events will be immediately recorded in the participant's medical record and in the case report form. The treating physiotherapist will immediately report the event to the site investigator who will alert the chief investigator within 24 h of the event for further investigation and classification. A significant adverse event (SAE) occurs where, in the opinion of the chief investigator, the event was directly related to the intervention or control treatments, was unexpected, and significantly impacted the participant's immediate health and/or delayed recovery. All SAE will be reported to the ethics committee.

Outcome measures

Primary outcome

The primary outcome is the first occurrence of a PPC within the first 14 postoperative hospital days. PPCs will be defined by the Melbourne Group Score (Table 3) which is reliable, valid [27, 28], sensitive to interventions [16], and has high inter-rater reliability [29]. It has eight clinical criteria: four factors relating to symptoms and four to diagnostic markers. A PPC will be diagnosed when four or more factors are present at any time from midnight to midnight on one postoperative day. The day a PPC is first diagnosed is the day of onset for purposes of time-to-event analysis.

Participants are assessed prospectively and daily for a PPC by a blinded assessor until the seventh postoperative day. From the 8th to the 14th postoperative day, additional PPC assessments are performed only as clinically suspected based on signs or symptoms of respiratory system deterioration reported within the medical record.

Table 3 PPC diagnostic criteria—Melbourne Group Score Version 3

When four or more of the following criteria* are present anytime in the 24-h period 00:01 to 24:00 on a single postoperative day:

1. New abnormal breath sounds on auscultation different to preoperative assessment⁺
2. Production of yellow, green, or brown sputum different to pre-morbid status⁺
3. Pulse oximetry oxygen saturation (SpO_2) < 90% on room air or FiO2 on 0.21 on more than one consecutive postoperative day**
4. Raised maximum tympanic temperature ≥ 38 °C on more than one consecutive postoperative day
5. Chest radiograph report of collapse/consolidation# ***
6. Presence of infective organisms on sputum culture report***
7. White cell count > 11 or < 3
8. Physician's diagnosis of postoperative pulmonary complication (e.g. atelectasis, pneumonia, AECOPD, respiratory failure, upper respiratory tract infection) OR prescription of an antibiotic specific for respiratory infection

Abbreviations: *PPC* postoperative pulmonary complications, *SpO2* pulse oximetry, *FiO2* fraction of inspired oxygen, *AECOPD* acute exacerbation of chronic obstructive pulmonary disease, *PEEP* positive end expiratory pressure, *CXR* chest X-ray

*If a blinded physiotherapist, nurse, or physician documents in the medical record the occurrence of a criterion, it can be taken as a positive finding. If no documentation present, a blinded assessor is required to assess this directly

⁺If no preoperative assessment or documentation assume normal at baseline

**For ventilated patients, if $FiO_2 \geq 0.5$ or PEEP ≥ 8, assume criterion 3 is present (do not alter FiO_2), for all other patients set FiO_2 to 0.21 and observe SpO_2 for 2 min. If SpO_2 drops below 90%, immediately reinstate previous FiO_2. If not permissible to alter ventilation parameters, assume positive

#If no written report for a CXR is available and a patient has three other positive signs, a masked senior physiotherapist or ward medical officer is to be contacted to report verbally on the available CXR

***When there are no daily measures of CXR or sputum sampling, carry over a positive finding to the next consecutive postoperative day

To reduce the potential for missing data, retrospective collection of PPC data from the medical record will be permitted when a patient or assessor is unavailable for PPC assessment. Diagnostic components (chest X-ray (CXR), white cell count, sputum microbiology) are recorded only if results are available. All medical officers are masked to group allocation, and these diagnostic tests are ordered only as clinically indicated, and not routinely for the purposes of the ICEAGE trial.

For this trial, modifications have been made to reduce delays to possible diagnosis of a PPC (Table 3). An automatic positive threshold for the hypoxemia criterion has been set for ventilated patients; a positive CXR and/or sputum sample finding can be carried over to the next postoperative day if serial testing was not performed; a CXR can be verbally reported by a blinded senior respiratory physiotherapist or physician, rather than awaiting a radiologist report; and when three factors (out of a possible eight) are present, the blinded site investigator or ward physiotherapist will discuss the option of further diagnostic testing to confirm PPC with the participant's treating physician. Additionally, patients with three out of eight criteria will be assessed twice daily for any clinical deterioration.

Any suspected PPC will be confirmed by a blinded senior physiotherapist, and the participant will then receive respiratory treatment as determined by the ward physiotherapist.

Secondary/exploratory trial outcomes

In hierarchical order:

1. Referral by the surgical team or other allied health professional within the first 14 postoperative days for additional acute-ward physiotherapy rehabilitation, sub-acute hospital rehabilitation, or community-based rehabilitation. On receipt of a referral, or by the 14th postoperative day if referral not received, a blinded senior physiotherapist will review the participant's current medical record and adjudicate for the requirement for rehabilitation services.
2. Discharge destination from the acute hospital ward (home, rehabilitation facility, nursing home, or other hospital);
3. Hospital LOS in days. This is defined as continuous days spent in any type of inpatient hospital service (i.e. acute care, sub-acute rehabilitation, or time at another hospital) from the day of admission for acute condition to the day of discharge to community. Hospital days will be sub-categorised into acute and sub-acute;
4. Incidence of a prolonged postoperative ileus (PPOI) anytime from the fourth to the 14th postoperative hospital day. A PPOI is defined if two or more of

the following criteria are met on or after the fourth postoperative day [30]: (i) nausea or vomiting, (ii) inability to tolerate an oral diet over last 24 h, (iii) absence of flatus over the last 24 h, (iv) abdominal distension, and (v) radiologic confirmation. The day which PPOI is first diagnosed is the day of PPOI onset for purposes of time-to-event analysis.

5. Diagnosis of pneumonia defined as the presence of new CXR infiltrates along with at least two of the following: temperature > 38 °C, dyspnoea, cough, and purulent sputum, altered respiratory auscultation, and white cell count > 14,000/ml or leukopenia < 3000/ml on any day within the first 14 postoperative hospital days;
6. Recovery of physical function and QOL
   i) Rate of change of the Modified Iowa Level of Assistance [31] (mILOA; Additional file 1) score over four measures taken second daily from the first postoperative day and a final score on the day of acute-ward discharge. The mILOA consists of four mobility tasks (supine to sitting on the edge of the bed, sit to stand, walking, and negotiation of one step), which are graded according to the level of assistance required, use of gait aid, and the distance that can be walked. Data will be extracted from the medical and physiotherapy records to score;
   ii) Rate of change in handgrip strength (kg) measured using a handheld dynamometer over four postoperative measures within the first 14 days. Measures will be taken at least 2 days apart;
   iii) Rate in change of the EuroQual QOL score [32] (EQ-5D; Additional file 2); measures to be taken directly from the patient over two consecutive measures separated by 48 h, within the first five postoperative days, and at 90 days following surgery;
   iv) Health-related QOL using World Health Organisation Disability Assessment Schedule V2 [33] (WHODAS; Additional file 3) change from self-rated status in the week prior to surgery, to day of discharge from acute care, and at 90 days following surgery;
   v) Physical capacity using Self-Assessment of Physical Activity Questionnaire [34] (SAQ; Additional file 4) from self-rated capacity regarding the week prior to surgery to 90 days following surgery;
   vi) Time in hours from end of operation to time able to achieve ambulation greater than 1 min;
   vii) Time in days from end of operation to achieve ambulation greater than 10 min;
7. ICU LOS in days;
8. Unplanned ICU admission during acute hospital stay;
9. Mortality—in-hospital, 30 and 90days, and at 1 year;
10. Sepsis within the first 7 days according to the Sequential Organ Failure Assessment (SOFA) for ICU patients and quick-SOFA for ward patients [35];
11. Time in days to discharge from physiotherapy as determined daily using the Post-Operative Physiotherapy Discharge Scoring Tool [18] (Additional file 1);
12. Time in days to readiness for hospital discharge within the first 14 postoperative days defined by standardised scoring criteria [36];
13. Patient reported complications at 90 days using a standardised semi-structured interview [16];
14. Hospital costs for the admission episode of care supplied by the participating centres', or health departments', costing data for each participant's admission episode.

WHODAS, EQ-5D, and SAQ measures will be via direct interview whilst in hospital and by phone interview when patient at home. At 90-day (± 14 days) follow-up, if participant is unable to be contacted for a period of five consecutive working days, a standardised cover letter, questionnaires, and self-addressed return paid envelope will be posted. Forms not returned within 2 weeks will be considered lost to follow-up for post-discharge secondary outcomes. Figure 3 describes the schedule of events, trial conduct, and outcome measurements.

Protocol endpoints

Treatment protocols will be ceased when:

1. Participant is discharged or transferred from the primary treating hospital.
2. Participant becomes deceased or death is expected within next 7 days.
3. Participants meet a threshold score to trigger discharge from physiotherapy treatment[18]. This criterion is delayed for the first five postoperative days for intervention participants.
4. A confirmed PPC diagnosis ceases the respiratory treatment protocol. Respiratory treatment is then provided at the discretion of the ward physiotherapist. Participants remain being treated with the rehabilitation protocol as per group allocation.
5. A confirmed referral for additional sub-acute rehabilitation services ceases the ambulation or early rehabilitation protocol. Rehabilitation is then provided at the discretion of the ward physiotherapist. Participants remain being treated with the respiratory treatment protocol as per group allocation.

Blinding

The recruiting and treating physiotherapists will be solely aware of group allocation. Assessments of primary and

		STUDY PERIOD					
		Eligibility Enrolment Allocation	Post-allocation				Close-out
		0	t_1 - t_7	$t_8 - t_{14}$	t_{15}	t_{16}	t_{17}
	TIMEPOINT	*Within 48h of surgery*	*POD 1 to POD 7*	*POD 8 to POD 14*	*D/C*	*90 days following surgery*	*1 year following surgery*
ENROLMENT	Enrolment	X					
	Eligibility screen	X					
	Informed consent		X				
	Random allocation	X					
INTERVENTIONS	*CONTROL: talk, walk, breathe*	X					
	INTERVENTION: Talk more, exercise more, breathe more	X					
VARIABLES	*Demographics, medical history, comorbidities*	X					
	Intraoperative variables	X					
	Postoperative variables		X ←—	—→ X			
OUTCOMES	*SAQ*	X				X	
	WHODAS	X			X	X	
	EQ-5D		X			X	
	Sepsis		X				
	PPC, including pneumonia		X ←—	—→ X			
	Referral for rehabilitation		X ←—	—→ X			
	PPOI		X ←—	—→ X			
	Time to ambulate >1min and >10min		X ←—	—→ X			
	Days to d/c from physiotherapy service		X ←—	—→ X			
	Handgrip strength		X ←—	—→ X			
	ICU admission and LOS, Hospital LOS		X ←—	———	—→ X		
	Discharge destination		X ←—	———	—→ X		
	mILOA		X ←—	———	—→ X		
	Hospital costs				X		
	Patient reported complications					X	
	Mortality				X	X	X

Fig. 3 ICEAGE schedule of events and timeline. Abbreviations: POD postoperative day, D/C hospital discharge, SAQ specific activity questionnaire, WHODAS World Health Organisation disability assessment score, EQ-5D EuroQuol five domains, PPC postoperative pulmonary complication, PPOI prolonged postoperative ileus, ICU intensive care unit, LOS length of stay, mILOA modified Iowa level of assistance

secondary outcomes and data collection will be performed by independent masked assessors not involved in the participant's care. Assessors will require access to the medical record. To ensure masking to group allocation, documentation of physiotherapy assessments and interventions will be written to a standardised format (Additional file 5) with treatment recorded 'Treatment provided as per ICEAGE protocol'. Documentation detailing physiotherapy treatment will be recorded separately and stored securely by the treating physiotherapist until the 14th postoperative day, the day of discharge, or until a defined endpoint is met, whichever occurs first, at which point the physiotherapy treatment documentation will be integrated into the medical record.

All doctors, surgeons, nurses, discharge coordinators, data analysts, and statisticians will be blinded to group allocation. If a participant inadvertently informs an assessor of their specific physiotherapy treatment, this will be reported, and a new assessor will be found for ongoing assessments.

It is anticipated that participants will be blinded to group allocations as both arms receive physiotherapy. A convenience sample of 30 consecutive participants will be asked which group they believed they had been allocated at the 90-day follow-up interview.

Data management

The data dictionary for ICEAGE is supplied in Additional file 6. Data will be collected from participants using a standardised electronic case report form (CRF) and stored in participating centres' password protected electronic hard drives. To ensure correct data entry, the CRF has been designed with extensive use of data entry limitation rules and on-screen prompts. Site investigators will be required to perform random covert audits of data collected by trial personnel during the trial for reliability and correctness against the medical record. There are no industrial contractual arrangements in relation to the de-identified data. On completion of the trial, the database will be made available for independent analysis or as an appendix in the publishing journal if requested.

Statistical analysis

Sample size

PPC rates previously reported following emergency abdominal surgery are between 30 and 40% [3, 4, 27]. A 2013 prospective audit (unpublished) of PPC incidence in 50 consecutive patients at the primary participating centre found a rate of 20% (95%CI 10–34%). A 60% relative risk reduction in PPC with timely physiotherapy can be achieved in the elective abdominal surgery population [16]. A total sample size of 262 completed participants (131 per group) is required to detect a reduction in PPC rate by 60% from an anticipated baseline of 20% (20% down to 8%) with an alpha 0.05 and power 80%. This is arbitrarily increased to compensate for a possible 10% drop out/withdrawal rate and uncertainty around baseline incidence and effect size. In total, a sample of 288 participants is required for this trial.

Statistical methods

Imbalances of potential confounding variables between trial groups at recruitment will be assessed. Adjustment covariates will be selected by backward stepwise regression from covariates that are anticipated to affect incidence of PPC. These include respiratory comorbidity, smoking history, age, gender, length of operation, operation category (upper gastrointestinal, colorectal, urological, other), and ICU admission immediately following the procedure.

Primary outcome The absolute and relative rates of PPC in the trial groups will be estimated using multivariate robust random effects Poisson generalised linear regression to allow assessment of binary outcomes with or without adjustment for potential confounding variables (incidence rates and rate ratios, 95% confidence intervals, p values). Treatment centre will be treated as a fixed variable in multi-level models. In addition, the effect of time from the end of surgery/anaesthesia to commencement of symptoms of PPC will be compared using Cox proportional hazards regression with and without covariate adjustment (hazards ratio, 95% confidence intervals, p values). A Kaplan-Meier graphic representation of this analysis will be performed.

Secondary outcomes

1. Binomial outcomes including rehabilitation referrals, pneumonia, PPOI, unplanned ICU admissions, patient-reported complications, and mortality will be analysed using multivariate robust random effects Poisson generalised linear regression.
2. Time-to-event binomial outcomes (e.g. PPC, pneumonia, PPOI, achievement of ambulation goals of 1 and 10 min; and hospital and ICU LOS; and mortality) will be compared by estimating hazard ratios using Cox proportional hazards regression, with and without covariate adjustment where necessary and graphically illustrated using Kaplan-Meier methods.
3. Measures involving estimation of rate of change over time (QOL and functional capacity) will be analysed using repeated-measures mixed effects linear regression or ordered logistic regression for rank-ordered scale measures.
4. Hospital costs will be compared using mixed effects linear regression. Log transformation of highly skewed cost data will be performed. Depending on the adequacy of the data for purposes of economic analysis, a cost-utility may be conducted.

All outcomes will be analysed on an intention-to-treat basis. An intention-to-protocol sensitivity analysis will be performed by identifying as a separate group participants who received more than 80% of planned protocol sessions as per group allocation. Other planned sensitivity analyses will be made according to age (> 65), surgery type (colorectal, upper gastrointestinal, other), preoperative self-reported physical capacity, and gender. Sensitivity of outcome estimates to missing data will be evaluated using multiple imputations. All analyses will be performed using Stata MP2 V14 (StataCorp, College Station, TX, USA).

Trial monitoring

The steering committee consists of the chief investigator, site investigators, and an academic investigator who contributed to the design and revision of the study protocol. The chief investigator is responsible for the study administrative management, communication with local investigators, and assists participating centres with trial conduct, record keeping, and data management. A planned interim analysis 1 year into trial, or at $n = 50$, whichever occurs first, will consider trial conduct, recruitment, adverse events, and adherence to trial protocol. The volume and duration of provided physiotherapy will be compared between groups. The trial will be amended or ceased due to futility if there are critical failures to recruitment rates, breaches to protocol, or minimal treatment separation between groups. Primary or secondary outcome differences will not be investigated at this interim analysis as this could lead to a subconscious bias in trial conduct.

Ethics and dissemination

Retrospective consent

Ethics approval has been granted for eligible patients to be randomised prior to consent. Patients within the first two postoperative days after emergency abdominal surgery are often unwell and in an emotionally vulnerable state. Initial ethics approval was granted with a traditional enrolment into the trial following gaining of consent. However, following a planned interim analysis of trial conduct on the 50th patient recruited into the trial (unpublished data), patients and next of kin reported feeling distressed when approached by researchers in the first two postoperative days to discuss the trial. Further detailed feedback on the consenting process was sought from patients ($n = 20$) at 1-week post-surgery. All patients reported feeling too unwell in the first few days after surgery and disliked having to consider participating in a trial that was comparing two forms of low-risk commonly provided care. All patients indicated that they would prefer to provide retrospective consent. They recommended approximately no earlier than the third postoperative day or when they were not feeling nauseated. The two comparison interventions had nil documented occasions of harm at that point in the trial. Adverse events are similarly very low (< 1%) in critically unwell patients who are provided with 30 min of daily rehabilitation therapy [25]. There is minimal clinical risk to the patient being provided with either two arms of the study. Randomisation immediately on eligibility also allows the physiotherapy protocol to be delivered without delay, possibly enhancing the clinical outcome for all participants. Additionally, the primary outcome measure is non-invasive, has minimal risk, and requires no additional participation from the patient outside of standard care. An application to all responsible ethics committees was placed to alter consent to a retrospective consent following randomisation and was granted.

The principal site investigator will approach the patient from the fourth postoperative day and describe the trial, including the potential risks and benefits, and involvement required from the patient. Written information will be provided, and the patient will be invited to participate in the trial. Any person not consenting following randomisation is withdrawn from the trial. If the patient consents to continue in the trial, they will sign a consent form as required by local ethics committees and in accordance with the Declaration of Helsinki. If the patient remains in a state where informed consent is unable to be provided, (i.e. unconscious, delirious, nauseated, pain, repeat surgery) the next of kin will be contacted for consent. If the patient or next of kin declines to participate, the patient will take no further part in the trial and all data will be withdrawn. Physiotherapy will then be provided to them at the discretion of the ward physiotherapist.

Trial participants will have the autonomy to decline any therapy session as per standard care provision and medico-legal requirements regardless of recruitment into the trial. Reasons for non-participation in therapy sessions will be documented.

Dissemination

This protocol is reported according to the SPIRIT guideline [37]. Trial results will be written in accordance with the CONSORT extensions for a pragmatic trial using a non-pharmacological intervention, published in a peer-reviewed journal, and presented at national and international meetings.

Trial status

This trial is currently active. First participant was recruited on 25 June 2015. It is anticipated that recruitment will be completed in late 2018.

Discussion

ICEAGE will provide the first high-level degree of evidence for the possible benefit of physiotherapy to reduce complications and improve physical recovery following emergency abdominal surgery. This trial involves three different types of hospitals: rural, regional, and metropolitan; includes most types of open major emergency abdominal surgery; and is conducted within a pragmatic framework where all other perioperative care is conducted without change. Our findings will be highly generalizable to most first-world hospitals.

In keeping with normal clinical practice and pragmatic trial methodology, it is unlikely that the interventions will be provided exactly as per protocol for every planned session; indeed, there will be many occasions where it will not be possible to treat a patient as planned due to extraneous circumstances (e.g. away at imaging, returned to theatre, refuses treatment, sudden deterioration). To ensure that our findings are relevant to practical real-life clinical situations in which our interventions are intended to be applied in, all patients entered in the trial will be analysed according to intention-to-treat principles, regardless of adherence to protocol. To determine if results are affected by adherence, we have planned a per-protocol sensitivity analysis of those patients who adhered to the protocol in more than 80% of intended occasions.

All assessors and patients will be masked to group allocation, and there is an active-placebo of current practice physiotherapy. This will ensure that any effects are independently associated with the additional therapy provided rather than the Hawthorne effect of health professional interaction. ICEAGE will include not only short-term clinical outcomes, but medium-term patient-reported QOL and physical recovery, and long-term mortality. The results of ICEAGE will inform the clinical provision of physiotherapy to millions of patients globally every year.

Additional files

Additional file 1: Postoperative Physiotherapy Discharge Scoring Tool. Table describing the discharge from physiotherapy scoring. (DOCX 15 kb)

Additional file 2: EQ-5D-5L. EuroQual 5 Domains scoring. (DOCX 90 kb)

Additional file 3: WHODAS. World Health Organisation disability assessment scale. (DOCX 20 kb)

Additional file 4: WHODAS. World Health Organisation disability assessment scale. (PDF 24 kb)

Additional file 5: Physiotherapist ward data collection and protocol form. Case report form for ward physiotherapists. (PDF 403 kb)

Additional file 6: ICEAGE Data Dictionary. Data fields for ICEAGE. (DOCX 18 kb)

Abbreviations

CRF: Case report form; CXR: Chest X-ray; DB&C: Deep breathing and coughing; EQ-5D: EuroQual five domains; ICEAGE: Incidence of Complications following Emergency Abdominal surgery—Get Exercising; ICU: Intensive care unit; LOS: Length of stay; mILOA: Modified Iowa level of assistance; PPC: Postoperative pulmonary complication; PPOI: Prolonged postoperative ileus; QOL: Quality of life; SAE: Serious adverse event; SAQ: Self-administered physical activity questionnaire; SOFA: Sequential organ failure assessment; VAS: Visual analogue scale; WHODAS: World Health Organisation disability assessment score

Acknowledgements

We would like to thank all physiotherapists and allied health assistants at the participating sites for providing the interventions and Prof Jenny Keating for providing early phase protocol review.

Funding

This study is an investigator-initiated trial funded by research grants from the Clifford Craig Foundation, Launceston, Australia (Project number 130, $80,000 AUD). The funding body has no influence on the study design, collection or data analysis, or publication of results.

Authors' contributions

IB and KS conceived and designed the study and devised the protocol. IB is the chief investigator, overseeing and coordinating trial conduct. IB, KS, CH, BW, and MM are site investigators. RL assisted in the study design and protocol development. IR and IB prepared the statistical analysis plan. IB prepared the first draft of the protocol manuscript and was responsible for the final manuscript. All authors (IB, KS, CH, BW, RL, MM, IR) revised all manuscript drafts, approved the final manuscript, and contributed intellectually important content. IB is the guarantor of the paper and takes responsibility for the integrity of the work as a whole, from inception to published article.

Competing interests

The authors declare that they have no competing interests.

Author details

[1]Physiotherapy Department, Launceston General Hospital, Charles St, Launceston, Tasmania 7250, Australia. [2]Department of Physiotherapy, The University of Melbourne, Melbourne, Victoria 3052, Australia. [3]School of Primary Health Care, Faculty of Nursing, Medicine and Health Science, Monash University, Frankston, Victoria 3199, Australia. [4]Department of Physiotherapy, Princess Alexandra Hospital, Woolloongabba, Queensland 4102, Australia. [5]Physiotherapy Department, Northeast Health Wangaratta, Green Street, Wangaratta, Victoria 3677, Australia. [6]School of Physiotherapy, Faculty of Health Sciences, Australian Catholic University, Ballarat, Victoria 3350, Australia. [7]Biostatistician, Clifford Craig Foundation, Launceston General Hospital, Charles Street, Launceston, Tasmania 7250, Australia. [8]College of Health Sciences, University of Tasmania, Locked Bag 1320, Launceston, Tasmania 7250, Australia.

References

1. Stewart B, Khanduri P, McCord C, Ohene-Yeboah M, Uranues S, Vega Rivera F, et al. Global disease burden of conditions requiring emergency surgery. Br J Surg. 2014;101:e9–22.
2. Smith M, Hussain A, Xiao J, Scheidler W, Reddy H, Olugbade K Jr, et al. The importance of improving the quality of emergency surgery for a regional quality collaborative. Ann Surg. 2013;257:596–602.
3. Tengberg LT, Cihoric M, Foss NB, Bay-Nielsen M, Gögenur I, Henriksen R, et al. Complications after emergency laparotomy beyond the immediate postoperative period—a retrospective, observational cohort study of 1139 patients. Anaesthesia. 2017;72:309–16.
4. Serejo LG, da Silva-Júnior FP, Bastos JP, de Bruin GS, Mota RM, de Bruin PF. Risk factors for pulmonary complications after emergency abdominal surgery. Respir Med. 2007;101:808–13.
5. Fernandez-Bustamante A, Frendl G, Sprung J, Kor DJ, Subramaniam B, Ruiz RM, et al. Postoperative pulmonary complications, early mortality, and hospital stay following noncardiothoracic surgery: a multicenter study by the perioperative research network investigators. JAMA Surg. 2017;152:157–66.
6. Thompson DA, Makary MA, Dorman T, Pronovost PJ. Clinical and economic outcomes of hospital acquired pneumonia in intra-abdominal surgery patients. Ann Surg. 2006;243:547–52.
7. Fleisher LA, Linde-Zwirble WT. Incidence, outcome, and attributable resource use associated with pulmonary and cardiac complications after major small and large bowel procedures. Perioper Med. 2014; https://doi.org/10.1186/2047-0525-3-7.
8. Arenal JJ, Bengoechea-Beeby M. Mortality associated with emergency abdominal surgery in the elderly. Can J Surg. 2003;46:111.
9. Aggarwal G, Peden CJ, Quiney NF. Improving outcomes in emergency general surgery patients: what evidence is out there? Anesth Analg. 2017; 125:1403–5.
10. Huddart S, Peden CJ, Swart M, McCormick B, Dickinson M, Mohammed MA, et al. Use of a pathway quality improvement care bundle to reduce mortality after emergency laparotomy. Br J Surg. 2015;102:57–66.
11. Tengberg LT, Bay-Nielsen M, Bisgaard T, Cihoric M, Lauritsen ML, Foss NB, et al. Multidisciplinary perioperative protocol in patients undergoing acute high-risk abdominal surgery. Br J Surg. 2017;104:463–71.
12. Patman S, Bartley A, Ferraz A, Bunting C. Physiotherapy in upper abdominal surgery—what is current practice in Australia? Arch Physiother. 2017;7:11.
13. Sullivan K, Reeve J, Boden I, Lane R. Physiotherapy following emergency abdominal surgery. In: Garbuzenko D, editor. Actual problems of emergency abdominal surgery. Rijeka: InTechOpen; 2016. https://doi.org/10.5772/63969.
14. Doig GS, Simpson F. Understanding clinical trials: emerging methodological issues. Intensive Care Med. 2014;40:1755–7.
15. Boden I, El-Ansary D, Zalucki N, Robertson IK, Browning L, Skinner EH, et al. Physiotherapy education and training prior to upper abdominal surgery is memorable and has high treatment fidelity: a nested mixed-methods randomised-controlled study. Physiotherapy. 2018;104:194–202.
16. Boden I, Skinner EH, Browning L, Reeve J, Anderson L, Hill C, et al. Preoperative physiotherapy for the prevention of respiratory complications after upper abdominal surgery: pragmatic, double blinded, multicentre randomised controlled trial. BMJ. 2018;360:j5916.
17. Boden I, Browning L, Skinner EH, Reeve J, El-Ansary D, Robertson IK, et al. The LIPPSMAck POP (lung infection prevention post surgery-major abdominal-with pre-operative physiotherapy) trial: study protocol for a multi-centre randomised controlled trial. Trials. 2015;16:1–15.
18. Brooks D, Parsons J, Newton J, Dear C, Silaj E, Sinclair L, et al. Discharge criteria from perioperative physical therapy. Chest. 2002;121:488–94.
19. Abadie B. Effect of viewing the RPE scale on the ability to make ratings of perceived exertion. Percept Mot Skills. 1996;83:317–8.
20. Wright SE, Thomas K, Watson G, Baker C, Bryant A, Chadwick TJ, et al. Intensive versus standard physical rehabilitation therapy in the critically ill (EPICC): a multicentre, parallel-group, randomised controlled trial. Thorax. 2018;73:213–21.
21. Hodgson CL, Bailey M, Bellomo R, Berney S, Buhr H, Denehy L, et al. A binational multicenter pilot feasibility randomized controlled trial of early goal-directed mobilization in the ICU. Crit Care Med. 2016;44:1145–52.
22. Kayambu G, Boots R, Paratz J. Early physical rehabilitation in intensive care patients with sepsis syndromes: a pilot randomised controlled trial. Intensive Care Med. 2015;41:865–74.

23. Nickels MR, Aitken LM, Walsham J, Barnett AG, McPhail SM. Critical Care Cycling Study (CYCLIST) trial protocol: a randomised controlled trial of usual care plus additional in-bed cycling sessions versus usual care in the critically ill. BMJ Open. 2017;7:e017393.
24. Parry SM, Berney S, Granger CL, Koopman R, El-Ansary D, Denehy L. Electrical muscle stimulation in the intensive care setting: a systematic review. Crit Care Med. 2013;41:2406–18.
25. Nydahl P, Sricharoenchai T, Chandra S, Kundt FS, Huang M, Fiscjill M, et al. Safety of patient mobilization and rehabilitation in the intensive care unit. Systematic review with meta-analysis. Ann Am Thorac Soc. 2017;14:766–77.
26. McComb A, Warkentin LM, McNeely ML, Khadaroo RG. Development of a reconditioning program for elderly abdominal surgery patients: the Elder-friendly Approaches to the Surgical Environment–BEdside reconditioning for Functional ImprovemenTs (EASE-BE FIT) pilot study. World J Emerg Surg. 2018;13:21.
27. Scholes RL, Browning L, Sztendur EM, Denehy L. Duration of anaesthesia, type of surgery, respiratory co-morbidity, predicted VO max and smoking predict postoperative pulmonary complications after upper abdominal surgery: an observational study. Aust J Physiother. 2009;55:191–8.
28. Haines KJ, Skinner EH, Berney S. Association of postoperative pulmonary complications with delayed mobilisation following major abdominal surgery: an observational cohort study. Physiotherapy. 2013;99:119–25.
29. Agostini P, Naidu B, Cieslik H, Rathinam S, Bishay E, Kalkat MS, et al. Comparison of recognition tools for postoperative pulmonary complications following thoracotomy. Physiotherapy. 2011;97:278–83.
30. Vather R, Trivedi S, Bissett I. Defining postoperative ileus: results of a systematic review and global survey. J Gastrointest Surg. 2013;17:962–72.
31. Kimmel LA, Elliott JE, Sayer JM, Holland AE. Assessing the reliability and validity of a physical therapy functional measurement tool, the modified Iowa level of assistance scale, in acute hospital inpatients. Phys Ther. 2015;96:176–82.
32. Badia X, Diaz-Prieto A, Gorriz M, Herdman M, Torrado H, Farrero E, et al. Using the EuroQol-5D to measure changes in quality of life 12 months after discharge from an intensive care unit. Intensive Care Med. 2001;27:1901–7.
33. Shulman MA, Myles PS, Chan MT, McIlroy DR, Wallace S, Ponsford J. Measurement of disability-free survival after surgery. Anesthesiology. 2015;122:524–36.
34. Rankin SL, Briffa TG, Morton AR, Hung J. A specific activity questionnaire to measure the functional capacity of cardiac patients. Am J Cardiol. 1996;77: 1220–3.
35. Singer M, Deutschman CS, Seymour CW, Shankar-Hari M, Annane D, Bauer M, et al. The third international consensus definitions for sepsis and septic shock (sepsis-3). JAMA. 2016;315:801–10.
36. Fiore JF Jr, Bialocerkowski A, Browning L, Faragher IG, Denehy L. Criteria to determine readiness for hospital discharge following colorectal surgery: an international consensus using the Delphi technique. Dis Colon Rectum. 2012;55:416–23.
37. Chan A, Tetzlaff JM, Altman DG, Laupacis A, Gøtzsche PC, Krleža-Jerić K, et al. SPIRIT 2013 statement: defining standard protocol items for clinical trials. Ann Intern Med. 2013;158(3):200–7.

19

IROA: International Register of Open Abdomen, preliminary results

Federico Coccolini[1*], Giulia Montori[1], Marco Ceresoli[1], Fausto Catena[2], Rao Ivatury[3], Michael Sugrue[4], Massimo Sartelli[5], Paola Fugazzola[1], Davide Corbella[6], Francesco Salvetti[1], Ionut Negoi[7], Monica Zese[8], Savino Occhionorelli[8], Stefano Maccatrozzo[8], Sergei Shlyapnikov[9], Christian Galatioto[10], Massimo Chiarugi[10], Zaza Demetrashvili[11], Daniele Dondossola[12], Yovcho Yovtchev[13], Orestis Ioannidis[14], Giuseppe Novelli[15], Mirco Nacoti[16], Desmond Khor[17], Kenji Inaba[17], Demetrios Demetriades[17], Torsten Kaussen[18], Asri Che Jusoh[19], Wagih Ghannam[20], Boris Sakakushev[21], Ohad Guetta[22], Agron Dogjani[23], Stefano Costa[24], Sandeep Singh[25], Dimitrios Damaskos[26], Arda Isik[27], Kuo-Ching Yuan[28], Francesco Trotta[29], Stefano Rausei[30], Aleix Martinez-Perez[31], Giovanni Bellanova[32], Vinicius Cordeiro Fonseca[33], Fernando Hernández[34], Athanasios Marinis[35], Wellington Fernandes[36], Martha Quiodettis[37], Miklosh Bala[38], Andras Vereczkei[39], Rafael L. Curado[40], Gustavo Pereira Fraga[40], Bruno M. Pereira[40], Mahir Gachabayov[41], Guillermo Perez Chagerben[42], Miguel Leon Arellano[43], Sefa Ozyazici[44], Gianluca Costa[45], Tugan Tezcaner[46] and Luca Ansaloni[1]

Abstract

Background: No definitive data about open abdomen (OA) epidemiology and outcomes exist. The World Society of Emergency Surgery (WSES) and the Panamerican Trauma Society (PTS) promoted the International Register of Open Abdomen (IROA).

Methods: A prospective observational cohort study including patients with an OA treatment. Data were recorded on a web platform (Clinical Registers®) through a dedicated website: www.clinicalregisters.org.

Results: Four hundred two patients enrolled. Adult patients: 369 patients; Mean age: 57.39±18.37; 56% male. OA indication: Peritonitis (48.7%), Trauma (20.5%), Vascular Emergencies/Hemorrhage (9.4%), Ischemia (9.1%), Pancreatitis (4.2%),Post-operative abdominal-compartment-syndrome (3.9%), Others (4.2%). The most adopted Temporary-abdominal-closure systems were the commercial negative pressure ones (44.2%). During OA 38% of patients had complications; among them 10.5% had fistula. Definitive closure: 82.8%; Mortality during treatment: 17.2%. Mean duration of OA: 5.39(±4.83) days; Mean number of dressing changes: 0.88(±0.88). After-closure complications: (49.5%) and Mortality: (9%). No significant associations among TACT, indications, mortality, complications and fistula. A linear correlationexists between days of OA and complications (Pearson linear correlation = 0.326 $p<0.0001$) and with the fistula development (Pearson = 0.146 $p=0.016$).

Pediatric patients: 33 patients. Mean age: 5.91±(3.68) years; 60% male. Mortality: 3.4%; Complications: 44.8%; Fistula: 3.4%. Mean duration of OA: 3.22(±3.09) days.

(Continued on next page)

* Correspondence: federico.coccolini@gmail.com
[1]General, Emergency and Trauma Surgery Department, Papa Giovanni XXIII Hospital, Piazza OMS 1, 24127 Bergamo, Italy
Full list of author information is available at the end of the article

(Continued from previous page)

Conclusion: Temporary abdominal closure is reliable and safe. The different techniques account for different results according to the different indications. In peritonitis commercial negative pressure temporary closure seems to improve results. In trauma skin-closure and Bogotà-bag seem to improve results.

Keywords: Open abdomen, IROA, Register, Peritonitis, Trauma, Ischemia, Vascular emergencies, Compartment, Negative pressure, Commercial, Non-commercial, Bogotà bag, Witmann, Skin, Barker

Background

Temporary abdominal closure technique (TACT) or open abdomen (OA) techniques were firstly described more than 120 years ago [1]. OA procedure is defined as intentionally leaving the fascial edges of the abdomen un-approximated (laparostomy). Since that moment, this technique has been utilized decade by decade more frequently. The "old" paradigm of closing the abdomen at "any cost" has been definitely overcome by the literature evidence. However, no definitive data about OA epidemiology and outcomes exist even if in many cases such as trauma, abdominal sepsis, severe acute pancreatitis, and more in general all those situations in which an intra-abdominal hypertension condition is present and/or when is necessary to prevent the development of abdominal compartment syndrome (ACS), the OA is applied. Moreover, patients treated with OA procedures are absolutely heterogeneous even within the same study and large cohorts of patients treated with the same procedures are rare [2–7]. To overcome this lack of high level of evidence data about the OA indications, management, definitive closure, and follow-up, the World Society of Emergency Surgery (WSES) and the Panamerican Trauma Society (PTS) promoted the International Register of Open Abdomen (IROA) [2].

The present study reports preliminary data from the first 16 months of IROA activity.

Methods

This is a prospective observational cohort study including patients with an open abdomen treatment. There were no exclusion criteria whereas the only inclusion criterion was the OA treatment. Data were recorded on a web platform (Clinical Registers®) through a dedicated website: www.clinicalregisters.org. Each center inserted data about its patients. Data were recorded according to the study protocol, approved by the coordinating center Ethical Committee (Papa Giovanni XXIII Hospital, Bergamo, Italy) and also registered to ClinicalTrials.gov (ClinicalTrials.gov Identifier: NCT02382770). For each patient, the following were recorded: demographical data, indication to the treatment, TACT, duration of the treatment and number of dressing changes, complications, enteric fistula and mortality before and after closure, according to the study protocol.

All the patients less than 14 years old were considered pediatric and were analyzed separately.

Indications were organized into seven groups (peritonitis, pancreatitis, ischemia, vascular emergencies and

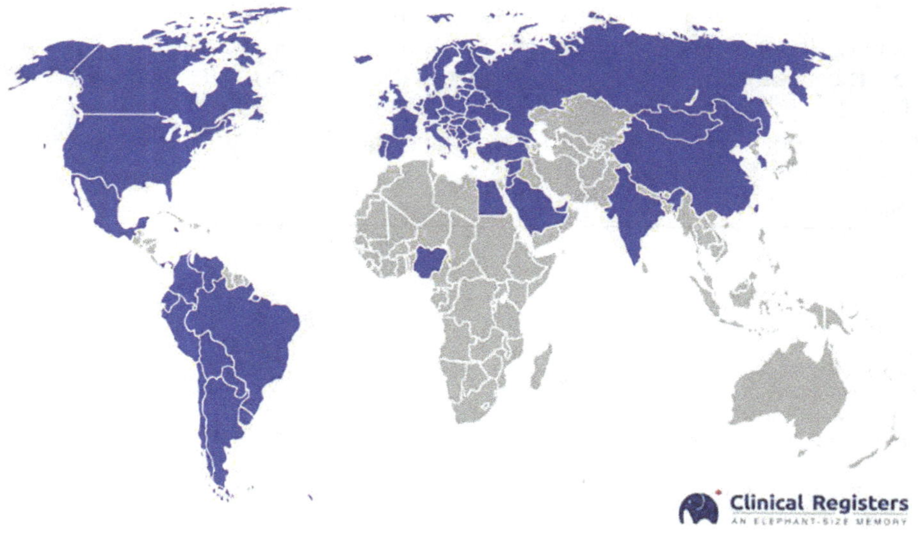

Fig. 1 IROA spread in the world

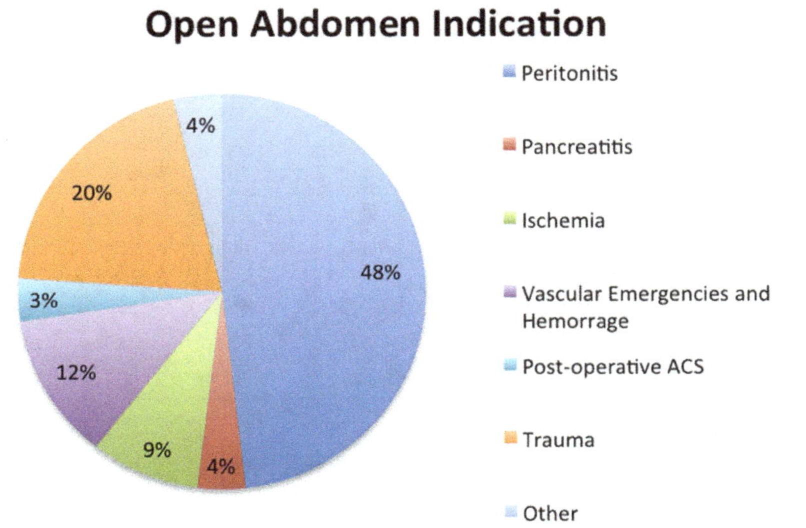

Fig. 2 Open abdomen treatment indications

hemorrhage, post-operative ACS, trauma and other). TACTs were summarized in four subgroups (Bogotà bag + skin closure, Barker vacuum pack, negative pressure wound therapy (NPWT) assisted and Wittmann patch) to allow an appropriate number of patients in each group.

Statistical analysis

Continuous variables were expressed as mean and standard deviation and were compared with the ANOVA test; categorical data were expressed as proportions and were compared with the chi square test. Linear associations were tested with the Pearson's linear correlation model. Data about mortality, definitive closure, and number of days with open abdomen were graphically plotted with the Kaplan-Meyer method for the different techniques and indications (patients who died during treatment were considered as never closed with a length of treatment = ∞).

All the statistical analyses were performed with IBM SPSS 20 (IBM Corp. Released 2011. IBM SPSS Statistics for Windows, Version 20.0. Armonk, NY: IBM Corp.).

Results

From May 1, 2015, to September 30, 2016, a total number of 402 patients were enrolled and recorded into the register. The IROA spread throughout the world as shown in Fig. 1.

Adult patients

A total of 369 adult patients were recorded; mean age was 57.39 ± 18.37 and 56% were male. The most frequent indication for open abdomen was peritonitis (48.7%) and the most adopted TACT was the commercial negative pressure wound therapy system (44.2%) (Fig. 2, Table 1). During the open treatment, 38% of patients had complications and 10.5% developed an enteric fistula. Definitive closure was achieved in 82.8% of the

Table 1 Outcomes divided for open abdomen treatment technique (TAC: temporary abdominal closure, NPWT: negative pressure wound therapy)

TAC technique	No. of patients [%] (total = 369)	Age [mean(SD)]	Male gender [%]	No. of dressing [*n*(SD)]	Days of open abdomen [*n*(SD)]	Definitive closure [%]	Fascia closure [%]	Complications during treatment [%]	Fistula [%]	Mortality during open [%]
Bogotà bag + skin closure	31.8	56.5 (18.9)	52.5	0.7 (1.1)	5.0 (4.4)	83.2	71.3	35.8	7.4	16.8
NPWT assisted	44.2	58.7 (17.9)	56.9	1.0 (1.6)	5.0 (4.1)	85.7	59.9	32.5	13.5	14.3
Barker vacuum pack	12.7	50.1 (19.9)	69.0	1.1 (1.6)	6.6 (7.2)	75.6	64.3	43.9	2.4	24.4
Wittmann patch	11.4	63 (14.8)	45.7	0.3 (0.6)	6.6 (4.8)	79.4	65.7	58.8	17.6	20.6
Total	100.0	57.4 (18.4)	55.8	0.9 (1.4)	5.4 (4.8)	82.8	64.7	38.2	10.5	17.2

Table 2 Outcomes divided for indication to open abdomen treatment

Indication	No. of patients [*n*(%)]	Age [mean(SD)]	Male gender [%]	No. of dressing [*n*(SD)]	Days of open abdomen [*n*(SD)]	Definitive closure [%]	Fascia closure [%]	Complications during treatment [%]	Fistula [%]	Mortality during open [%]
Peritonitis	178 (48.7%)	61.9 (14.6)	49.3	0.9 (1.4)	5.2 (4.0)	79.9	59.3	43.2	14.4	20.1
Pancreatitis	14 (4.2%)	60.9 (15.3)	69.2	2.1 (2.2)	12.1 (7.1)	76.9	53.8	53.8	7.7	23.1
Ischemia	32 (9.1%)	69.8 (11.9)	57.1	0.9 (0.9)	5.7 (3.4)	92.9	78.6	39.3	14.3	7.1
Vascular emergencies and hemorrhage	44 (9.4%)	64.6 (12.6)	41.4	0.4 (0.8)	3.7 (3.4)	88.5	72.4	23.1	0.0	11.5
Post-operative ACS	13 (3.9%)	46.8 (20.1)	25.0	0.4 (0.7)	3.9 (2.6)	66.7	50.0	58.3	8.3	33.3
Trauma	74 (20.5%)	39.5 (18.3)	79.4	0.9 (1.6)	5.4 (6.2)	86.4	73.0	20.3	6.8	13.6
Other	14 (4.2%)	57.3 (19.3)	53.8	1.4 (1.8)	5.9 (5.5)	75.0	46.2	41.7	8.3	25.0

patients with a mortality during treatment of 17.2%. The mean duration of the open treatment was 5.39(±4.83) days with a mean number of dressing changes of 0.88(±0.88). After-closure complications were recorded in 49.5% of the patients and mortality was 9%.

Tables 1 and 2 show data in detail divided for indication and TACT. Table 3 shows data in details for peritonitis and trauma patients.

There were no significant associations among TACT, indications, mortality, complications, and fistula formation. Figures 3, 4, and 5 show the incidence of complications and enteric fistula.

There was a linear correlation between days of open abdomen and complications (Pearson linear correlation = 0.326 $p < 0.0001$) and with the development of fistula (Pearson = 0.146 $p = 0.016$) (Figs. 6 and 7).

Among the indications, the duration of open treatment was longer for pancreatitis ($p < 0.0001$); no differences were found among different TACTs.

Figures 8, 9, and 10 plotted the days of open abdomen together with the definitive closure rate, shown with the Kaplan-Meyer method, for different TACTs and respectively overall, in peritonitis and in trauma patients.

Pediatric patients

A total number of 33 pediatric patients were enrolled: mean age was 5.91 ± (3.68) years and 60% were male. Table 4 shows data in detail. The indications for open abdomen were missing for the majority of patients; the most common indicated were various (other), peritonitis, and post-operative ACS. Mortality was recorded in only one patient (3.4%) and complications were recorded in 44.8%; one patient (3.4%) developed enteric fistula. The open treatment had a mean duration of 3.22(±3.09) days.

Discussion

Present data, even if preliminary, explain clearly the worldwide diffusion of such techniques. The most part of cases registered are from adult patients where promising results can be extracted: first of all, the usefulness of OA in acute care in managing severe peritonitis. Acosta et al. in 2011 [8] already described the OA use in Europe

Table 3 Outcomes in peritonitis and trauma patients (TAC: temporary abdominal closure, NPWT: negative pressure wound therapy)

Indication	TACT	No. of patients [%] (total = 178)	Male gender [%]	Definitive closure [%]	Fascia closure [%]	Complications during treatment [%]	Fistula [%]	Mortality during open [%]
Peritonitis	Bogotà bag + skin closure	28.7	46.5	72.5	62.8	40.0	12.5	27.5
	NPWT assisted	46.0	49.3	85.7	53.6	33.3	14.3	14.3
	Barker vacuum pack	7.3	63.6	80.0	72.7	70.0	0.0	20.0
	Wittmann patch	18.0	48.1	76.9	63.0	61.5	23.1	23.1
	Total	100.0	49.3	79.9	59.3	43.2	14.4	20.1
Trauma	Bogotà bag + skin closure	49.2	71.0	92.9	74.2	25.0	7.1	7.1
	NPWT assisted	28.6	94.4	88.2	77.8	17.6	11.8	11.8
	Barker vacuum pack	22.2	78.6	71.4	64.3	14.3	0.0	28.6
	Total	100.0	79.4	86.4	73.0	20.3	6.8	13.6

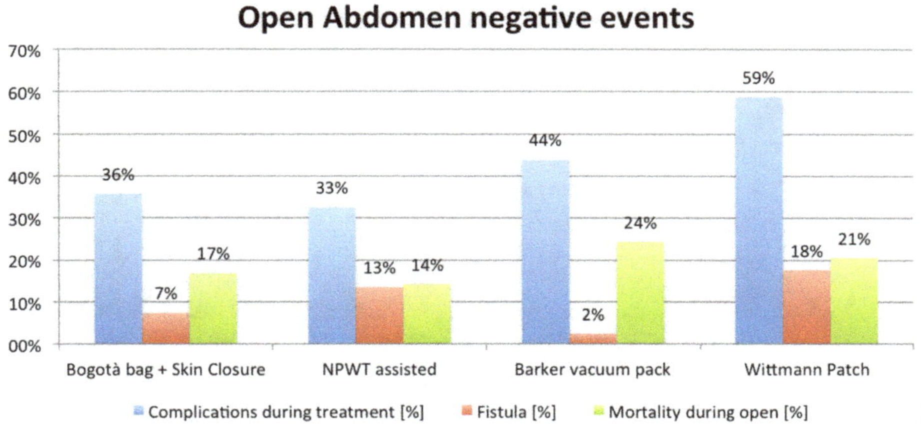

Fig. 3 Overall negative event rate (NPWT: negative pressure wound therapy)

demonstrating as more than the 50% of cases of OA were derived from peritonitis patients. Trauma patients represent the second cohort in terms of numerosity. Other interesting results are emerging regarding the different techniques adopted. The most diffused are the commercial negative pressure techniques. As a counterpart, skin closure and Bogotà bag are used in more than 20% of patients with interesting results especially in trauma patients. As recently demonstrated by Kirkpatrick et al., the commercial negative pressure systems obtain better results in term of survival especially in those patients with intra-abdominal infections or contamination [9], or at least in case possibly associated to pro-inflammatory cytokines increased release. The most effective is the removal of infected and cytokine-loaded fluids the better seems to be survival results. Even with no definitive data regarding the effect on the circulating load of cytokines and toxins, maybe the negative pressure will be found to be useful also in reducing these values. Kirkpatrick et al. tried to demonstrate this with their randomized trial in a mixed court of patients [9]. Their results offered one possible way to understand the OA effect related to the utilized TACT. As clearly demonstrated by present data, the different OA techniques are differently useful in each indication. In fact in patients affected by peritonitis the negative pressure systems seem to be the most effective in reducing the mortality rate; moreover, considering the commercial and not commercial systems, the commercial ones seem to be the best in improving survival results (Fig. 9) (see figure legend). As a counterpart in trauma patients, the non-negative pressure systems seem to provide better results if compared to the negative pressure ones (Fig. 10) (see figure legend). This can be partially explained with the relative absence of infection and cytokines to be cleared. Moreover, the closure time is positively influenced by the most appropriate TACT in the different indications (Figs. 9 and 10). In fact closure times differ within the indications and can be partially considered as strictly linked to the utilized TACT.

In terms of complication rate, the different techniques differ one from each other. In absolute, the less the

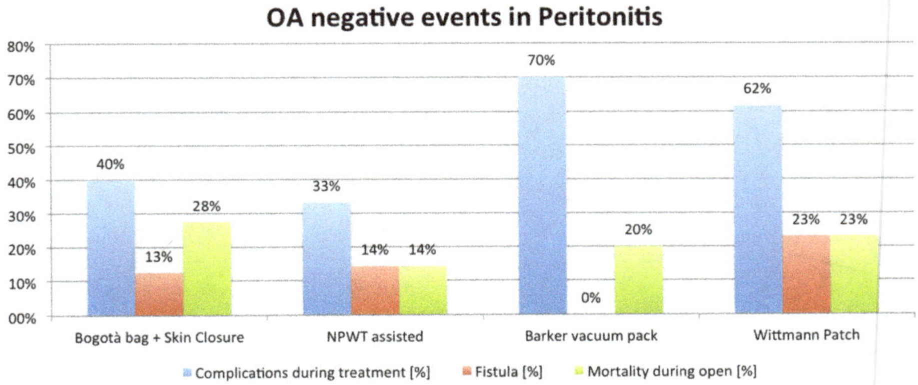

Fig. 4 Negative event rate in peritonitis (NPWT: negative pressure wound therapy)

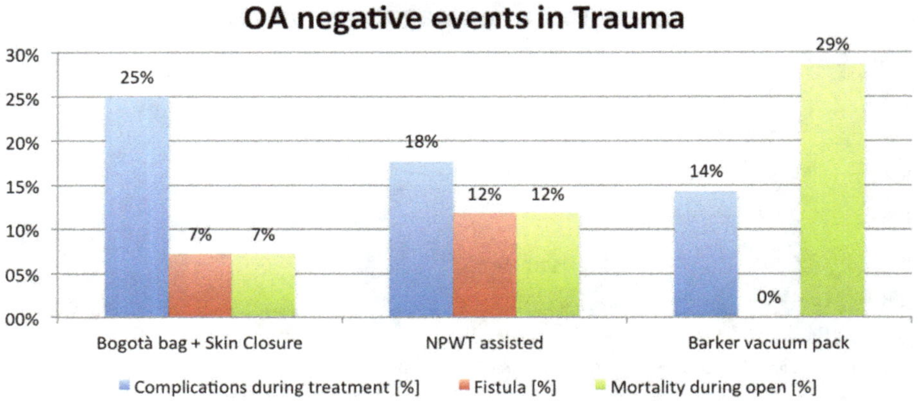

Fig. 5 Negative event rate in trauma (NPWT: negative pressure wound therapy)

abdomen remains opened the lesser the complication rate. Miller et al. in a big cohort study showed that 8 days of OA represents a cutoff in the complication rate [10]. Present data clearly show that no cutoff can be posed in the complication rate, it progressively increases day by day. The longer the period of OA the higher the number of complications and fistula, starting directly from the very first days of treatment (Figs. 6 and 7). This result is important if analyzed in association with the different outcomes related to the technique of OA and the indications. In fact, analyzing Figs. 8, 9, and 10 (see figure legend), it is possible to see how the two variables are intrinsically connected to the time of closure; the OA technique influences the survival and the time to closure in the different indications, as a counterpart, the indication (i.e., the cause of OA) plays a fundamental role in survival and closure decisions. Both by influencing the time to closure determine part of the causes of the complication insurgence. So it is becoming progressively more evident as it is necessary to reanalyze the TACTs under a different view. The different indications have completely different underlying physiopathology; as a consequence, they maybe are not to be treated with the same TACT. In fact the different techniques possess different characteristic allowing managing different situations. Maybe the application of one technique instead than one-other should not be based only on the availability of the most advanced systems but also on the consideration that each technique has a proper effect on the physiopathology. If these preliminary results will be confirmed by subsequent data, this will lead also to an optimization of the resources located to OA management. Moreover, it would promote future development and researches also regarding the "less technological techniques".

Within the different indications, the different TACT systems account for different complication rates. As showed in Table 1 and Figs. 3, 4, and 5, the several

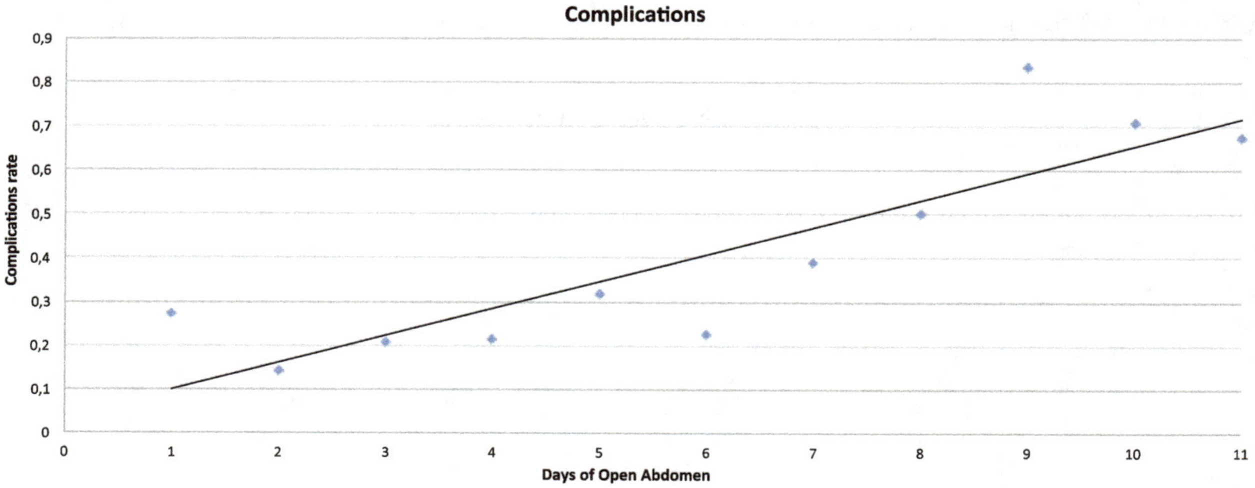

Fig. 6 Time distribution of overall complication

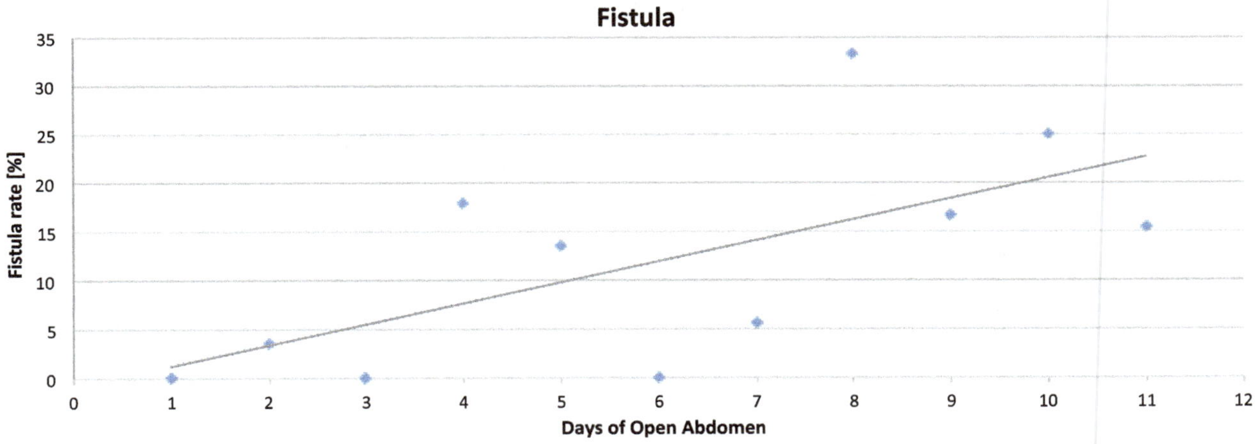

Fig. 7 Time distribution of fistula

TACTs seem to lead to different incidence of complication. In evaluating these data however, the underlying cause of OA and the consequent physiopathology conditioning of the outcome should be kept in mind. The technique alone is not completely responsible for all the complications. Some complications such as fistula, however, seem to be more related to the TACT than others.

The incidence of fistula in OA has been reported variously depending on the indication for the OA varying from 4.5 to 25% in trauma [11] and from 5.7 and 17.2% in non-trauma patients [12]. Fistula increase considerably mortality, length of stays, and costs [13]. Present paper confirms data of the literature. The difference in fistula incidence depends also from the adopted TAC technique used. As shown, some techniques account for a higher fistula incidence but as also showed by data different indication have different time of OA and the longer the OA the higher the overall complication and fistula rate. Again, the correlation between TACT, indication, and underlying physiopathology must be kept in mind.

The use of OA in pediatric setting is diffused but not sufficiently studied. Present register is trying to overcome this lack of data. The pediatric data recruitment however must be improved. In fact from the pediatric cohort, no conclusion can be obtained.

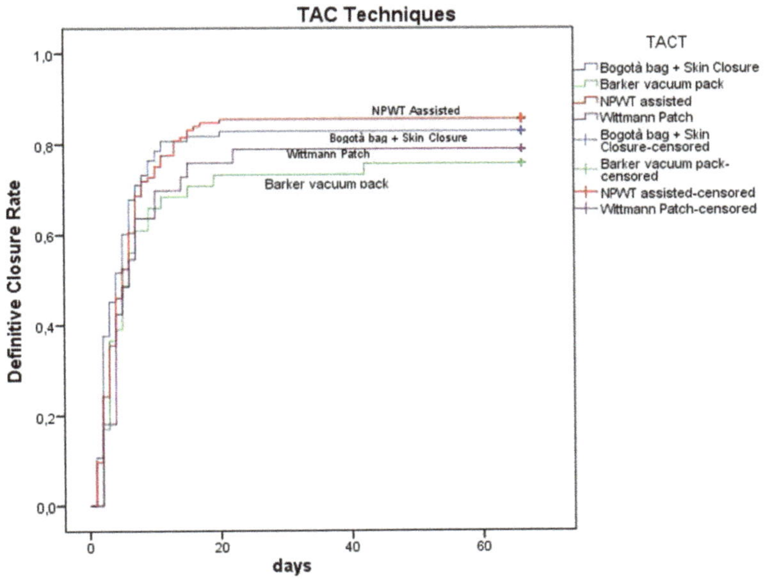

Fig. 8 Definitive closure rate and days of open abdomen among different TAC techniques. Those patients died during treatment never achieved definitive closure and had a duration of treatment = infinite (as a consequence asymptotic curve indicates also survival). (TAC: temporary abdominal closure, NPWT: negative pressure wound therapy)

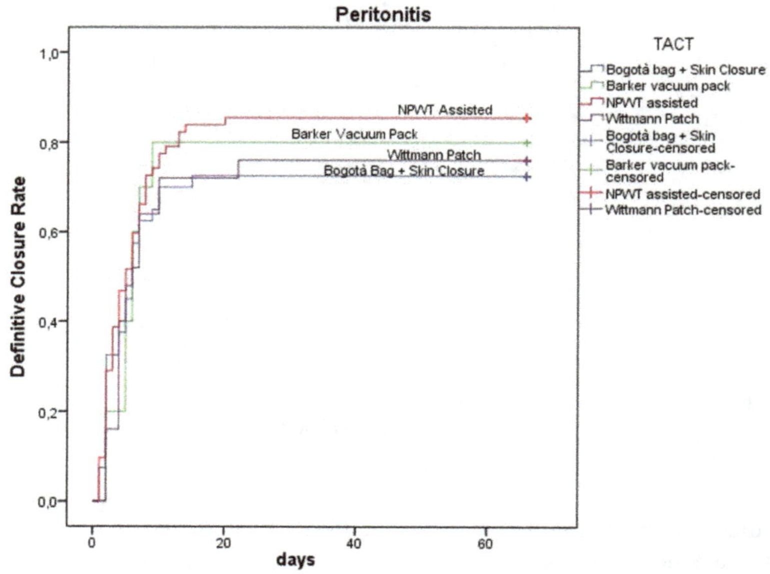

Fig. 9 Definitive closure rate and days of open abdomen among different TAC techniques in patients treated for peritonitis. Those patients died during treatment never achieved definitive closure and had a duration of treatment = infinite (as a consequence asymptotic curve indicates also survival). (TAC: temporary abdominal closure, NPWT: negative pressure wound therapy)

One last consideration should be done regarding the limitation of using clinical registries data for evaluating the outcome of rare diseases or those conditions such as emergency interventions in which a randomized controlled trial is rather difficult or even impossible to realize. Results from registries as any non-randomized comparison are affected by the same methodological limitations. Specifically, the comparability of selected patient groups is not ensured. As a counterpart, the only way to obtain wide and trustful results in these situations is the use of dedicated registries; a strong attempt should be done in projecting them to make included patients as much uniform as possible.

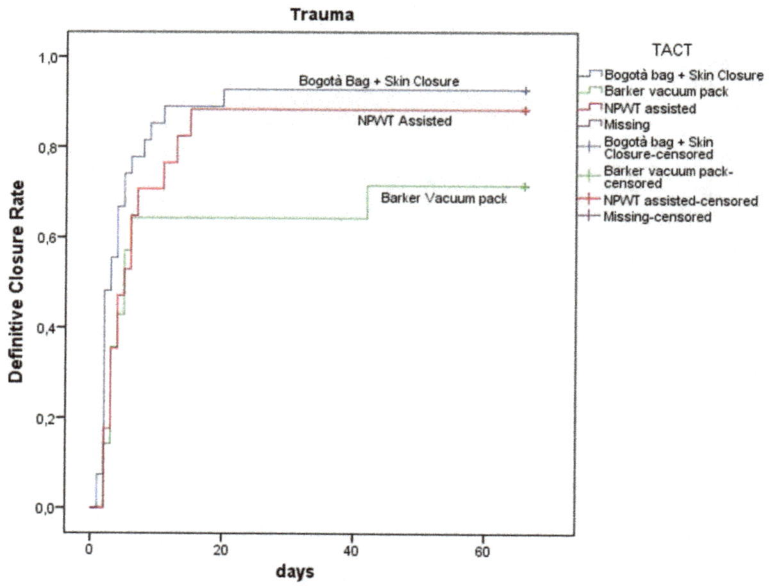

Fig. 10 Definitive closure rate and days of open abdomen among different TAC techniques in patients treated for trauma. Those patients died during treatment never achieved definitive closure and had a duration of treatment = infinite (as a consequence asymptotic curve indicates also survival). (TAC: temporary abdominal closure, NPWT: negative pressure wound therapy)

Table 4 Outcomes in pediatric patients (TAC: temporary abdominal closure, NPWT: negative pressure wound therapy)

Open abdomen in pediatrics	
No. of patients	33
Age	5.9 (3.7)
Male gender	60.6%
Indications	
Peritonitis	12%
Pancreatitis	6%
Vascular emergencies and hemorrhage	6%
Post-operative ACS	12%
Other	15%
Missing	48%
No. of dressings	0.3 (0.9)
Days of open abdomen	3.2 (3.1)
Fistula	3.4%
Mortality during treatment	3.4%
Definitive closure	96.6%
Complications post closure	53.6%
Mortality post closure	0.0%
TAC techniques	
Bogotà bag + skin closure	30%
Barker vacuum pack	35%
NPWT assisted	35%

Conclusions

Temporary abdominal closure is reliable and safe in treating severely injured and acute care surgery patients. The different techniques account for different results according to the different indications. In peritonitis, commercial negative pressure temporary closure seems to improve results. In trauma, skin closure and Bogotà bag seem to improve results.

Abbreviations

ACS: Abdominal compartment syndrome; IROA: International Register of Open Abdomen; NPWT: Negative pressure wound therapy; OA: Open abdomen; PTS: Panamerican Trauma Society; TACT: Temporary abdominal closure technique; WSES: World Society of Emergency Surgery

Acknowledgements

None

Funding

None

Authors' contributions

FC and LA are responsible for the manuscript conception and draft; FC, GM, MC, FCa, RI, MS, MS, PF, DC, FS, IN, MZ, SO, SM, SS, CG, MC, ZD, DD, YY, OI, GN, NM, DK, KI, DD, TK, ACJ, WG, BS, OG, AD, SC, SS, DD, AI, KCY, FT, SR, AMP, GB, VCF, FH, AM, WF, MQ, MB, AV, RC, GPF, BMP, MG, GPC, MLA, SO, GC, TT, and LA are responsible for the patients accrual and data insertion; FC, LA, and MC are responsible for the data analysis critically revised the manuscript, all authors gave the final approval.

Competing interests

The authors declare that they have no competing interests.

Author details

[1]General, Emergency and Trauma Surgery Department, Papa Giovanni XXIII Hospital, Piazza OMS 1, 24127 Bergamo, Italy. [2]Emergency Surgery Department, Parma University Hospital, Parma, Italy. [3]Virginia Commonwealth University, Richmond, VA, USA. [4]General Surgery, Letterkenny Hospital, Donegal, Ireland. [5]General and Emergency Surgery Department, Macerata Hospital, Macerata, Italy. [6]Neuro Intensive Care Unit Department, Papa Giovanni XXIII Hospital, Bergamo, Italy. [7]Emergency Surgery Hospital, Bucharest, Romania. [8]Emergency Surgery Department, Ferrara University Hospital, Ferrara, Italy. [9]Science Research of Emergency Care N. A., Djanelidze, Russia. [10]Azienda Ospedaliera Universitaria Pisana, Pisa, Italy. [11]Kipshidze Central University Hospital, Kipshidze, Georgia. [12]HPB Surgery, Fondazione IRCCS Cà Granda Ospedale Maggiore Policlinico, Milano, Italy. [13]University Hospital "Prof Stoian Kirkovich" AD, Stara Zagora, Bulgaria. [14]Fourth Surgical Department, Hospital George Papanikolau, Aristotle University, Thessaloniki, Greece. [15]General Surgery, Infermi Hospital, Rimini, Italy. [16]Pediatric Intensive Care Unit, Papa Giovanni XXIII Hospital, Bergamo, Italy. [17]LAS + USC Medical Centre, Los Angeles California, USA. [18]Pediatric Intensive Care Unit, Hannover University Hospital, Hannover, Germany. [19]Khuala Krai Hospital, Kuala Krai, Malaysia. [20]Mansoura Faculty of Medicine, Mansoura, Egypt. [21]Medical University of Plovdiv, Plovdiv, Bulgaria. [22]Soroka Medical Centre, Beersheba, Israel. [23]University Hospital of Trauma, Tirana, Albania. [24]Emergency and General Surgery, Fondazione IRCCS Cà Granda Ospedale Maggiore Policlinico, Milano, Italy. [25]Oxford University Hospital, Oxford, UK. [26]John Radcliffe Hospital, Oxford, UK. [27]Erzincan University Faculty of Medicine Mengucek Gazi Training Research Hospital Erzincan, Erzincan, Turkey. [28]Chang Gung Memorial Hospital, Taoyuan, Taiwan. [29]Ospedale Maggiore, Lodi, Italy. [30]Ospedale di Circolo e Fondazione Macchi, University of Insubria, Varese, Italy. [31]Hospital Universitario Doctor Peset, Valencia, Spain. [32]S.S. Annunziata Hospital, Taranto, Italy. [33]Hospital Santa Virgínia, São Paulo, Brazil. [34]Hospital Central Militar, Mexico City, Mexico. [35]Tzaneio General Hospital of Piraeus, Piraeus, Greece. [36]Hospital Regional de Sao Jose, San Jose, Brazil. [37]Hospital Santo Tomás, Panama City, Panama. [38]Hadassah Hebrew University Medical Center, Jerusalem, Israel. [39]Department of Surgery, Medical School University Pécs, Pécs, Hungary. [40]Hospital De Clinicas Da Unicamp, Campinas, Brazil. [41]Vladimir City Clinical Hospital of Emergency Medicine, Vladimir City, Russia. [42]University Hospital, Cuenca, Ecuador. [43]Hospital La Paz, Madrid, Spain. [44]Adana Numune Training and Research Hospital, Department of Surgery, Adana, Turkey. [45]Ospedale Sant' Andrea University Hospital Sapienza, Rome, Italy. [46]Baskent University School of Medicine, Ankara, Turkey.

References

1. McCosh II AJ. The treatment of general septic peritonitis. Ann Surg. 1897;25:687–97.
2. Coccolini F, Catena F, Montori G, Ceresoli M, Manfredi R, Nita GE, et al. IROA: the International Register of Open Abdomen: an international effort to better understand the open abdomen: call for participants. World J Emerg Surg. 2015;10:37.
3. Balogh ZJ, Lumsdaine W, Moore E, Moore FA. Postinjury abdominal compartment syndrome: from recognition to prevention. Lancet. 2014; 384(9952):1466–75.
4. Malbrain ML, Cheatham ML, Kirkpatrick A, Sugrue M, Parr M, De Waele J, et al. Results from the international consensus of experts on intra-abdominal hypertension and abdominal compartment syndromel. I. Definitions. Intensive Care Med. 2006;32:1722–32.
5. Kirkpatrick AW, Roberts DJ, De Waele J, Jaeschke R, Malbrain MLNG, De Keulenaer B, et al. Intra-abdominal hypertension and the abdominal compartment syndrome: updated consensus definitions and clinical practice guidelines from the World Society of the Abdominal Compartment Syndrome. Intensive Care Med. 2013;39:1190–206.

6. Sugrue M, Jones F, Janjua KJ, Deane SA, Bristow P, Hillman K. Temporary abdominal closure: a prospective evaluation of its effects on renal and respiratory physiology. J Trauma. 1998;45:914–21.
7. Bosscha K, Hulstaert PF, Hennipman A, Visser MR, Gooszen HG, van Vroonhoven TJMV, et al. Fulminant acute pancreatitis and infected necrosis: results of open management of the abdomen and "planned" reoperations. J Am Coll Surg. 1998;187:255–62.
8. Acosta S, Bjarnason T, Petersson U, Pålsson B, Wanhainen A, Svensson M, Djavani K, Björck M. Multicentre prospective study of fascial closure rate after open abdomen with vacuum and mesh-mediated fascial traction. Br J Surg. 2011;98(5):735–43.
9. Kirkpatrick AW, Roberts DJ, Faris PD, Ball CG, Kubes P, Tiruta C, Xiao Z, Holodinsky JK, McBeth PB, Doig CJ, Jenne CN. Active negative pressure peritoneal therapy after abbreviated laparotomy: the intraperitoneal vacuum randomized controlled trial. Ann Surg. 2015;262(1):38–46.
10. Miller RS, Morris Jr JA, Diaz Jr JJ, Herring MB, May AK. Complications after 344 damage-control open celiotomies. J Trauma. 2005;59(6):1365–71.
11. Atema JJ, Gans SL, Boermeester MA. Systematic review and meta-analysis of the open abdomen and temporary abdominal closure techniques in non-trauma patients. World J Surg. 2015;39:912–25.
12. Teixeira PGR, Inaba K, Dubose J, Salim A, Brown C, Rhee P, et al. Enterocutaneous fistula complicatingtrauma laparotomy: a major resource burden. Am Surg. 2009;75:30–2.
13. Martinez JL, Luque-De-Leon E, Mier J, Blanco-Benavides R, Robledo F. Systematic management of postoperative enterocutaneous fistulas: factors related to outcomes. World J Surg. 2008;32:436–43.

20

A meta-analysis of resuscitative endovascular balloon occlusion of the aorta (REBOA) or open aortic cross-clamping by resuscitative thoracotomy in non-compressible torso hemorrhage patients

Ramiro Manzano Nunez[1], Maria Paula Naranjo[1], Esteban Foianini[2*], Paula Ferrada[3], Erika Rincon[1], Herney Andrés García-Perdomo[4], Paola Burbano[7], Juan Pablo Herrera[6], Alberto F. García[4,5] and Carlos A. Ordoñez[4,5]

Abstract

Background: The objective of this systematic review and meta-analysis was to determine the effect of REBOA, compared to resuscitative thoracotomy, on mortality and among non-compressible torso hemorrhage trauma patients.

Methods: Relevant articles were identified by a literature search in MEDLINE and EMBASE. We included studies involving trauma patients suffering non-compressible torso hemorrhage. Studies were eligible if they evaluated REBOA and compared it to resuscitative thoracotomy. Two investigators independently assessed articles for inclusion and exclusion criteria and selected studies for final analysis. We conducted meta-analysis using random effect models.

Results: We included three studies in our systematic review. These studies included a total of 1276 patients. An initial analysis found that although lower in REBOA-treated patients, the odds of mortality did not differ between the compared groups (OR 0.42; 95% CI 0.17–1.03). Sensitivity analysis showed that the risk of mortality was significantly lower among patients who underwent REBOA, compared to those who underwent resuscitative thoracotomy (RT) (RR 0.81; 95% CI 0.68–0.97).

Conclusion: Our meta-analysis, mainly from observational data, suggests a positive effect of REBOA on mortality among non-compressible torso hemorrhage patients. However, these results deserve further investigation.

Keywords: Injuries, Non-compressible torso hemorrhage, REBOA, Resuscitation strategies, Traumatic shock, Endovascular procedures

Background

Resuscitative endovascular balloon occlusion of the aorta (REBOA) is a procedure that involves placement of an endovascular balloon in the aorta to obtain proximal control of hemorrhage [1]. In recent years, REBOA has become increasingly popular amongst trauma surgeons [2] for the management of traumatic non-compressible torso hemorrhage (NCTH) [3–5]. Although the use of REBOA in the trauma setting has been studied, most of the information comes from series of patients with blunt or penetrating trauma [6] and clear evidence on its effectiveness for improving mortality rates is lacking. Furthermore, little is known about the comparative effectiveness of REBOA and resuscitative thoracotomy (RT) on mortality in NCTH trauma patients.

The objective of this systematic review and meta-analysis was to determine the effect of REBOA, compared to RT, on mortality among NCTH trauma patients.

* Correspondence: ruralcirugiatrauma@gmail.com; efoianini@hotmail.com
[2]Clinical Foianini, Santa Cruz de La Sierra, Bolivia

Methods

This systematic review was conducted following Cochrane recommendations [7] and PRISMA guidelines [8].

Our PICO strategy was as follows: Patients: patients with non-compressible torso hemorrhage, intervention: REBOA, comparison: resuscitative thoracotomy, and outcomes: mortality and REBOA deployment complications. For this strategy, the proposed systematic review will answer the following questions:

1. In patients with non-compressible torso hemorrhage, does REBOA in comparison with RT result in reduced mortality?
2. What is the type and frequency of complications related to REBOA deployment in included studies?

Inclusion criteria

We included studies involving patients that suffered blunt or penetrating injuries to the torso. Studies were eligible if they assessed the effect of resuscitative endovascular balloon occlusion of the aorta (REBOA) on relevant outcomes among NCTH patients and compared it to traditional open aortic occlusion by resuscitative thoracotomy. Studies without comparison group were excluded.

Outcomes

Mortality and complications related to REBOA deployment were the outcomes of interest. Only those studies with sufficient information on the outcomes (effect size and associated precision) were included in the meta-analysis.

Search methods

We built a highly sensitive search strategy (search strategies are available in Additional file 1) following established recommendations [9, 10]. The literature search was performed in MEDLINE and EMBASE from inception to May 2017 using and combining terms and synonyms related to our condition of interest (trauma, injuries, non-compressible torso hemorrhage, etc.) and our intervention of interest (resuscitative endovascular balloon occlusion of the aorta). We also searched key journals (Journal of Trauma and Acute Care Surgery, World Journal of Emergency Surgery, European Journal of Trauma and Emergency Surgery and the Scandinavian Journal of Trauma Resuscitation and Emergency Surgery). Finally, references from previous relevant narrative and systematic reviews were examined.

Study selection and data collection

Two individuals independently examined the titles and abstracts identified in the searches. Articles that appeared relevant were selected for full-text review. Two researchers independently reviewed full-text articles for final eligibility. A third reviewer, an experienced trauma surgeon of our review team, resolved disagreements in both phases. The following information was independently extracted using a standardized data form: author, year of publication, the region of origin, trauma characteristics, patient demographics and clinical characteristics, type of operative interventions performed, number and type of complications, mortality, and measures of association for mortality reported.

Risk of bias

The internal validity of each non-randomized study included in this systematic review was critically evaluated for bias according to the Methodological Index for Non-randomized studies (MINORS) [11]. MINORS evaluate 12 methodological items by scoring each one as 0 (red) if not reported (high risk of bias); 1 (yellow), reported but inadequate (unclear risk of bias); and 2 (green), reported and adequate (low risk of bias). Moreover, we evaluated three additional domains through which bias can be introduced in a study and that are important in trauma outcomes research. Those were as follows: the risk of indication bias, the risk of survival bias, and the risk of reporting bias (selective reporting) [7, 12]. Two independent investigators made the evaluation of the risk of bias as previously mentioned and computed a graphic representation of potential bias in a visual table where high, unclear, and low risks of bias were represented by the colors red, yellow, and green, respectively.

Data analysis

A meta-analysis was performed to assess the effect of REBOA on mortality, compared it to open aortic cross-clamping by resuscitative thoracotomy. The meta-analysis was restricted to available measures of associations with their correspondent confidence intervals (CIs).

Unadjusted ORs and their CIs were calculated in a 2 × 2 table using data provided in studies. Adjusted ORs and CIs were extracted as provided. Unadjusted and adjusted odds ratios were pooled using a random-effects (DerSimonian and Laird) meta-analysis. The results were reported in forest plots of the estimated effects of the included studies with a 95% confidence interval (95% CI). Heterogeneity was evaluated using the I^2 test, which corresponded to low ($I^2 < 25\%$), medium ($I^2 = 25–75\%$), and high ($I^2 > 75\%$) heterogeneity.

Sensitivity analysis

The risk ratio is thought to be a better measure of effect to communicate research findings [13]. Moreover, the odds ratio may overestimate a risk association or a treatment effect when the outcome of interest is common in the study population [14, 15]. In this case, our outcome of interest was mortality, which is a very common outcome in patients suffering severe torso trauma and NCTH. Therefore, we decided to convert adjusted odds ratios (ORs) extracted from the studies to risk ratios (RRs) using an inverse probability weighted binomial model [16]. The model used the following equation to convert an OR to an RR:

$$RR = \frac{OR}{[1\text{-}(q\text{-}(OR \times q))]}$$

In this equation, q is the incidence of the outcome of interest in the unexposed (control group). For this analysis, the unexposed were those groups who underwent open aortic cross-clamping by resuscitative thoracotomy. The transformed measures of effect were pooled using a random effect model.

All analyses were done in Stata statistical software.

Results

We identified 1084 records from our searches, of which 13 studies were eligible to be included in our systematic review. These articles were retrieved as full texts and reviewed. After applying inclusion and exclusion criteria, three studies were included in the systematic review, all of them in both the qualitative and quantitative synthesis (meta-analysis). Figure 1 shows the flowchart for the selection of the studies.

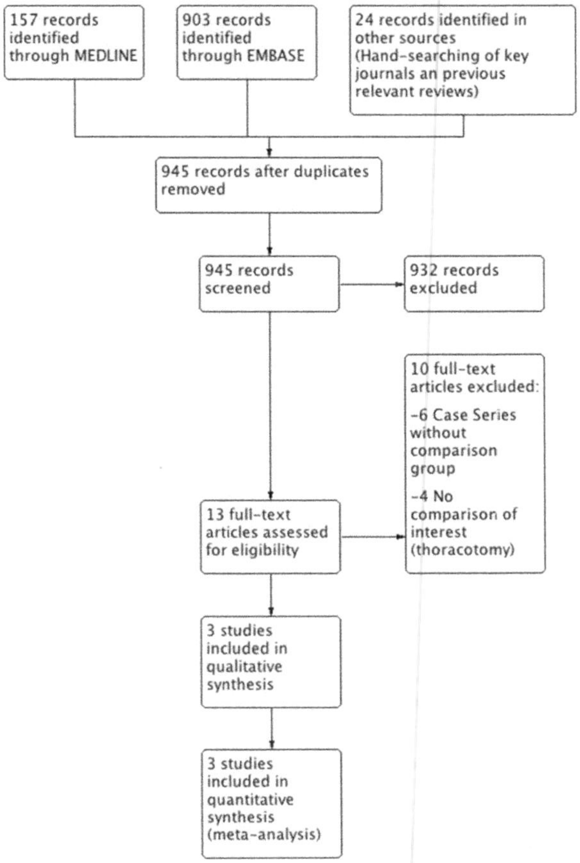

Fig. 1 Flowchart according to PRISMA guidelines

Characteristics of included studies

Included studies were published in 2016 [17, 18] and 2017 [19]. These studies included a total of 1276 patients. Two were retrospective cohort studies [17, 19] and one was a prospective cohort [18].

Characteristics of participants

A total of 1276 participants were analyzed in the included studies. Overall, REBOA was deployed in 873 (68%) patients while open aortic cross-clamping by resuscitative thoracotomy was performed in 403 (32%).

An overview of patients' characteristics by interventions is presented in Table 1. The majority was male ($n = 851/1276$), and all were victims of torso trauma by blunt or penetrating mechanisms. Age structure was heterogeneous and included both young and elderly patients. Two studies reported information on injury severity. In these studies, patients suffered severe trauma and presented primarily with moderate (AIS = 2) and/or serious (AIS = 3) injuries.

Data on operative interventions was captured. Overall, 494 (38%) and 271 (21%) patients underwent exploratory laparotomy and arterial embolization, respectively. Two studies reported data on splenic and hepatic procedures; these included different damage control strategies such as packing and resections. The same studies reported information on operative interventions for pelvic fractures management, which included the use of packing, external fixation, and surgery.

Differences between REBOA and resuscitative thoracotomy patients

Two studies reported data on initial blood pressure and injury severity. In these studies, RT patients were more likely to present with significantly lower values systolic blood pressure (SBP: median (IQR): DuBose: REBOA = 23 (105) vs. RT = 0 (80), $p = 0.01$; Abe: REBOA = 89 (46) vs. RT = 87 (45), $p < 0.001$). However, REBOA and RT patients were similar in severity of injuries as reflected by reported AIS and ISS. One study reported the probability of survival for both groups. This study showed that patients that underwent REBOA had a significantly higher probability of survival on admission (TRISS (probability of survival), mean (SD): Abe: REBOA = 0.43 (0.36) vs. RT = 0.27 (0.30), $p < 0.001$].

Resuscitation strategies, including transfusions requirements, were reported in all studies. Two studies

Table 1 Characteristics of participants

	DuBose 2016		Abe 2016		Aso 2017 [a]	
	REBOA (n = 46)	RT (n = 68)	REBOA (n = 636)	RT (n = 267)	REBOA (n = 191)	RT (n = 68)
Age [a]	43.2 (19.6) [b]	39.2 (16.7) [b]	52.5 (21.2) [b]	56.7 (21.1) [b]	15–49 years = 75 50–79 years = 95 ≥80 years = 21	15–49 years = 26 50–79 years = 35 ≥80 years = 7
Gender (male), n (%)	32 (69.6%)	60 (88.2%)	417 (66%)	194 (73%)	114 (59.7%)	44 (64.7%)
SBP	23 (105) [c]	0(80) [c]	89 (46) [c]	87 (45) [c]	NR	NR
Hypotension (SBP <90), n (%)	21 (45.6%)	47 (69.1%)	NR	NR	NR	NR
Trauma mechanism						
Blunt, n (%)	35 (76.1%)	36 (53.9%)	591 (93%)	247 (93%)	NR	NR
Penetrating, n (%)	11 (23.9%)	32 (47.1%)	45 (7%)	20 (7%)	NR	NR
Cardiac arrest on admission, n (%)	16 (34.8%)	35 (51.5%)	212 (33%)	216 (81%)	42 (22%)	42 (61%)
TRISS (PS)	NR	NR	0.43 (0.36) [b]	0.27 (0.30) [b]	NR	NR
Injury severity						
ISS	31 (30) [c]	31.5 (22) [c]	34 (25) [c]	34 (20) [c]	NR	NR
Head AIS	2.0 (5) [b]	1.5 (4) [b]	3.6 (1.2) [b]	3.3 (1.1) [b]	NR	NR
Chest AIS	1.0 (4) [b]	3.0 (4) [b]	3.8 (0.9) [b]	4.3 (1.1) [b]	NR	NR
Abdomen AIS	2.5 (3) [b]	2.0 (5) [b]	3.6 (1.1) [b]	3.8 (1.5) [b]	NR	NR
Procedures						
Laparotomy, n (%)	25 (54.3%)	40 (58.8%)	301 (47%)	99 (37%)	17 (8.9%)	12 (17.6%)
Embolization, n (%)	3 (6.5%)	3 (4.4%)	153 (24%)	18 (6.7%)	76 (39.8%)	18 (26.5%)
Surgery for liver injury, n (%)	7 (15%)	16 (23%)	NR	NR	14 (7.3%)	5 (7.4%)
Spleen resection, n (%)	4 (8.7%)	7 (10.3%)	NR	NR	18 (9.4%)	9 (13.2%)
Operative procedures for pelvic fractures	PP 3 (6.5%); PB 4 (8.7%); PEF 3 (6.5%)	PP 10 (14.7%); PB 4 (5.9%); PEF 0 (0%)	NR	NR	OS 15 (7.9%); CS 4 (2.1%)	OS 7 (10.3%); CS 3 (4.4%)
In-hospital mortality, n (%)	33 (71.7%)	57 (83.8%)	405 (67%)	210 (90%)	90 (47.1%)	48 (70.6%)
Adjusted measures of association for mortality (REBOA vs. thoracotomy) [d]	OR 0.263 (95% CI 0.043–1.609) [e]		OR 0.261 (95% CI 0.130–0.523) [f]		HR 0.94 (95% CI 0.60–1.48) [g]	

SBP systolic blood pressure, *NR* not reported, *PS* probability of survival, *ISS* Injury Severity Score, *AIS* Abbreviate Injury Score, *PP* pelvic packing, *PB* pelvic binder, *PEF* pelvic external fixation, *OS* open surgery, *CS* closed surgery, *OR* odds ratio, *HR* hazard ratio
Adjusted by:
[a]Patients were categorized in age groups
[b]Mean (SD)
[c]Median (IQR)
[d]As reported in studies
[e]Not reported
[f]Propensity Score Matching by age, gender, mechanism of injury, cause of injury, transport type, pre-hospital treatment, vital signs at emergency department, and injury severity score
[g]Propensity Score Matching by age, sex, body mass index, etiology, Japanese coma scale, presence of head injury, presence of cardiopulmonary arrest on admission, TMPM (Trauma Mortality Prediction Model), and annual number of patients receiving resuscitative thoracotomy (RT) at each hospital

reported transfusions requirements as a continuous variable. In these studies, no significant differences were found regarding the amounts of transfusions in first 24 h. The study by Abe et al. reported the number of patients that required transfusions. They found that a significantly higher proportion of patients required transfusions in the REBOA group (Abe: required transfusion, n (%): REBOA = 542/636 (85%) vs. RT = 197/267 (74%), $p < 0.001$].

Among operative interventions, overall, REBOA patients underwent arterial embolization more often than RT patients (arterial embolization, n (%): REBOA = 232/873 (26%) vs. RT = 39/403 (9.6%), $p < 0.01$). Finally, mortality was significantly higher in patients that underwent RT (mortality, n (%): REBOA = 528/873 (60.4%) vs. RT = 315/403 (78.1%), $p < 0.01$].

Risk of bias

A summary of the risk of bias is presented in Fig. 2 (a detailed description on how studies were evaluated is available in Additional file 1). Studies were prone to biases present in retrospective studies. However, included studies

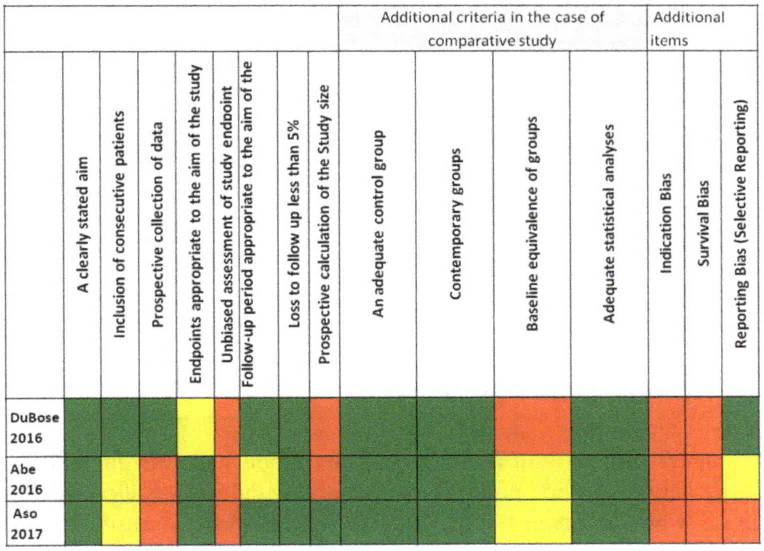

Fig. 2 Risk of bias within studies

were rated as having high risk of indication and survival bias. The study by Aso [19] had a high risk of selective reporting.

Outcomes

Mortality

Our primary outcome was mortality. All studies reported information on this outcome. Data captured included the proportion of deaths in each group and the adjusted measures of association for in-hospital mortality. Table 1 provides an overview of the primary outcome information extracted from each study.

REBOA-related complications

Only the study by DuBose et al. [18] reported complications related to REBOA deployment. In this study, three patients of those in the REBOA group ($n = 46$) suffered complications, which included one pseudoaneurysm and two cases of distal arterial embolism.

Quantitative synthesis results

Meta-Analysis of unadjusted odds ratios showed that the odds of mortality were lower in patients that underwent REBOA compared to those that were taken to RT (OR 0.45; 95% CI 0.34–0.61) (Fig. 3).

To be able to pool the adjusted odds ratios in a meta-analysis, the hazard ratio reported in the study by Aso [19] was converted to an odds ratio. For the procedure, we assumed that the hazard ratio is a type of relative risk and, thus, is asymptotically similar to a relative risk [14]. Then, using the inverse probability weighted binomial model (10) we transformed the adjusted hazard ratio of mortality reported in the study by Aso [19] to an odds ratio. Following this approach, we obtained an adjusted odds ratio of mortality (Aso: OR 0.821; 95% CI 0.306–1.234). After combining adjusted odds ratios using a random effect model, we found that, although lower in REBOA patients, the odds of mortality did not significantly differ between compared groups (OR 0.42; 95% CI 0.17–1.03) (Fig. 4).

Sensitivity analyses

When the outcome of interest (mortality) is common, the OR can jeopardize a risk association or a treatment effect by producing biased estimates of the underlying risk ratio (7)(8). In this systematic review, mortality was high in all groups (RT, REBOA) with rates ranging from 47 to 90% (Tables 1 and 2). Therefore, we decided to convert reported ORs to RRs as proposed in the "Methods" section.

Using the inverse probability weighted binomial model, we obtained the transformed risk ratios of in-hospital mortality for the studies by Abe [17] (RR 0.796; 95% CI 0.624–0.924) and DuBose [18] (RR 0.687; 95% CI 0.217–1.06). For the hazard ratio reported by Aso, we assumed the asymptotical similarity between the hazard ratio and the risk ratio and combined it with the transformed risk ratios using a random effect model. This analysis showed that the risk of mortality was significantly lower among torso trauma patients who underwent REBOA, compared to those who underwent RT (RR 0.81; 95% CI 0.68–0.97) (Fig. 5).

Further sensitivity analyses were performed by methods of adjustment used in individual studies. Therefore, we conducted a meta-analysis of risk ratios from the studies where a propensity score method was used

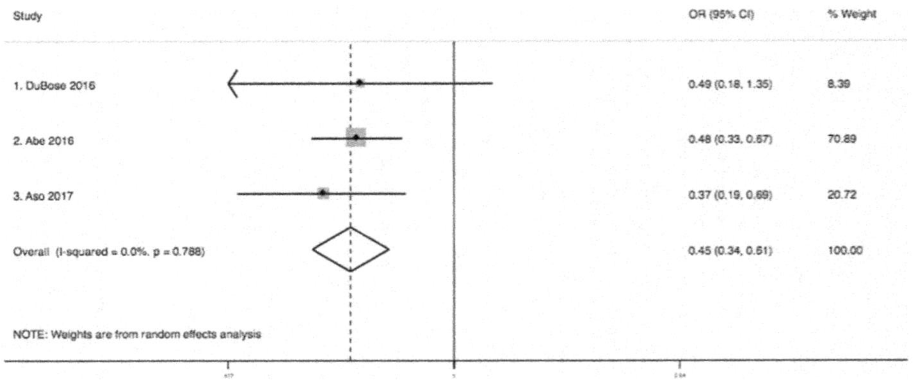

Fig. 3 Meta-analysis of unadjusted odds ratios of mortality (REBOA vs RT)

(Aso, Abe) [17, 19]. In this analysis, the risk of mortality was significantly lower in patients who underwent REBOA, compared to those who underwent RT (RR 0.818; 95% CI 0.683–0.979; $I^2 = 0.0\%$).

A final sensitivity analysis that took into account the evaluation of risk of bias was performed. We ranked the study by Aso [19] with a high risk of selective reporting. They did not report important baseline trauma characteristics such as those related to initial vital signs, physiological status, and injury severity. Not reporting these variables and, furthermore, not including them in the multivariate model analysis could have introduced further indication bias. Therefore, we decided to exclude the study by Aso [19] and to run a random effect model of the remaining studies. This analysis found that the risk of death was significantly lower among REBOA patients (RR 0.79; 95% CI 0.653–0.956; $I^2 = 0.0\%$).

Discussion

To our knowledge, this is the first systematic review and meta-analysis assessing the comparative effectiveness of REBOA and resuscitative thoracotomy on mortality among trauma patients suffering NCTH. Our initial analysis found that although lower in REBOA patients, the odds of mortality did not significantly differ between the compared groups. Although sensitivity analyses showed consistent results on the positive effect of REBOA on mortality, results could be comprised by the presence of survival and indication bias within individual studies.

Non-compressible torso hemorrhage (NCTH) is a life-threatening condition defined as shock associated with hemorrhage due to vascular disruption secondary to pulmonary or solid organ injury, major vascular trauma or pelvic fracture [20]. Concerning this, patients included were primarily victims of serious and severe injuries as reflected by the abbreviated injury scale scores and the procedures for hemorrhage control reported. The need for hemostatic procedures is a fundamental component in the definition of NCTH. These comprise mainly open surgery and endovascular interventional procedures. We found that patients included underwent different aggressive surgical and endovascular procedures for immediate hemorrhage control. Therefore, patients analyzed in this systematic review can be classified as suffering wounds that ultimately ended in a pattern of injury consistent with NCTH anatomic definition.

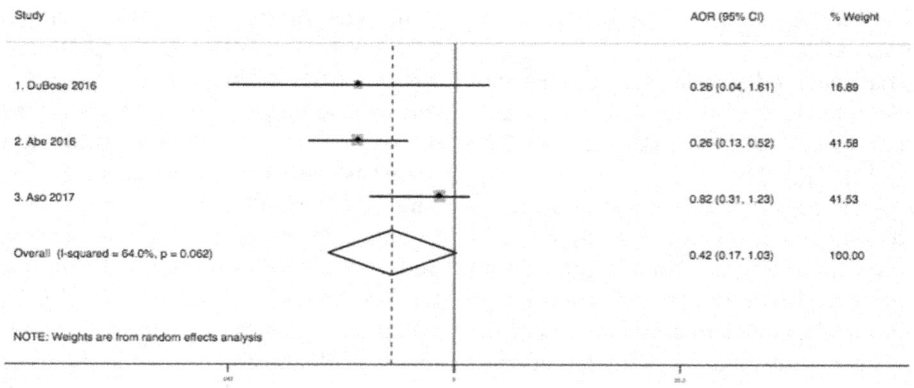

Fig. 4 Meta-analysis of adjusted odds ratios of mortality (REBOA vs. RT)

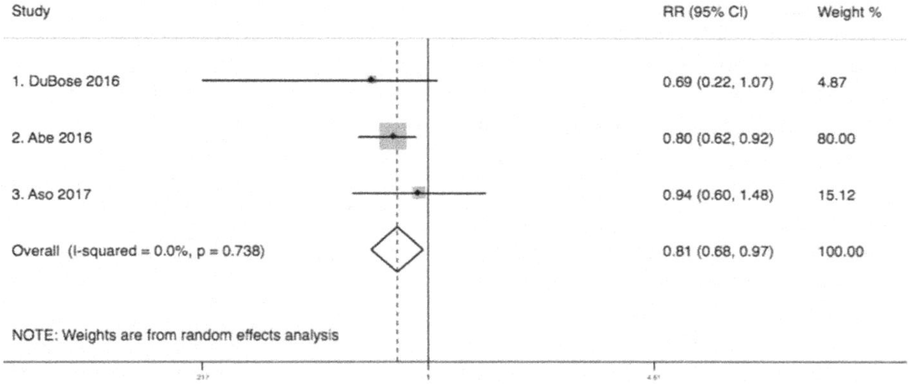

Fig. 5 Sensitivity analysis. Meta-analysis of transformed risk ratios of mortality (REBOA vs. RT)

Shock secondary to NCTH is associated with higher mortality rates. However, a proportion of NCTH-related deaths are potentially preventable [20, 21]. Therefore, research on new technologies such as REBOA for further progress in the principles of damage control resuscitation is of paramount importance for improving survival among NCTH patients. Although we found that the risk of death was lower in NCTH REBOA-treated patients, other reports have shown an increased mortality with the use of REBOA in this population. For example, Norii et al. [22] and Inoue et al. [23] showed that among similarly ill trauma patients, the use of REBOA was associated with higher odds of mortality compared to patients who did not receive REBOA.

In this systematic review, REBOA-treated patients underwent endovascular angioembolization more often than RT patients (Arterial embolization, n (%): REBOA = 232/873 (26%) vs. RT = 39/403 (9.6%), $p < 0.01$). This result further supports the concept that in patients suffering torso trauma in which NTCH is suspected, early REBOA deployment could aid in hemodynamic stabilization while hemorrhage control is achieved by endovascular procedures. To date, one study reported the use of REBOA followed by arterial embolization [24]. In this study, seven patients with severe hepatic and splenic blunt injuries were managed following damage control resuscitation strategies which included early massive transfusion followed by REBOA deployment for hemodynamic support and angioembolization for definitive hemorrhage control. Six of seven patients survived demonstrating the feasibility of REBOA in these scenarios.

Although our quantitative synthesis shows that REBOA is associated with lower mortality, these results could be flawed by the presence of indication and survival bias within individual studies [12]. Indication bias arises when patients are classified on the basis of the non-randomized intervention they received during the natural course of their medical treatment. Survival bias appears when comparing groups in which patients may die before treatment is initiated [12]. As shown in Table 1, patients that underwent RT were more likely to present with cardiac arrest and lower values of systolic blood pressure. Furthermore, the study by Abe [17] reported that REBOA patients had a significantly higher probability of survival on arrival. These facts could increase the risk of significant indication and survival bias, which are selection biases and are a primary evil in observational studies of non-randomized interventions. The main trouble with these biases is that their presence may produce biased effect estimates, thus comprising validity of results.

Traditionally, RT has been used in severely ill trauma patients as the last effort for resuscitation of the moribund patient [25]. REBOA is thought to emulate RT with the advantage of being a less invasive procedure. However, the fact that RT was performed in patients with a higher physiological exhaustion and with a lower probability of survival illustrates a lack of concrete indications for REBOA use in trauma patients. Moreover, it poses the question if REBOA is a comparable intervention to RT or if it is an intervention aimed to prevent hemodynamic collapse in non-agonal unstable patients.

Knowing the balance of benefits and harms of interventions is a paramount component of evidence-based health care. Therefore, we acknowledge that only the study by DuBose et al. [18] reported complications related to REBOA deployment and that was one main reason to rate the studies by Aso [19] and Abe [17] as having a high and unclear risk of selective reporting respectively. Although the severity and proportion of complications related to REBOA deployment were low in the DuBose series, another report by Saito et al. [26] documented serious adverse events that ultimately ended in lower limb amputations in 2 of 14 patients. However, REBOA is an evolving endovascular technology, and new strategies such as improvements in endovascular skills training [27, 28] and the advent of smaller diameter catheters [29] may improve the safety related to its deployment [30].

Although we found a benefit of REBOA over RT in NCTH patients, our results can be comprised by the biases present in primary studies. Future studies must address specific indications for REBOA to know which population could benefit from its use. Furthermore, trauma researchers should determine if REBOA is a comparable intervention to RT. Therefore, prospective evaluation with specific inclusion and exclusion criteria that ameliorates noise and biased results should be undertaken.

Conclusion

Our meta-analysis mainly from observational data suggests that the use of REBOA is associated with lower mortality. However, our findings deserve further investigation.

Acknowledgements

Dedicated to the memory of Isabel C. Muñoz Chavez MD.

Funding

No funding. This article received no specific grant from any funding agency in the public, commercial, or non-for-profit sectors.

Authors' contributions

RMN, MPN, EF, PF, ER, HAG, PB, JPH, AFG, and CAO contributed equally to this work. RMN and CAO designed the research. RMN, MPN, EF, PF, ER, HAG, PB, JPH, AFG, and CAO performed the research, analyzed the data, and wrote the paper. All authors read and approved the final manuscript.

Competing interests

The authors declare that they have no competing interests.

Author details

[1]Clinical Research Center, Fundación Valle del Lili, Cali, Colombia. [2]Clinical Foianini, Santa Cruz de La Sierra, Bolivia. [3]Virginia Commonwealth University, Richmon, VA, USA. [4]Universidad del Valle, Cali, Colombia. [5]Division of Trauma and Acute Care Surgery, Fundación Valle del Lili, Cali, Colombia. [6]Department of Surgery, Brigham and Women's Hospital, Boston, MA, USA. [7]School of Medicine, Universidad Javeriana Cali, Cali, Valle del Cauca, Colombia.

References

1. Stannard A, Eliason JL, Rasmussen TE. Resuscitative endovascular balloon occlusion of the aorta (REBOA) as an adjunct for hemorrhagic shock. J Trauma Acute Care Surg [Internet]. 2011;71:1869–72. Available from: http://journals.lww.com/jtrauma/Fulltext/2011/12000/Resuscitative_Endovascular_Balloon_Occlusion_of.62.aspx.
2. Belenkiy SM, Batchinsky AI, Rasmussen TE, Cancio LC. Resuscitative endovascular balloon occlusion of the aorta for hemorrhage control: Past, present, and future. J. Trauma Acute Care Surg. [Internet]. 2015;79: S236–S242. Available from: http://journals.lww.com/jtrauma/Fulltext/2015/10001/Resuscitative_endovascular_balloon_occlusion_of.29.aspx .
3. Gupta BK, KHANEJA SC, FLORES L, EASTLICK L, LONGMORE W, Shaftan GW. The role of intra-aortic balloon occlusion in penetrating abdominal trauma. J Trauma Acute Care Surg [Internet]. 1989;29:861–5. Available from: http://journals.lww.com/jtrauma/Fulltext/1989/06000/The_Role_of_Intra_aortic_Balloon_Occlusion_in.26.aspx.
4. Moore LJ, Brenner M, Kozar RA, Pasley J, Wade CE, Baraniuk MS, et al. Implementation of resuscitative endovascular balloon occlusion of the aorta as an alternative to resuscitative thoracotomy for noncompressible truncal hemorrhage. J Trauma Acute Care Surg. 2014;79:523–32.
5. Morrison JJ, Galgon RE, Jansen JO, Cannon JW, Rasmussen TE, Eliason JL, et al. A systematic review of the use of resuscitative endovascular balloon occlusion of the aorta in the management of hemorrhagic shock. J Trauma Acute Care Surg. 2015;80:324–34.
6. Brenner ML, Moore LJ, DuBose JJ, Tyson GH, McNutt MK, Albarado RP, et al. A clinical series of resuscitative endovascular balloon occlusion of the aorta for hemorrhage control and resuscitation. J. Trauma Acute Care Surg. [Internet]. 2013;75:506–511. Available from: http://journals.lww.com/jtrauma/Fulltext/2013/09000/A_clinical_series_of_resuscitative_endovascular.24.aspx.
7. Higgins JP, Green S. Cochrane Handbook for Systematic Reviews of Interventions: Cochrane Book Series. Cochrane Handb. Syst. Rev. Interv. Cochrane B. Ser. John Wiley and Sons; 2008.
8. Liberati A, Altman DG, Tetzlaff J, Mulrow C, Gøtzsche PC, Ioannidis JPA, et al. The PRISMA statement for reporting systematic reviews and meta-analyses of studies that evaluate health care interventions: explanation and elaboration. PLOS Med [Internet]. 2009;6:e1000100. Public Library of Science. Available from: http://journals.plos.org/plosmedicine/article?id=10.1371/journal.pmed.1000100.
9. Robinson KA. Development of a highly sensitive search strategy for the retrieval of reports of controlled trials using PubMed. Int J Epidemiol. 2002;31:150–3.
10. McGowan J, Sampson M, Salzwedel DM, Cogo E, Foerster V, Lefebvre C. PRESS Peer Review of Electronic Search Strategies: 2015 Guideline Statement. J Clin Epidemiol. 2016;75:40-6.
11. Slim K, Nini E, Forestier D, Kwiatkowski F, Panis Y, Chipponi J. Methodological index for non-randomized studies (MINORS): development and validation of a new instrument. ANZ J Surg. 2003;73:712–6. Blackwell Science Pty.
12. del Junco DJ, Fox EE, Camp EA, Rahbar MH, Holcomb JB. Seven deadly sins in trauma outcomes research: an epidemiologic post-mortem for major causes of bias. J Trauma Acute Care Surg. 2013;75:S97–103.
13. Grant RL. Converting an odds ratio to a range of plausible relative risks for better communication of research findings. BMJ Br Med J. 2014;348: f7450.
14. Nurminen M. To use or not to use the odds ratio in epidemiologic analyses? Eur J Epidemiol. 1995;11:365–71.
15. Zhang J, Yu KF. What's the relative risk? A method of correcting the odds ratio in cohort studies of common outcomes. JAMA. 1998;280:1690–1.
16. Popham F. Converting between marginal effect measures from binomial models. Int J Epidemiol. 2016;45:590–1.
17. Abe T, Uchida M, Nagata I, Saitoh D, Tamiya N. Resuscitative endovascular balloon occlusion of the aorta versus aortic cross clamping among patients with critical trauma: a nationwide cohort study in Japan. Crit Care. 2016;20:400.
18. DuBose JJ, Scalea TM, Brenner M, Skiada D, Inaba K, Cannon J, et al. The AAST prospective Aortic Occlusion for Resuscitation in Trauma and Acute Care Surgery (AORTA) registry: data on contemporary utilization and outcomes of aortic occlusion and resuscitative balloon occlusion of the aorta (REBOA). J Trauma Acute Care Surg [Internet]. 2016;81:409–19. Available from: http://journals.lww.com/jtrauma/Fulltext/2016/09000/The_AAST_prospective_Aortic_Occlusion_for.1.aspx.
19. Aso S, Matsui H, Fushimi K, Yasunaga H. Resuscitative endovascular balloon occlusion of the aorta or resuscitative thoracotomy with aortic clamping for noncompressible torso hemorrhage: A retrospective nationwide study. J. Trauma Acute Care Surg. 2017;82(5):910-914.
20. Kisat M, Morrison JJ, Hashmi ZG, Efron DT, Rasmussen TE, Haider AH. Epidemiology and outcomes of non-compressible torso hemorrhage. J Surg Res. 2013;184:414–21.
21. Kauvar DS, Wade CE. The epidemiology and modern management of traumatic hemorrhage: US and international perspectives. Crit Care. 2005;9:S1.
22. Norii T, Crandall C, Terasaka Y. Survival of severe blunt trauma patients treated with resuscitative endovascular balloon occlusion of the aorta compared with propensity score-adjusted untreated patients. J Trauma Acute Care Surg. 2015;78(4):721-8.
23. Inoue J, Atsushi S, Ayako Y, Koichi H, Hiroki M, Yasuhiro O. Resuscitative endovascular balloon occlusion of the aortamight be dangerous in patients with severe torso trauma: a propensity score analysis. J Trauma Acute Care Surg. 2016;80:559–67.
24. Ogura T, Lefor AT, Nakano M, Izawa Y, Morita H. Nonoperative management of hemodynamically unstable abdominal trauma patients with angioembolization and resuscitative endovascular balloon occlusion of the aorta. J Trauma Acute Care Surg. 2015;78:132–5.
25. Moore EE, Knudson MM, Burlew CC, Inaba K, Dicker RA, Biffl WL, et al. Defining the Limits of Resuscitative Emergency Department Thoracotomy:

A Contemporary Western Trauma Association Perspective. J. Trauma Acute Care Surg. 2011;70(2):334-9.
26. Saito N, Matsumoto H, Yagi T, Hara Y, Hayashida K, Motomura T, et al. Evaluation of the safety and feasibility of resuscitative endovascular balloon occlusion of the aorta. J Trauma Acute Care Surg. 2015;78:897–904.
27. Villamaria CY, Eliason JL, Napolitano LM, Stansfield RB, Spencer JR, Rasmussen TE. Endovascular skills for trauma and resuscitative surgery (ESTARS) course: curriculum development, content validation, and program assessment. J Trauma Acute Care Surg. 2014;76:929–35. discussion 935–6.
28. Brenner M, Hoehn M, Pasley J, Dubose J, Stein D, Scalea T. Basic endovascular skills for trauma course: bridging the gap between endovascular techniques and the acute care surgeon. J Trauma Acute Care Surg. 2014;77:286–91.
29. Teeter WA, Matsumoto J, Idoguchi K, Kon Y, Orita T, Funabiki T, et al. Smaller introducer sheaths for REBOA may be associated with fewer complications. J Trauma Acute Care Surg. 2016;81:1.
30. Taylor JR, Harvin JA, Martin C, Holcomb JB, Moore LJ. Vascular complications from resuscitative endovascular balloon occlusion of the aorta (REBOA). J. Trauma Acute Care Surg. 2017;83(1):S120-S123.

21

What is the treatment of tracheal lesions associated with traditional thyroidectomy?

Nicola Tartaglia, Roberta Iadarola*, Alessandra Di Lascia, Pasquale Cianci, Alberto Fersini and Antonio Ambrosi

Abstract

Aim: The aim of this study is to review the literature focusing on various treatments based on time of tracheal injury and on different surgeons' personal experience.

Methods: We retrospectively reviewed all cases of total thyroidectomy performed at the University Surgical Department of Ospedali Riuniti of Foggia from 2006 to 2017. Only a single case of tracheal lesion due to traditional total thyroidectomy was found. An extensive search of the relevant literature was carried out using MEDLINE (PubMed). We included articles that reported article type, patient number, sex, age, reasons for surgery, time of tracheal perforation intraoperatively or delayed rupture, symptoms, diagnosis, type of surgical procedure, pathological report and follow-up.

Results: A total of 156 published studies were screened from the sources listed. Of these, 15 studies were included in the present study. We introduced our case in the analysis. A total of 16 patients were totally analysed. There were seven males (43.7%) and seven females (43.7%), and for two patients, gender was not available. The mean patient age was 41.6 years.

Conclusions: The literature review showed very few cases treated differently. However, it would be good to standardise treatments. Tracheal perforation, if encountered, needs to be managed appropriately in centres of expertise with a high volume of thyroidectomies.

Keywords: Total thyroidectomy, Tracheal injury, Tracheal surgery, Tracheal lesion, Tracheal laceration, Tracheostomy

Background

Thyroidectomy is one of the most common surgical operations performed in endocrine surgery for benign and malignant thyroid disease. Complication rates from total thyroidectomy are low. At present, mortality for this procedure is approximately 0%, and the overall complication rate is less than 3% [1]. These most commonly include vocal fold paresis or paralysis, hypoparathyroidism, hypocalcaemia, haematoma and wound infection [1, 2]. Tracheal injury associated with thyroidectomy is rare (less than 1%) [3]. The trachea may be perforated or lacerated intraoperatively, often recognised and repaired immediately with little patient morbidity. However, unrecognised injury or delayed rupture secondary to tracheal necrosis can present up to 2 weeks postoperatively [2]. Because this complication occurs in less than one patient for most thyroid surgeons, it is unlikely that any individual will gather sufficient data to report the management in a series [3]. There are no published reports describing the management of inadvertent tracheal perforation during thyroid surgery [3]. Nevertheless, tracheal perforation, if encountered, needs to be managed appropriately. The aim of the present study was to review the literature with a focus on the various treatments based on time of injury and on different surgeons' personal experience.

Materials and methods

From 2006 to 2017, approximately 2150 total thyroidectomies were carried out at the University Surgical Department of Ospedali Riuniti of Foggia. We can report only a single case of tracheal injury.

* Correspondence: robertaiadarola@gmail.com
Department of Surgery, University of Foggia, Luigi Pinto Street, No. 1, 71122 Foggia, Italy

Literature review

An extensive search for relevant literature was carried out using MEDLINE (PubMed). The keywords used for the search were Tracheal injuries after thyroidectomy, Tracheal injury, Tracheal laceration, Tracheal lesion, used with the Boolean operator 'AND' total thyroidectomy. Exclusion criteria were thyroidectomy performed by approaches other than traditional (for example robotic, MIVAT or laser) and other causes of tracheal laceration (for example, perforation due to intubation). Languages were restricted to English and Italian. We included articles that reported article type, patient number, gender, age, reasons for surgery, time of tracheal perforation intraoperatively or delayed rupture, symptoms, diagnosis, type of surgical procedure, pathological report and follow-up.

Results

A total of 156 published studies were screened from the sources listed. After examination of all titles, 120 papers were excluded as 'not relevant'. Among the remaining 36 studies, the following were excluded: 4 articles were in other languages, 7 described injury due to thyroidectomy performed by approaches other than the traditional one and 10 analysed other causes of tracheal laceration. Finally, 15 studies were included in the present study (Table 1). We introduced our case in the analysis. A total of 16 patients were analysed. There were seven males (43.7%) and seven females (43.7%), and for two patients, gender was not available. The mean patient age was 41.6 years.

Case report

A 44-year-old Romanian woman underwent elective total thyroidectomy in our department for Grave's disease. Euthyroidism was preoperatively achieved with methimazole and Lugol's solution. At the time of the surgical procedure, due to Grave's disease, a fibrotic and vascular thyroid gland was found. Total thyroidectomy was performed with the use of a combination of electrocautery and shears. During mobilisation of the thyroid gland, all four parathyroid glands and both recurrent laryngeal nerves were identified and carefully preserved. Because of the fibrotic nature of the gland, the use of a bipolar device (Enseal) was necessary for management of the right Gruber ligament. Immediately after, thermal damage to the anterior-lateral surface of the trachea (I/II tracheal ring) was found (1.5 cm, Fig. 1). This was repaired primarily using non-absorbable sutures (Prolene 3/0). A muscle flap was used for reinforcement, and a suction drain was left at the surgical site. The patient was subsequently transferred to intensive care for delayed extubation that occurred on postoperative (PO) day 5. On the same day, because of her respiratory condition, the patient underwent bronchoscopy and subsequent tracheostomy because the wound remained open. On PO day 7, she was readmitted to our department with tracheostomy, spontaneously breathing and with good cardio-circulatory parameters. The ear, nose and throat consultant diagnosed adduction vocal cord paralysis for which she started phonation and swallowing training. The patient was discharged on PO day 26, euthyroid on substitution treatment. At follow-up, 6 months later, she had no vocal cord paralysis. However, she still had the tracheostomy. Subsequently, the patient returned to her country for personal reasons and was lost to follow-up.

Discussion

Complication rates from total thyroidectomy are low. At present, mortality for this procedure is approximately 0%, and the overall complication rate is less than 3% [1, 2, 4]. Major complications include wound infection (0.02–0.5%), haematoma (0.3–4.3%), transient recurrent laryngeal nerve palsy (1–2%), permanent recurrent laryngeal nerve palsy (< 1%), transient hypoparathyroidism (1.6–50%) and permanent hypoparathyroidism (0–13%) [1]. During the period between 1997 and 2016, we performed 2150 thyroidectomies with the following percentage of complications: wound infection (0.002%), haematoma (1.3%), transient recurrent laryngeal nerve palsy (1.5%), permanent recurrent laryngeal nerve palsy (0.2%), transient hypoparathyroidism (5.9%) and permanent hypoparathyroidism (0.3%).

Risk factors

It is possible to identify several preoperative, intraoperative and postoperative risk factors. Female gender and thyrotoxic goitre are commonly considered risk factors [2]. Golger et al. [5] and Conzo et al. [6] suggest that long-term tracheal compression by a large goitre may cause local tracheal wall weakening and subsequent tracheomalacia. Intraoperative risk factors include prolonged intubation and elevated cuff pressure because of reduction of blood supply to the trachea with subsequent damage [2]. Gosnell et al. [3] report frequent exceeding difficulty to define the plane of dissection in patients with multi-nodular goitre that is characterised by repeated cycles of hyperplasia, degeneration and fibrosis. These often contain dense fibrotic thyroid tissue that is contiguous with surrounding fibrous tissues, including the trachea. This condition is associated, as in our case, with considerable use of a device. The use of a device for diathermy can be dangerous with respect to tracheal lesions. When dissecting around the trachea, the lateral pedicles should be carefully preserved to maintain the blood supply to the upper segments, and thyroid branches should be ligated close to the capsule.

Table 1 Literature review and our case

Author	Article type	No. of cases	Reason of TT	Age gender	I setting Y/N	II setting Y/N (day PO)	Size/place trauma	Necrosis/bacterial involvement	Treatment	Posttreatment follow-up
Gosnell [3]	Retrospective 11,917 cases	7/11917 (0.06%)	4 multinodular goitre 1 Hurthle adenoma 1 Grave's 1 Anaplastic tumour	na	Yes	No	PI	No	Primarily absorbable sutures with muscle strap in two patients	1 subcutaneous emphysema 1 bilateral pneumothorax
Iacconi [7]	Letter to editor	7	Grave's disease	na	Yes	No	na	na	na	2 died 1 respiratory distress 2 mediastinitis
Our case	Case report	1	Grave's disease	44 F	Yes	No	AI	No	Primarily not absorbable sutures with muscle flap	Tracheostomy in VI PO
Damrose [2]	Case report	1	Grave's disease	20 F	No	Yes (7 days PO)	1–2 mm/A/I ring	No	Primarily absorbable sutures	No
Golger [5]	Case report	1	Grave's disease	30 F	No	Yes (8 days PO)	A/II-III-IV rings	Yes/*Beta-haemolytic Streptococcus*	Montgomery T-tube with the trap muscles.	T-tube removed 3 months after
Conzo [6]	Case report and review	1	Bilateral adenoma	65 M	No	Yes (15 days PO)	1.5-mm/AL	No	Conservative treatment*	No
Mazeh [8]	Case report and review	1	Grave's disease	17 F	No	Yes (9 days PO)	2.5-cm/A/II-III-IV rings	No	Conservative treatment*	Primarily suture
Toe Ew [9]	Case report	1	Papillary thyroid carcinoma	62 M	No	Yes (10 days PO)	A	No	na	na
Jacqmin [10]	Case report	1	Grave's disease	53 F	No	Yes (8 days PO)	A/III ring	Yes/*Streptococcus mitis*	Circumferential tracheal excision with anastomosis	No
Chauhan [11]	Case report	1	Medullary carcinoma thyroid	65 M	No	Yes (7 days PO)	5 mm/A II ring	Yes	Debridement tracheostoma drain	Chauhan [11]
Benjamin [12]	Case report	1	Papillary thyroid carcinoma	55 M	No	Yes (4 days PO)	na	na	Primarily absorbable sutures	No
Bertolaccini [13]	Case report	1	Papillary thyroid carcinoma	45 M	No	Yes (4 days PO)	AL/IV ring	*Staphylococcus aureus*	Primarily absorbable sutures with muscle flap	No
Sanna [4]	Case report and review	1	Papillary thyroid carcinoma	17 F	No	Yes (7 days PO)	3 cm/AL/II–V rings	No	A muscular flap, rounded on the tracheal defect	No
Rosato L [14]	Case report	1	na	na	No	Yes (10 days PO)	na	na	Primarily sutures with patch of fibrinogen-thrombin collagen	No
Escott [15]	Case report	1	na	29 M	No	Yes (14 days PO)	2.5-mm PL	na	Conservative treatment*	After 48 h with a myovascular transposition flap with Tisseel tissue-bonding agent.
Xinwei Han [16]	Case report	1	Nodule	39 F	no	Yes (1 PO)	na	na	Covered tracheal stent	Abscess removed with drainage stent was removed 55 days after

F female, *M* male, *TT* total thyroidectomy, *L* lymphadenectomy, *PR* primarily repair, *MF* muscolar flap, *D* drains, *PO* postoperative, *I setting* trachea may be perforated or lacerated intraoperatively, *II setting* unrecognised injury, or delayed rupture secondary to tracheal necrosis, can present up to 2 weeks postoperatively, *PL* posterolateral surface of trachea, *AL* anterolateral, *A* anterior, *na* not applicable
*Conservative treatment (bed rest, antibiotic and cough suppressants)

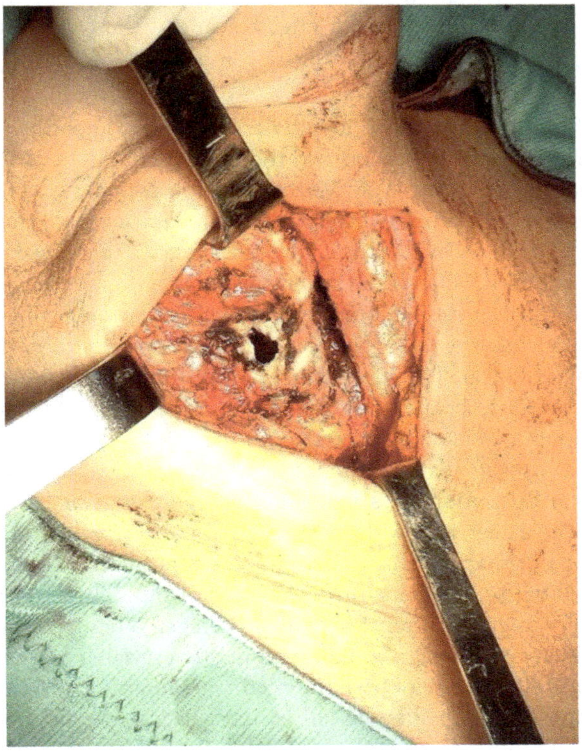

Fig. 1 Trachea injury identified during the surgery

Furthermore, extended operating time always increases the risk of complications [5]. In addition, Lugol's solution may reduce the amount of intraoperative cautery required for control of haemorrhage. In the postoperative period, persistent uncontrolled cough can be another risk factor.

A review of the literature identified two distinct settings for tracheal injury associated with thyroid surgery (Table 1). In the first setting, the trachea may be perforated or lacerated intraoperatively. In the second, unrecognised injury or delayed rupture secondary to tracheal necrosis can present up to 2 weeks postoperatively.

First scenario: trachea injury identified during the surgery

To our knowledge, we described the third case reported in the literature [3, 7]. In this setting, a full-thickness thermal injury to the trachea can occur and is typically identified when the endotracheal tube is observed through the tracheal defect. This type of tracheal injury is usually associated with either excision of large and bulky tumours or technical errors and is almost always repaired primarily, with no further consequences [8]. Assessment of the actual rate of such tracheal injuries is difficult because they are underreported. In one study, Gosnell et al. [3] reviewed 11,917 thyroidectomies performed during a 45-year period and identified tracheal perforations in 0.06%. In that report, all perforations were located at the posterolateral surface of the trachea, either following attempted suture ligation of vessels in the region of the ligament of Berry or with the use of diathermy adjacent to the trachea (Table 1). The same author reported that most perforations were recognised as they occurred, but smaller inadvertent injuries were identified at the conclusion of the procedure. Because visual inspection of the trachea may miss small perforations when an injury is suspected during the surgical procedure, saline surrounding the trachea may be used to test for an air leak. This is more sensitive and is recommended routinely for all thyroid surgeries [2, 3]. Once identified, the defect must be repaired by single absorbable suture [3] or non-absorbable. Subsequently, a muscle flap can be used for reinforcement. Placement of drains and the use of postoperative antibiotics are dictated by surgeon preference.

Second scenario: trachea injury identified after the surgery

The second setting, which includes delayed tracheal rupture after a thyroid surgical procedure, seems to be less rare, but it too has only been described in case reports [2, 4–6, 8–16]. As reported by Mazeh et al. [8], in this setting, the thermal injury during the initial procedure is not recognised by the surgeon, and over the course of several days, tracheal necrosis surrounding the thermal injury results in an air leak to the surrounding tissues [8]. These can lead to extensive subcutaneous and mediastinal emphysema and severe dyspnoea. It can also adversely affect venous return to the heart. In addition, tracheal rupture may cause neck infections, which may lead to mediastinitis, mediastinal abscess and death [16, 17]. In addition to the above mentioned generic risk factors, the damage to the tracheal wall and possible development of a haematoma may create an environment in which bacteria can seed, resulting in infection and necrosis [5]. Careful elicitation of history may reveal strenuous coughing or sneezing as a precipitating factor [8]. Typically, these patients present on varying postoperative days with either subcutaneous emphysema or wound infection. Other symptoms may include neck or facial swelling, haemoptysis, retrosternal pain or hoarseness [2, 5]. Respiratory compromise may follow. The diagnosis is clinical and should be confirmed with a CT scan that rules out other causes of subcutaneous emphysema (such as spontaneous pneumothorax). CT may demonstrate the tracheal defect and provide localization. Of importance, a normal tracheal outline does not exclude the diagnosis [8]. Flexible or rigid bronchoscopy may also locate the tracheal rupture. Nevertheless, some injuries may not be identified [2, 10]. Airway control should be a priority. Equipment should be on hand for performing an emergent tracheostomy if necessary. Rapid sequence induction of anaesthesia and orotracheal intubation with placement of the cuff distal to the site of injury is usually sufficient to control the airway [13]. The management of delayed tracheal rupture after thyroidectomy should not differ from that of any other delayed tracheal injury. Despite past assumptions that surgical treatment is indicated in all cases, recent studies have identified a subset of patients who could and should be managed conservatively [18, 19]. If necessary, surgery must not be delayed [13]. Potential patient morbidity can include neck abscess, mediastinitis, pneumothorax, cardiac tamponade and tension pneumomediastinum. Mortality has been reported [2]. By review of literature data in this setting, we found 15 case reports [2, 4–6, 8–16] (Table 1). Five case reports reported patients affected by Grave's disease. The other five patients were affected by malignant disease of the thyroid gland and only one by bilateral adenoma. The diagnosis of tracheal injury occurred between the 1st and 15th postoperative day [6, 16]. In most of these patients, necrosis was found, and culture revealed bacterial infection in 3/15 patients by *Beta-haemolytic Streptococcus* [5], *Streptococcus mitis* [10] and *Staphylococcus aureus* [13]. The management depends on the authors and was very different among them. In all cases where necrosis was present, debridement of the devitalized trachea was necessary. Primary conservative treatment (bed rest, antibiotic and cough suppressants) was attempted by Conzo et al. [6] with success and by Mazeh et al [8] with failure. The first [6] was a very small laceration (1.5 mm). Primary closure of the wound with absorbable suture, with or without drains, was attempted first by different authors [2, 12] and Mazeh et al. [8] after conservative treatment failure. Bertolaccini et al [13] and Sanna et al [4] opted for a muscle flap stitched with an absorbable suture on the defect. There was no necrosis or infection in these patients, and this procedure was successful. Other authors reported good results with primary sutures with a patch of fibrinogen-thrombin-coated collagen [14] or a myovascular transposition flap in conjunction with a Tisseel tissue-bonding agent after conservative treatment failure [15]. In contrast, large extension of a tracheal tear and a wide necrosis or infection contraindicated a primary repair. Golger et al [5], after debridement, chose to partially close the trachea around a no. 11 Montgomery T-tube with adjacent strap muscles that were removed after 3 months. Jacqmin et al [10] preferred circumferential tracheal excision with anastomosis. Chauhan et al [11], after debridement, chose tracheostomy (removed 14 days postoperative) and a drain. Finally, Han et al. [16] proposed a tracheal stent that was implanted to cover the entire lesion complicated by abscess. Use of a covered tracheal stent for treatment of tracheal rupture represents a minimally invasive technique that can be performed under local anaesthesia by interventional radiologists. The procedure is likely to be especially suited to patients with poor general condition. The implantation can be performed quickly (usually 3–5 min) and results in effective and instant coverage of the site of tracheal rupture.

Some authors try to identify a precise treatment based on the size of the lesion and the clinical condition of the patient. As reported by Mazeh et al [8], patients with no respiratory distress who have stable or improving symptoms and no evidence of infection may be observed as in-patients while receiving intravenous antibiotic coverage. An aggressive surgical approach is warranted in all other patients. Other authors proposed different criteria. Kaloud et al. [20], for example, reported that surgical repair is indicated for transmural tears with a length exceeding 1 cm. In contrast, Kuhne et al. [21] reported that conservative treatment may be indicated for tracheal disruptions less than 2 cm. Large extension of the tracheal tear and wide necrosis or infection contraindicated primary repair. In several case reports, the authors used cultures obtained from the neck wound intraoperatively to guide future antibiotic coverage. When possible, primary repair should be attempted over viable tracheal edges. Repairs may be reinforced with muscle flaps, and a suction drain may be left at the surgical site for possible future ongoing leaks. The rationale for use of a muscle flap is to reinforce the repair with viable muscle tissue, which may help to prevent postoperative leaks. This tissue plastically adheres to the airway lesion and permits to maintain its rigidity, obtaining a good result. This potentially prevents further complications because of its vascular feeding [8, 13]. No published studies have assessed the utility of such a flap. Similarly, the use of suction drains is not supported by any high-quality studies [22].

Conclusion

Tracheal injury associated with thyroidectomy is very rare, but when it occurs, it can be dangerous. Tracheal perforation is generally not considered a complication as such but rather a technical occurrence during surgery that requires expeditious attention. A literature review revealed very few cases treated in different ways. Nevertheless, it would be good to standardise the treatments. Tracheal perforation, if encountered, needs to be managed appropriately in centres of expertise with a high volume of thyroidectomies.

Acknowledgements
Not applicable.

Funding
No funding was provided for this study.

Authors' contributions

NT and RI made substantial contributions to the study conception and design and were responsible for acquisition of data, analysis and interpretation of data. RI and AF were involved in drafting the manuscript. DLA and PC critically revised the manuscript for important intellectual content. AA and RI gave final approval of the version to be published. All authors read and approved the final manuscript.

Competing interests

The authors declare that they have no competing interests.

References

1. Lombardi CP, Raffaelli M, De Crea C, Traini E, Oragano L, Sollazzi L, Bellantone R. Complications in thyroid surgery. Minerva Chir. 2007;62(5):395–408.
2. Damrose EJ, Damrose JF. Delayed tracheal rupture following thyroidectomy. Auris Nasus Larynx. 2009;36:113–5.
3. Gosnell JE, Campbell P, Sidhu S, Sywak M, Reeve TS, Delbridge LW. Inadvertent tracheal perforation during thyroidectomy. Br J Surg. 2006;93(1):55–6.
4. Sanna S, Monteverde M, Taurchini M, Mengozzi M, Genestreti G, Grossi W, Argnani D, Bettini D, Dell'Amore D. It could suddenly happen: delayed rupture of the trachea after total thyroidectomy. A case report. G Chir. 2014; 35(n. 3/4):65–6.
5. Golger A, Rice LL, Jackson BS, Young JE. Tracheal necrosis after thyroidectomy. Can J Surg. 2002;45:463–4.
6. Conzo G, Fiorelli A, Palazzo A, Stanzione F, Della Pietra C, Santini M. An unpredicted case of tracheal necrosis following thyroidectomy. Ann Ital Chir. 2012;83:55–8.
7. Iacconi P. Inadvertent tracheal perforation during thyroidectomy. Br J Surg. 2006;93:770–1.
8. Mazeh H, Suwanabol PA, Schneider DF, Sippel RS. Late manifestation of tracheal rupture after thyroidectomy: case report and literature review. Endocr Pract. 2012;18:e73–6.
9. To EW, Tsang WM, Williams MD, Lai EC, Chan M. Tracheal necrosis and surgical emphysema: a rare complication of thyroidectomy. Ear Nose Throat J. 2002;81:738–41.
10. Jacqmin S, Lentschener C, Demirev M, Gueroult S, Herman P, Ozier Y. Postoperative necrosis of the anterior part of the cervical trachea following thyroidectomy. J Anesth. 2005;19:347–8.
11. Chauhan A, Ganguly M, Saidha N, Gulia P. Tracheal necrosis with surgical emphysema following thyroidectomy. J Postgrad Med. 2009;55:193–5.
12. Heavrin BS, Benjamin S, et al. Tracheal perforation after thyroidectomy. J Emerg Med. 2012;43(4):e259–60.
13. Bertolaccini L, Lauro C, Priotto R, Terzi A. It sometimes happens: late tracheal rupture after total thyroidectomy. ICVTJ. 2012;14:500–1.
14. Rosato L, Ginardi A, Mondini G, Sandri A, Oliaro A, Filosso PL. Efficacy of fleece-bound sealing system (TachoSil®) in delayed anterior tracheal lacerations secondary to ischemic tracheal necrosis after total thyroidectomy. Minerva Chir. 2012;67(3):271–5.
15. Escott AB, Pochin RS, Escott BJ. Repair of a posterior perforation of the trachea following thyroidectomy with a muscle transposition flap. Ear Nose Throat J. 2016;95(2):E14–7.
16. Xinwei Han MD, Qingchun Mu MD, Chao Liu MD, Xiubo Lu MD, Detao Yin MD, Kewei Ren MD, Gang Wu MD. Covered stent implantation in the treatment of tracheal rupture after thyroidectomy. J Vasc Interv Radiol. 2016;27(11):1758–61.
17. Tartaglia N, Cianci P, Iadarola R, Di lascia A, Fersini A, Ambrosi A, Neri V. Acute suppurative thyroiditis after fine needle aspiration. Case report and literature review. Chirurg. 2017;30(3):89–94.
18. Mullan GP, Georgalas C, Arora A, Narula A. Conservative management of a major post-intubation tracheal injury and review of current management. Eur Arch Otorhinolaryngol. 2007;264:685–8.
19. Conti M, Porte H, Wurtz A. Conservative management of postintubation tracheobronchial ruptures [with author reply]. J Thorac Cardiovac Surg. 2007;134(3):821–2.
20. Kaloud H, Smolle-Juettner FM, Prause G, List WF. Iatrogenic ruptures of the tracheobronchial tree. Chest. 1997;112:774–8.
21. Kuhne CA, Kaiser GM, Flohe S, Beiderlinden M, Kuehl H, Stavrou GA, Waydhas C, Lendemanns S, Paffrath T, Nast-Kolb D. Non operative management of tracheobronchial injuries in severely injured patients. Surg Today. 2005;35:518–23.
22. Grillo HC. Surgery of trachea and bronchi. BC Decker; 2004. p. 249–70.

22

Acute appendicitis, inflammatory appendiceal mass and the risk of a hidden malignant tumor

Frederico José Ribeiro Teixeira Jr[1], Sérgio Dias do Couto Netto[2,3,6*], Eduardo Hiroshi Akaishi[4], Edivaldo Massazo Utiyama[5], Carlos Augusto Metidieri Menegozzo[7]and Marcelo Cristiano Rocha[8]

Abstract

Introduction: Acute appendicitis is significantly common. Despite the increased use of computed tomography, the number of perforated cases has been stable in the past three decades. Between 2% and 6% of patients with acute appendicitis present appendiceal mass, often described as inflammatory phlegmon or abscess. Malignant tumors are confirmed by pathological analysis in 0.9–1.4% of all appendectomies performed to treat acute appendicitis. However, recent series demonstrate an elevated incidence of malignancies, ranging from 5.9 to 12%, in patients with inflammatory appendiceal mass.

Methods: The analysis was based on a systematic review of the literature. The articles were searched in PubMed for the period from 1987 to 2016. Articles presenting the incidence of the hidden malignancy among patients with appendiceal inflammatory mass were selected. Variables as age, interval appendectomy rate, the incidence of neoplasm, time to surgery, minimally invasive assessment, histology, right colectomy rate and morbidity were analyzed.

Results: A total of 13.244 patients were described as presenting acute appendicitis. Appendiceal tumor is present in approximately 1% of the appendectomies, while the rate of neoplasm varies from 10 to 29% in patients presenting appendiceal inflammatory mass. Interval appendectomies, despite been the minority of the procedures, disregard the higher morbidity associated with right sided colectomies. The review of literature also describes oncologic, histologic and clinical aspects of patients presenting appendiceal neoplasm, describing the most frequent histologic subtypes of this illness.

Conclusion: Hidden appendiceal neoplasm in acute appendicitis are rare, fortunately. However, its incidence is much higher in patients presenting appendiceal inflammatory mass. Hence, interval appendectomy should be considered in this subgroup of patients.

Keywords: Appendiceal inflammatory mass, Acute appendicits, Appendiceal neoplasms, Appendiceal neuroendocrine tumors, Pseudomixoma peritonei, Interval appendectomy

* Correspondence: sergiodcnetto@gmail.com
[2]Surgical Oncology Group from the III Surgical Clinic Division, Hospital das Clínicas of the University of São Paulo (USP), School of Medicine, Rua Dr. Ovídio Pires de Campos, 255, 8 th floor, room 8131, Cerqueira César 05403-010, São Paulo, Brazil
[3]Emergency Surgical Service, Hospital das Clínicas of the University of São Paulo (USP), School of Medicine, Rua Dr. Ovídio Pires de Campos, 255, 8 th floor, room 8131, Cerqueira César 05403-010, São Paulo, Brazil
Full list of author information is available at the end of the article

Background

The incidence of appendicitis demanding emergency surgical treatment is significantly common, with appendectomy being used as the standard treatment since 1889 [1]. Only in the US, appendicitis generates about 300,000 annual hospital admissions [2].

Despite the increased use of computed tomography to evaluate acute abdominal pain and diagnose appendicitis, and of laparoscopic appendectomy, the number of perforated cases has been stable in the past three decades. Between 2 and 6% of patients with acute appendicitis present appendiceal mass, often described as inflammatory phlegmon or abscess [3]. In these cases, the ideal approach is still controversial, since there are proposals to an indirect, non-surgical treatment.

When conservative treatments have a positive result at first, there is often a dilemma whether or not to perform an interval appendectomy or maintain nonoperative approach. However, the real disadvantage of the latter is not having the appendix submitted to histological analysis. In a meta-analysis and systematic review of 2771 patients diagnosed with inflammatory appendiceal mass (phlegmon or abscess), Andersson and collaborators found 31 with malignant tumors [4].

These lesions are detected in 0.9 to 1.4% of the appendectomies performed to treat acute appendicitis [5, 6].

Although rare, appendiceal tumors represent about 1% of malignancies of the large intestines. Acute appendicitis is the initial presentation of primary neoplasms of the appendix in more than 50% of the cases, causing an unpleasant surprise to both the doctor and the patient [7].

It's reported that 2 to 6% of acute appendicitis cases consist in inflammatory appendiceal mass [8], and recent series demonstrate an elevated incidence of malignant tumors in this organ, between 5.9 and 12% [9, 10].

Methods

The present analysis was made through a Medline search with the profiles "acute appendicitis AND (conservative OR interval appendectomy OR mass OR abscess OR phlegmon)", and identified references, written in English, between 1987 and 2016.

Inclusion criteria for review consisted in searching articles describing patients older than 18 years-old treated for acute appendicitis with abdominal abscess or phlegmon who underwent, or not, interval appendectomy, with pathological analysis of the appendix described.

Based on the title and the abstracts, potential articles were selected, and the full text was analyzed to identify original studies that reported results from this treatment. Variables as age, interval appendectomy rate, the incidence of neoplasm, time to surgery, minimally invasive assessment, histology, right colectomy rate and morbidity were analyzed.

A review of the literature regarding the main clinical presentation, oncologic, histopathologic features was made. In this context, surgical management of appendiceal neoplasms was also highlighted.

Results

A total of 40 initial reports were identified. Four were excluded because they described interval appendectomy in children. Seventeen studies were excluded because, despite being systematic reviews or retrospective case series, they did not contemplate histologic features from operated patients. Two other papers were excluded because they were case reports of only one patient. A total of nine uncontrolled retrospective series fulfilled the inclusion criteria (Fig. 1). A total of 13.244 patients were described as presenting acute appendicitis.

Eight studies reported the mean ages of patients showing appendicitis [8, 11–17]. Patients presenting with appendiceal abscess who underwent interval appendectomy were older than those submitted to an upfront appendectomy. The mean age of patients with usual appendicitis was 49.7 ± 6 years old (ranging from 41 to 57 years-old). Of those with inflammatory mass, average age was 52.4 ± 5.9 years old (ranging from 46 to 62 years-old) and 52% of them were male. The majority of patients was initially managed with immediate appendectomy or conservative treatment (77,5 and 16% respectively). Only a few patients were subjected to an interval appendectomy, in a mean of 6.5% in pooled analysis [8, 11–16, 18]. Six papers reported interval appendectomy rates that varied from 1.5% to 28% [8, 16], and five of them addressed less than 10% of patients been treated by interval procedure [8, 11, 13, 14]. Even Tingstedt B. et al [16] states the changes in treatment choices throughout the decades. Interval appendectomy was very common before 1995, in up to 46% of the patients, showing a reduction to 8% after that period.

Laparoscopic appendectomy was less frequent for interval appendectomy; only two papers [8, 11] were describing surgical technique. Minimally invasive approach for appendiceal mass ranged from 54 to 78% compared to 99%, from the same author, when treating noncomplicated appendicitis. The rates of conversion to open procedures were also higher in appendiceal mass than usual, varying from 8 to 29% [11, 18].

Four articles [8, 11, 13, 14] described the time to surgery, which ranged from 52 to 78 days, with a mean of 63 ± 11 days.

No patient had appendiceal neoplasm diagnosed preoperatively, and overall incidence was extremely low. From 13.244 patients operated from appendicitis, 206 were submitted to interval appendectomy, 24 underwent

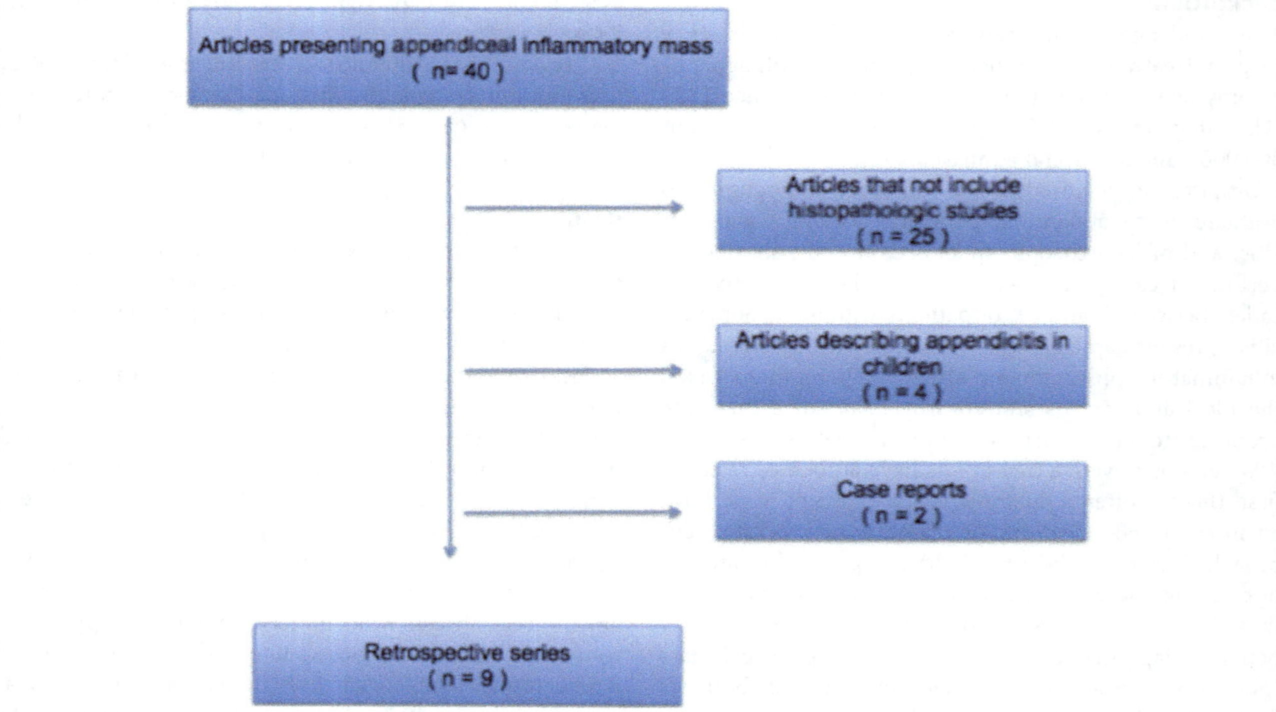

Fig. 1 Diagram of study selection

right colectomy, and 130 (0.9%) had the histopathological analysis demonstrating tumor [8, 11–16, 18]. The incidence ranged from 0.3 to 3.2%. However, in patients presenting with appendiceal inflammatory mass the rate of neoplasm was much higher, from 10 to 29%, as stated in Table 1. The incidence of tumor's histological subtypes is described in Table 2.

Interval appendectomy shows morbidity varying from 6 to 11% [8, 13, 14]. The most frequent complications were assigned as minor representing wound infections, but there were post-operative abscesses, colocutaneous fistulas and hemorrhage [8]. Right-side hemicolectomy was employed in 7 to 25% of the cases [8, 12], and there was one fatal complication due to anastomotic leakage [8].

Table 1 Articles considering incidental neoplasm findings among appendiceal abscess

Author	Year	Appendicitis (N)	Abscess	Neoplasm N (%)
Carpenter S.G. et al.	2012	315	18	5 28
Lee W.S. et al.	2011	3744	(–)	28 (–)
Roberts J.K. et al.	2008	876	41	4 10
Wright G.P. et al.	2015	6038	82	11 12
Deelder J.D. et al.	2014	(–)	119	12 10
Lai H.W. et al.	2006	1873	70	7 10
Furman M.J. et al.	2013	376	17	5 29
Cerame M.A. et al.	1987	305	192	56 29
Tingstedt B. et al.	2002	93	30	3 10
Sum		13.244	569	131 23%

Review of the literature

Classifying and staging cecal appendix tumors

Recognizing the differences in the clinical presentation and the prognosis of appendiceal primary tumors is essential. When the tumor presents a signet-ring cell formation, the average survival is 6 months. Meanwhile, when histology shows a low-grade mucinous neoplasm, the median overall survival increases to 8 years [17].

Recently, a study based in the database produced by the Surveillance, Epidemiology and End Results (SEER) of the National Institute of Cancer of Bethesda revealed different survival rates for 5655 patients diagnosed with a primary appendiceal tumor, depending on the histology. The same study also showed an increased number of accidental diagnosis, which can be explained by a boost in the number of patients submitted to computed tomography and by the substantial use of laparoscopy, improving the sight of the abdominal cavity [19] (Fig. 2).

The overall survival rate related to the disease in the five coming years changed in line with the histologic subtype [19] (Fig. 3; Table 3).

Table 2 Incidence among histologic subtypes

Author	Histologic subtypes	% (N)
Carpenter S.G. et al. [11]	LGMN	0%
	Mucinous AdenoCa	20% (1)
	In situ AdenoCa	20%(1)
	Adenocarcinoma	40%(2)
	Carcinoid	20%(1)
Lee W.S. et al. [12]	LGMN	50%(14)
	Mucinous AdenoCa	11%(3)
	In situ AdenoCa	0%
	Adenocarcinoma	7%(2)
	Carcinoid	32%(9)
Wright G.P. et al. [8]	LGMN	
	Mucinous AdenoCa	55%(6)
	In situ AdenoCa	0%
	Adenocarcinoma	9%(1)
	Carcinoid	36%(4)
Lai H.W. et al. [13]	LGMN	80%(5)
	Mucinous AdenoCa	0%
	In situ AdenoCa	0%
	Adenocarcinoma	20%(2)
	Carcinoid	
Furman M.J. et al. [14]	LGMN	100%(5)
	Mucinous AdenoCa	
	In situ AdenoCa	
	Adenocarcinoma	
	Carcinoid	
Cerame M.A. et al. [15]	LGMN	0%
	Mucinous AdenoCa	40%(79)
	In situ AdenoCa	1%(2)
	Adenocarcinoma	59%(117)
	Carcinoid	
Tingstedt B. et al. [16]	LGMN	33%(1)
	Mucinous AdenoCa	0%
	In situ AdenoCa	0%
	Adenocarcinoma	66%(2)
	Carcinoid	0%

The World Health Organization (WHO) classifies appendiceal tumors in two main groups: appendiceal carcinomas and neuroendocrine neoplasia (Table 4).

Appendiceal neuroendocrine (NET) tumors

Oberndorfer first described NET tumors in the ileum and appendix in 1907, with mention to an indolent course, although some of them, with a different phenotype, had a more unfavorable outcome [20]. The two sub-groups of carcinoids based on their histological characteristics are Enterochromaffin cell serotonin producing carcinoid and its tubular variation with L-cell glucagon-like peptide, and PP/PPY producing tumor.

Therefore, carcinoid is a definition mostly used for tumors with more favorable histological characteristics while neuroendocrine is a broader description, which includes more aggressive attributes of the disease.

Epidemiology and prognosis

NETs have approximately 0.15 per 100,000/year incidence, according to the SEER registry. The frequency is similar to other populations, based on European databases [21–24].

Those NETs are frequent when considering only neuroendocrine gastroenteropancreatic tumors. There is slight prevalence among women, affecting mostly Caucasians, and its incidence could be underestimated, since most of the cases, which are incidentally diagnosed, may not be notified in tertiary centers. The frequency of appendectomies performed without any particular reason is 3–9 per 1000 inhabitants [25, 26].

Appendiceal NET belongs to a sub-group of neoplasia with a significant number of incidental diagnosis, representing about 80% of the neoplasia, including benign and malignant tumors. The average age of the diagnosis varies from 38 to 51 years old [27–29].

In most cases, the prognosis is excellent, with 100% of overall 5-year survival rate for localized disease and 85–100% for regional disease. Nevertheless, when including staging, the 5-year survival rates vary between 70 and 85%. Advanced disease has unfavorable prognosis with a 5-year survival rate of 12 and 28%. Tumors with more aggressive histology, such as Goblet cell carcinoids and mixed adenoneuroendocrine carcinomas, were not included in this study [27].

For NETs, Location, tumor depth, dimensions and possible invasion of the mesoappendix are important factors to calculate disease recurrence. In 70% of the cases, the tumors are located at the tip of the appendix, leading to a lower recurrence rate (Fig. 4). About its length, tumors with 1 cm (60 to 80% of the cases), invading through the subserosa or into the mesoappendix for 3 mm also have a lower recurrence rate. However, tumors with positive margins, located in the appendicular base, larger than 2 cm, or deeply invading the mesoappendix, have a higher recurrence rate, suggesting the need to perform additional resection [30–32].

The presentation of the disease is usually associated with acute appendicitis. It rarely evolves into a metastatic disease and hardly ever develops carcinoid syndrome.

Because there is no suspicion of NET before an appendectomy is performed, preoperative exams do not offer additional information. Computed tomography or

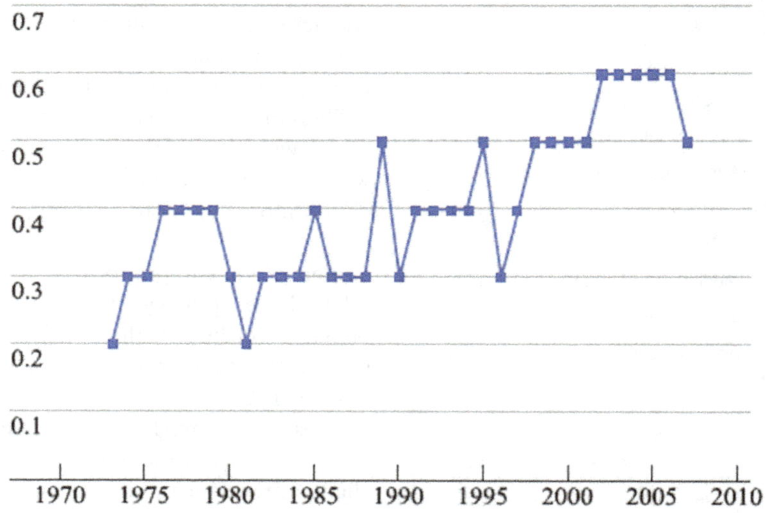

Fig. 2 The number of appendix tumors, adjusted by age, from 1997 to 2007, according to SEER database (per 100,000 inhabitants)

nuclear magnetic imaging could be used in postoperative exams, to clinically stage the regional (lymph nodes) or metastatic disease. Usually, colonoscopy will not reveal the tumor, since in 70% of the time it occurs in the tip of the appendix, rarely invading the caecum. Metabolic studies, such as Octreo Scan and gallium 68 PET-CT, are unusually performed. Laboratory tests, such as serum chromogranin A and 5-hydroxyndoleaticeticacid, are used selectively in the follow-up, or for suspicion of possible carcinoid syndrome, respectively. A well--differentiated NET, smaller than one centimeter and treated with R0 resection, usually do not evolve into a metastatic or regional disease in follow-up. Postoperative computed tomography and MRI are justified when tumors measure 1 to 2 cm. In cases of larger tumors, deep invasion of the mesoappendix or angiolymphatic invasion, image-led exams and metabolic tests, such as OctreoScan and gallium 68 PET-CT, are often required.

The histopathological test should be revised and must describe location of the tumor, grade, mitotic index, Ki-67 rate, dimension of the tumor, potential multifocal/multicentric disease, vascular invasion, perineural invasion, presence of non-endocrine component, presence

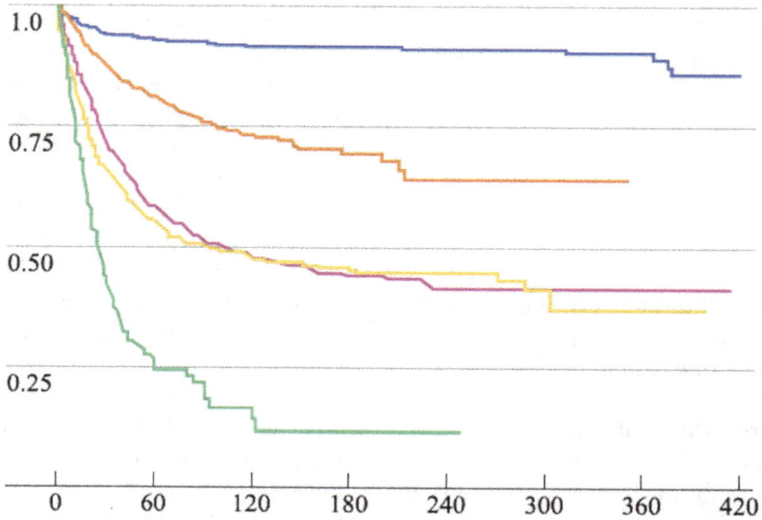

Fig. 3 Survival according to the histological type. Modified by Turaga et cols, Ann SurgOncol (2012) 19:1379–1385

Table 3 Specific survival rate of the disease in the coming five years according to its histologic subtype

Histologic subtype.	Survival rate per specific disease in 5 years %.
Carcinoid tumor	91%
Globet cell carcinoid	81%.
Mucinous adenocarcinoma	58%
Non-specificadenocarcinoma	55%
Signet-ring cell formation.	27%

and number of lymph nodes, margin status, and TNM system (Table 5).

Individual immunohistochemical studies could be included to detect neuroendocrine markers, including chromogranin A, synaptophysin, specific peptides and others.

Tumor grade is determined by the mitotic index and Ki-67 (Table 6).th=tlb=

A major factor in the grading risk is the accurate staging of T in the TNM system since the diagnosis is usually incidental. For tumors T1a (UICC/AJCC), a simple appendectomy is appropriate treatment, also in the pediatric population. The overall survival in this group is 100% [33, 34].

Tumors larger than 2 cm (T2) are rare (<10%), but carry a risk of becoming a metastatic disease in 25 to 40% of the cases. Because of such previous data, radical resection is indicated, with follow-up for high-risk disease [35–39].

Table 4 The World Health Organization classification (2010)

Appendiceal carcinomas.

- Adenocarcinoma 8140/3
- Mucinous adenocarcinoma 8480/3
- Low-grade mucinous neoplasia 8480/1
- Signet-ring cell formation carcinoma 8490/3
- Undifferentiated carcinoma 8020/3

Neuroendocrine appendix neoplasias.

- Neuroendocrine tumors (NET).
- NET G1 (carcinoid) 8240/3
- NET G2 8249/3
- Neuroendocrine carcinomas (NEC) 8246/3
- NEC large cells type 8013/3
- NEC smal cells type 8041/3
- Mixed tumor:
- Mixed Adenoneuroendocrine carcinomas 8244/3
- Serotonin-producing endocrine carcinoma 8241/3
- Globet cell carcinoid 8243/3
- Tubular carcinoid 8245/1
- Peptide-producing/ Glucagon-producing large cell tumor PP/PYY 8152/1

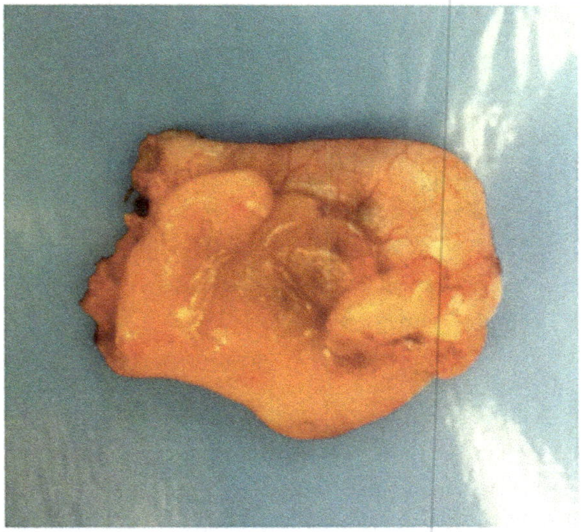

Fig. 4 Well-differentiated neuroendocrine neoplasia, with 1 to 2 cm, located in the tip of the appendix. Degree I (WHO) (Courtesy of Andre Bouzas, MD – Oncology Institute - Santa Paula Hospital, São Paulo

Other criteria also considered is the location of the tumor in the cecal appendix. Most of the tumors (60 to 75%) are located in the tip of the appendix, 5 to 20% in the middle third and less than 10% in the appendiceal base. It has been suggested metastasis frequently appear in tumors located at the base, suggesting additional resection when the tumors have 1 to 2 cm length.

The decision to perform additional resection depends on the extent of mesoappendix invasion, if present. Up to 20% of the adults and 40% of the children undergo further resection. It is possible that the invasion of the mesoappendix be greater than initially reported. Despite not being considered in the TNM staging, the invasion of the mesoappendix could be related to a higher appearance of lymphatic invasion. When the malignancy compromises more than 3 mm, there is increased risk of nodal metastasis, and additional resection should be considered [40, 41].

Surgical treatment

Resection options for NET are appendectomy, ileocolectomy, and right colectomy. For T1a tumors with no invasion of the mesoappendix or not located in the appendiceal base, an appendectomy should suffice. When the tumor has invaded the mesoappendix in more than 3 mm, or the tumor is located in the base, an ileocolectomy and right colectomy should be indicated. However, there is not enough data to support the

Table 5 TNM staging

Neuroendocrine tumors:

T:

Tx: Primary tumor which cannot be evaluated.

T0: No primary tumor was found in the appendix.

T1: Tumor with up to 2 cm dimension.

T1a: Up to one centimeter.

T1b: Up to 2 cm.

T2: Greater than two up to 4 cm or with extensions to the caecum.

T3: Greater than 4 cm or extension to the ileum.

T4: Tumor invades abdominal wall or adjacent organs or perforated tumor

N:

NX: Nodal staging could not be evaluated for lack of information.

N0: Absence of metastasis in regional lymph nodes

N1: Presence of metasis in regional lymph nodes

M:

M0: Absence of distant metastasis

M1: Presence of distant metastasis

Stadium I: T1N0M0.

Stadium II: T2/T3N0M0.

Statium III: TN1M0 / T4N0M0.

Statium IV: TNM1.

hypothesis that an additional resection will increase patient survival and its morbidity should also be considered.

When tumors have dimensions greater than 2 cm, the ileocolectomy or right colectomy should be performed. For those between 1 and 2 cm, other criteria are considered before performing additional resection, including age, extension of mesoappendix invasion, and location. However, there is scarce long-term follow-up information of the patients. Angioinvasion or G2 could also be taken into consideration when deciding for additional resection. However, there is even less evidence published about such criteria. Nevertheless, additional resection has been used based on the consensus of the European Neuroendocrine Tumor Society and when certain histologic characteristics are present.

Table 6 Grade of NET tumors according to the World Health Organization (WHO), considering the Mitotic index and Ki-67

Grade	NETs appendix	Tumor differentiation
Low grade (G1)	<2 mitoses /10 high power fields (HPF) or < Ki-67 < 3%.	Well-differentiated
Intermediate grade (G2)	2–10 mitoses / 10 HPF or Ki-67 between 3 and 20%.	Well-differentiated
High grade (G3)	>10 mitoses / 10 HPF or Ki-67 > 20%.	Poorly differentiated

Carcinoid/Globet cell carcinoid

It is a mixed phenotype tumor, with goblet cell morphology and neuroendocrine features more or less pronounced. The incidence of such tumor is extremely rare, representing less than 5% of primary appendiceal tumors. The disease is common among Caucasians, who represent 80% of the studied population [42].

The overall 5-year survival rate is lower than well-differentiated NET and varies between 40% and 75%. The disease can behave as adenocarcinomas with more or less pronounced phenotype of goblet cells or neuroendocrine tumors [43]. In two-thirds of the goblet cell tumor patients, the diagnosis is incidental, resulting from an appendectomy for acute appendicitis, which represents 50 to 60% of the initial presentation. Ten to 20% of them present peritonitis resulting from perforation [44, 45].

In 50% of the cases, the tumor invades the serosa and the mesoappendix. In 15 to 30% of the patients, there is the occurrence of distant metastasis, commonly in the ovaries, or in the lymph nodes. However, when measurement is possible, the progression of the disease is increased when tumors have more than 2 cm in length.

Other parameters foreseeing the aggressive behavior of the illness include high mitotic counts (more than two mitoses per 10 high-power fields); a Ki-67 greater than 3%; invasion into the serosa and into the mesoappendix; angioinvasion; increased number of Paneth cells; enhanced production of mucin; production of pancreatic polypeptide and lymph node involvement [46, 47].

In a retrospective series of 63 patients with carcinoid/goblet cell carcinoid, Tang and collaborators demonstrated the correlation between the pathological analysis and the, aggressiveness of the disease. According to the morphologic characteristics, three subgroups were found [48]:

Group A –Typical Goblet cell carcinoid. Tumors had minimum cellular atypia, rare mitoses and minimum stromal invasion. The overall survival rate in 5 years was 100%.

Group B – Goblet cell adenocarcinoid and signet-ring cell formation. Tumors presenting an evident cellular atypia, prominent desmoplasia and structural distortion of the appendiceal wall. Overall survival rate in 5 years was 36%.

Group C – Undifferentiated Adenocarcinoma with goblet cell carcinoid. The overall survival rate in 5 years was 0%.

Epithelial tumors of the appendix

Merling published the first reference to appendiceal neoplasms in 1838. In 1903, Elting published a series of patients with tumors emerging from preexisting adenomas in the appendix, assuming a growth pattern with cystic dilatation of the appendix (mucinous tumors). He realized that sometimes it could exhibit a growth pattern similar to primary colon tumors (colonic-types), these are either polypoid or ulcerative, emerging from tubular or tubulovillous adenomas [49].

The mucinous-type is inclined to rupture and mucin extravasation, with or without mucin epithelia into the abdominal cavity, resulting into Pseudo myxoma Peritonei [42, 50]. The Colonic-type is similar to colon adenocarcinomas and results in lower overall survival rate than mucinous-type tumors [51].

In an analysis based on the SEER registry between 1973 and 2004, 2791 patients with malignant appendiceal neoplasm were studied. Adenocarcinomas were more frequent, responding for 65.4% of the cases. While neuroendocrine tumors have presented a regular occurrence in the same period, there was a 260% increase in carcinoma rates. The overall 5-year survival rate for those patients was 46.5%. When considering mucinous cystadenocarcinoma, it rose to 59% in all stages, and in signet-ring cell formation tumors, to 20.3% [52].

Mucinous appendiceal tumors

Although appendiceal mucinous tumors are recognized as benign, as per their histology, those tumors can progress to peritoneal dissemination.

Ronnet and collaborators, in 1995, published a classification based on 109 patients who presented peritoneal dissemination caused by mucinous epithelial tumor in appendix [53].

- Disseminated Peritoneal Adenomucinosis (DPAM): Peritoneal lesions composed of abundant extracellular mucin, with minimum cytologic atypia and rare mitoses. In all the cases, the appendix tumor was an adenoma
- Peritoneal Mucinous Carcinomatosis (PMCA): Peritoneal lesions composed of more abundant mucinous epithelium with the architectural and cytologic features of carcinoma. The primary tumor was mucinous appendix carcinoma, with prominent cytologic atypia and, in some cases, with signet-ring cell formation. The distinct subgroup can potentially evolve to metastatic disease to other organs or lymph nodes.

In 2003, Misdraji and collaborators reclassified mucinous disease to low-grade mucinous neoplasia (LGMN) and mucinous adenocarcinoma (Figs. 5 and 6) [10].

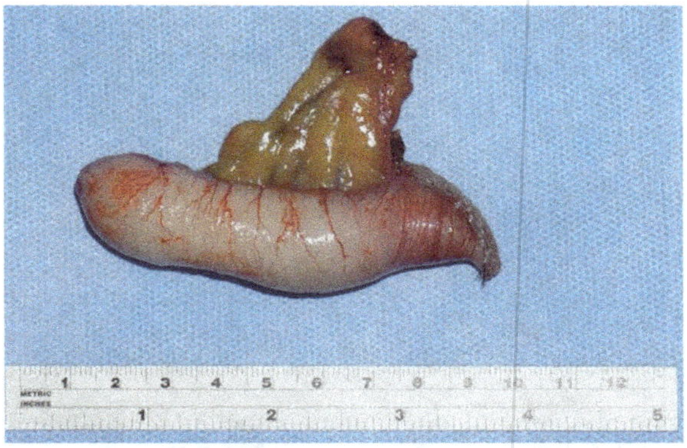

Fig. 5 Low-grade mucinous neoplasia (LAMN – Grade 1 WHO), measuring 2 cm, invading the distal third with free margin

Clinical presentation and prognosis

Performance and patient prognosis vary, and the diagnosis can be incidental, in a case of complicated acute appendicitis. However, preoperative diagnosis can be made by abdominal ultrasound with the finding of an appendix mucocele, indicating a dilated appendix filled with mucinous content (Figs. 7 and 8).

Eventually, in a similar clinical scenario, there is a condition in which the disease is located and restricted to the right lower quadrant of the abdomen. In those cases, mucin deposits can be found in the serosa, in the mesoappendix or extending to right iliac fossa. Those mucin lakes do not contain any neoplastic cells when submitted to pathological analysis [54].

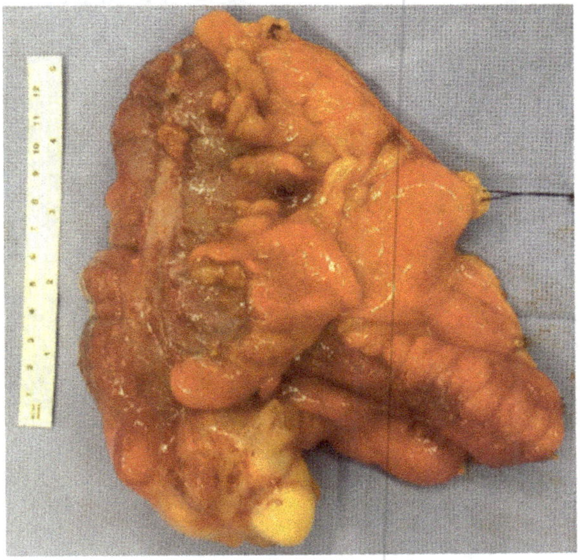

Fig. 6 Surgical specimen from ileocolectomy to treat perforated appendiceal mucinous adenocarcinoma

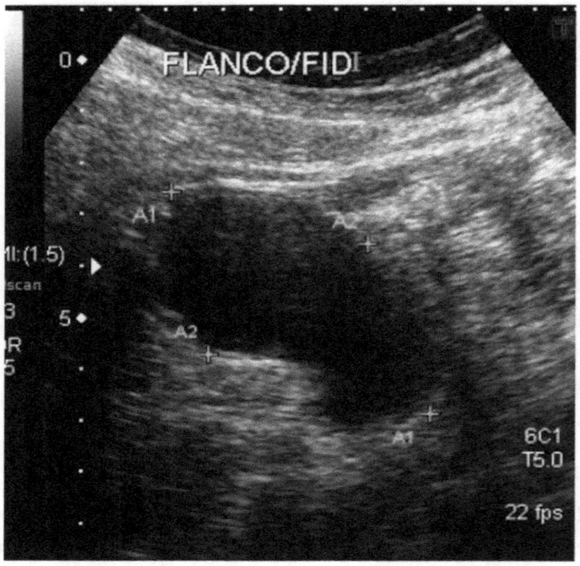

Fig. 7 Dilated appendix, with a diameter of 3.5 cm compatible with appendiceal mucocele, in ultrasound

Yantiss and collaborators have studied the prognosis of patients with appendiceal mucinous neoplasms and mucin deposits in the right lower quadrant. Of 65 patients, 77% did not present cells in the mucin lakes while 23% had low-grade mucin epithelial cells. In follow-up after 52 months, 96% of the patients without cells in the mucin lakes were free the disease. In that group of patients showing no extra-appendicular mucinous epithelium, two of them developed peritoneal dissemination, but the appendix of those two individuals was not analyzed in the study [55]. Regarding patients presenting extra-appendicular mucinous epithelium, 33% evolved to pseudomyxoma peritonei. The study demonstrated excellent prognosis for patients with mucin dissemination in the right lower quadrant and no extra-appendicular mucinous epithelium [55] (Figs. 9 and 10).

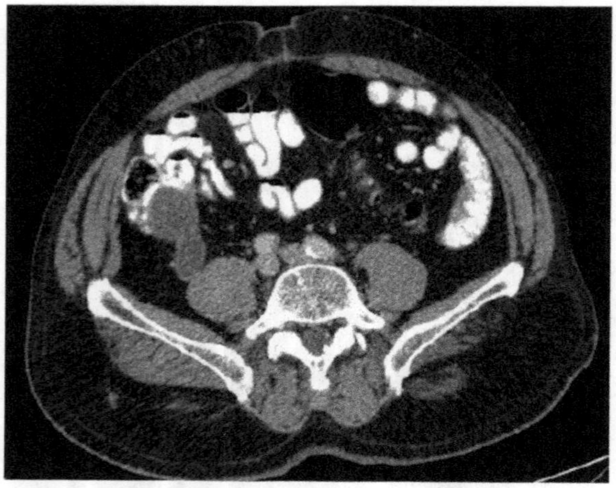

Fig. 8 Axial computerized tomography view of a burst cecal appendix (up to 3.5 cm), with thin and regular walls, and no signs of densification of adjacent adipose tissue. This corresponds to the cystic formation already described in the ultrasound, compatible with mucocele of undetermined etiology. Appendectomy revealed well-differentiated mucinous adenocarcinoma, with invasion into of the muscularis mucosae

Pseudomyxoma peritonei is considered by the UICC/AJCC and the WHO a malignant disease secondary to a carcinoma [56, 57].

The extension of a disease with extra-appendicular mucinous epithelium significantly affects patient prognosis. In a series of 184 patients, Carr and collaborators observed that mucinous disease restricted to the appendix has an indolent course. When the neoplasia is limited to the muscular mucosa, which is intact, it is called adenoma. When there is invasion of deeper layers or extra-appendicular extension, it is called carcinoma. Tumors that do not invade the muscular mucosa, but develop mucin deposits in the serosa without cells, are referred as uncertain potential for malignity [58].

Tumors characterized by neoplastic mucinous epithelium invading the muscular mucosa should be considered as high risk of peritoneum dissemination and classified and staged according to WHO and AJCC. Mucinous tumors with extra-appendicular dissemination of mucinous epithelium are considered by WHO low or high-grade mucinous adenocarcinoma, depending on the cytoarchitecture atypia.

Miner and collaborators analyzed histologic characteristics of appendiceal mucinous tumors presenting with peritoneal dissemination treated with surgical cytoreduction. In a retrospective series of 97 patients, complete cytoreduction was possible in 53% of the patients. Low--grade cytology was independently associated with longer disease-free survival. Some 90% of patients who lived an

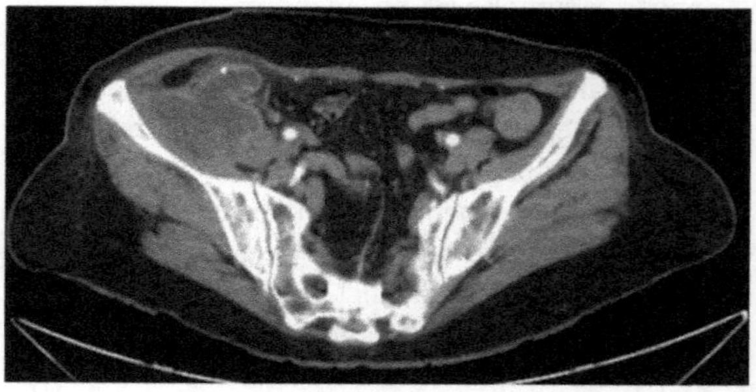

Fig. 9 Axial computerized tomography view showing mucin lakes in a patient with low-grade appendiceal mucin adenocarcinoma limited to the right iliac fossa. Pathological analysis revealed extra-appendicular mucin without the presence of mucinous epithelium

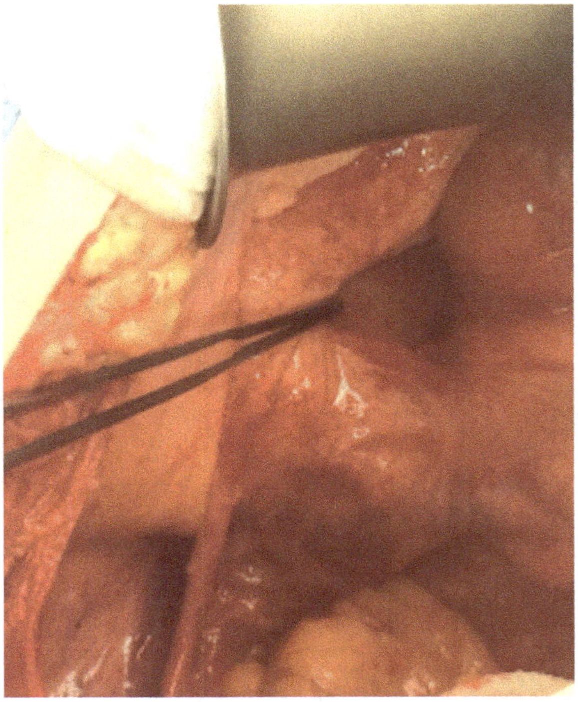

Fig. 10 Intraoperative view of pericecal and retrocecal mucin. The disease was limited to the right iliac fossa. Pathological analysis analysis revealed no cells in the mucin

additional 10 years were diagnosed with low-grade tumors [59].

Traditional treatment for pseudo myxoma peritonei is composed of surgical cytoreduction associated with hyperthermic intraperitoneal chemotherapy (HIPEC) [60].

A retrospective analysis based on 2289 patients diagnosed with pseudo myxoma peritonei resulting from perforated appendiceal mucinous tumors showed the importance of associating complete macroscopic cytoreduction and HIPEC. The study reported 10 and 15 years survival in 63 and 59% of the cases respectively, with perioperative mortality of 2% [61].

Appendiceal adenocarcinoma – Colonic-type

There are few studies on Colonic-type appendiceal adenocarcinoma. In a recent German multi-centric study about primary appendiceal carcinomas, 99 patients, with an average age of 64 years old, were identified. Those tumors had an average length of 3.27 cm, 72% were T3/T4 tumors, and 36.4% of them had lymph node metastasis. More than 60% were moderately differentiated, and more than 20% were poorly differentiated. Stage IV disease represented 23.2% of the cases, and overall survival was 47.5% for all stages. When compared to other more frequent primary appendiceal tumors (carcinoid and mucinous adenocarcinoma), the colonic-type has the higher incidence of lymph nodes metastasis [62, 63].

Such information reinforces the indication of any surgical intervention (appendectomy/ileocolectomy) required to treat and appendiceal inflammatory mass after conservative treatment (Figs. 11 and 12).

Literature is scarce when discussing patients diagnosed with adenocarcinomas with signet-ring cell formation or undifferentiated. The effects of therapeutic interventions (cytoreduction and systemic chemotherapy) in this group are unknown. In a series analyzing 142 patients diagnosed with undifferentiated tumors or with signet-ring cell formation (defined by the WHO as more than 50% of the cells in the tumor in a signet-ring formation), the average age was 52 years old, and 75% presented metastatic disease. In patients with metastatic disease, all of them had peritoneum involvement, and 36% also had it in the ovaries. The median survival rate was 2 years for patients diagnosed with undifferentiated adenocarcinomas and 2.5 years for those with adenocarcinomas with signet-ring cell formation. Patients who were submitted to surgical cytoreduction had a median recurrence-free survival of 1.2 years, and an overall

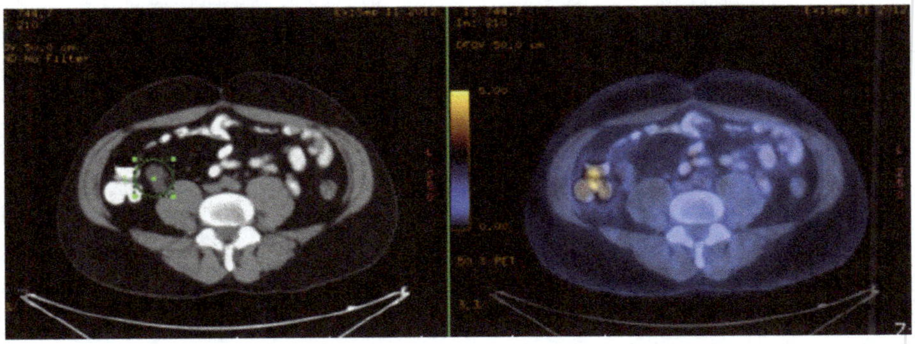

Fig. 11 PET-CT of a patient subjected to appendectomy to treat acute appendicitis with incidental diagnosis of appendiceal tubular adenocarcinoma with signet-ring cell formation T3NXMX. In postoperative follow-up, CEA was elevated and the PEC-CT revealed pericecal lymphadenopathy

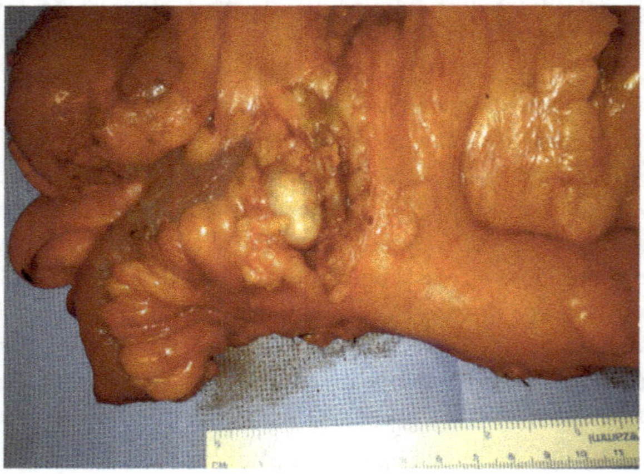

Fig. 12 Product of ileocolectomy and/or right colectomy performed in same patient of Fig. 11, revealing pericecal lymphadenopathy. Margins in the caecum showed a 2.5 cm adenocarcinoma with signet-ring cell formation and metastasis in nine of the 14 dissected lymph nodes. pT3pN2

survival of 4.2 years was achieved when patients underwent a complete cytoreduction. This surgical approach is also improves overall survival of patients with A oligometastatic peritoneal disease. Unfortunately, complete cytoreduction was only achieved in 21% of the patients [64].

Conclusion

Hidden appendiceal neoplasm findings in post-operative appendectomy for acute appendicitis is a rare event, fortunately. However, its incidence in acute appendiceal inflammatory mass is not negligible. In our point of view all patients submitted upfront to a more conservative treatment (percutaneous drainage and antibiotics) should be submitted to interval appendectomy.

Acknowledgements
There is no other contributor for acknowledgements.

Funding
Not applicable

Authors' contributions
FJRTJr. carried out the manuscript writing, SDCN. was responsable for data/article collection. EHA. participated in the article design, and EMU. coordinated and helped with article review. All authors read and approved the final manuscript. CAMM and MCR, both contributed to English spelling corrections and paper formatting. Without their help, this article could not be possible.

Competing interests
The authors declare that they have no competing interests.

Author details
[1]Surgical Oncology Group from the III Surgical Clinic Division, Hospital das Clínicas of the University of São Paulo (USP), School of Medicine, Rua Dr. Ovídio Pires de Campos, 255, 8 th floor, room 8131, Cerqueira César 05403-010, São Paulo, Brazil. [2]Surgical Oncology Group from the III Surgical Clinic Division, Hospital das Clínicas of the University of São Paulo (USP), School of Medicine, Rua Dr. Ovídio Pires de Campos, 255, 8 th floor, room 8131, Cerqueira César 05403-010, São Paulo, Brazil. [3]Emergency Surgical Service, Hospital das Clínicas of the University of São Paulo (USP), School of Medicine, Rua Dr. Ovídio Pires de Campos, 255, 8 th floor, room 8131, Cerqueira César 05403-010, São Paulo, Brazil. [4]Sarcoma and Melanoma Surgery group - São Paulo Cancer Institute, University of São Paulo, School of Medicine, Cerqueira César, Brazil. [5]General and Trauma Surgery - III Surgical Clinic Division, Hospital das Clínicas of the University of São Paulo (USP), School of Medicine, Rua Dr. Ovídio Pires de Campos, 255, 8 th floor, room 8131, Cerqueira César 05403-010, São Paulo, Brazil. [6]850, Francisco Matarazzo Avenue, apt 181, Bloco 2, Zip Code 05001-200 Perdizes, São Paulo, Brazil. [7]General Surgery Senior Resident - III Surgical Clinic Division, Hospital das Clínicas of the University of São Paulo, School of Medicine, São Paulo, Brazil. [8]Chief of Staff of the Emergency Surgical Service - III Surgical Clinic Division, Hospital das Clínicas of the University of São Paulo, School of Medicine, São Paulo, Brazil.

References

1. McBurney C. Experience with early operative interference in cases of disease of the vermiform appendix. N Y Med J. 1889;50:676–84.
2. De Frances CJ, Cullen KA, Kozak LJ. National Hospital Discharge Survey: 2005 annual summary with detailed diagnosis and procedure data. Vital Health Stat. 2007;1:209.
3. Buckius MT. Changing epidemiology of acute appendicitis in the United States: study period 1993–2008. J Surg Res. 2012;175:185–90.
4. Andersson RE. Nonsurgical treatment of appendiceal abscess or phlegmon: a systematic review and meta- analysis. Ann Surg. 2007;246:741–8.
5. Collins DC. 71,000 human appendix specimens. A final report, summarizing forty years of study. Am J Proctol. 1963;14:265–81.
6. Livingston EH. Disconnect between incidence of nonperforated and perforated appendicitis: implications for pathophysiology and management. Ann Surg. 2007;245:886–92.
7. Connor SJ. Appendiceal tumors: retrospective clinicopathologic analysis of appendiceal tumors from 7,970 appendectomies. Dis Colon Rectum. 1998;41:75–80.
8. Wright GP. Is there truly an oncologic indication for interval appendectomy? Am J Surg. 2015;209:442–6.
9. Deelder JD. How to treat an appendiceal inflammatory mass: operatively or nonoperatively? J Gastrointest Surg. 2014;18:641–5.
10. Misdraji J. Appendiceal mucinous neoplasms: controversial issues. Arch Pathol Lab Med. 2010;134:864–70.
11. Carpenter S. Increased risk of neoplasm in appendicitis treated with interval appendectomy: single-institution experience and literature review. Am Surg. 2012;78:339–43.
12. Lee WS. A retrospective clinicopathological analysis of appendiceal tumors from 3,744 appendectomies: a single-institution study. Int J Colorectal Dis. 2011;26:617–21.
13. Lai HW. Interval appendectomy after conservative treatment of an appendiceal mass. World J Surg. 2006;30:351–7.
14. Furman MJ. Increased risk of mucinous neoplasm of the appendix in adults undergoing interval appendectomy. JAMA Surg. 2013;148(8):703–6.
15. Cerame MA. A 25-year review of adenocarcinoma of the appendix a frequently perforating carcinoma. Dis Colon Rectum. 1988;31(2):145–50.
16. Tingstedt B. Management of appendiceal masses. Eur J Surg. 2002;168: 579–82.
17. McCusker ME. Primary malignant neoplasms of the appendix: a population-based study from the Surveillance, Epidemiology and End-Results program, 1973–Cancer. 2002;94:3307 –12.
18. Roberts JK. Macroscopic findings at appendicectomy are unreliable: implications for laparoscopy and malignant conditions of the appendix. Int J Surg Pathol. 2008;16(4):386–90.
19. Turaga KK, Pappas SG, Gamblin T. Importance of histologic subtype in the staging of appendiceal tumors. Ann Surg Oncol. 2012;19:1379–85.
20. Oberndorfer S. Karzinoide Tumoren des Dünndarms. Frankf Z Pathol. 1907;1:426.
21. Ellis L. Carcinoid tumors of the gastrointestinal tract: trends in incidence in England since 1971. Am J Gastroenterol. 2010;105:2563–9.
22. Hauso O. Neuroendocrine tumor epidemiology: contrasting Norway and North America. Cancer. 2008;113:2655–64.

23. Quaedvlieg PF. Epidemiology and survival in patients with carcinoid disease in the Netherlands. An epidemiological study with 2,391 patients. Ann Oncol. 2001;12:1295–300.
24. Perez EA. 7,201 carcinoids: increasing incidence overall and disproportionate mortality in the elderly. World J Surg. 2007;31:1022–30.
25. Moertel CG. Carcinoid tumors of the vermiform appendix. Cancer. 1968;21:270–8.
26. Groth SS. Appendiceal carcinoid tumors: predictors of lymph node metastasis and the impact of right hemicolectomy on survival. J Surg Oncol. 2011;103:39–45.
27. García-Carbonero R. Incidence, patterns of care and prognostic factors for outcome of gastro-enteropancreatic neuroendocrine tumors (GEP-NETs): results from the National Cancer Registry of Spain (RGETNE). Ann Oncol. 2010;21:1794–803.
28. Lepage C. Incidence and management of primary malignant small bowel cancers: a well-defined French population study. Am J Gastroenterol. 2006;101:2826–32.
29. Ploeckinger U. The German NET registry: an audit on the diagnosis and therapy of neuroendocrine tumours. Neuroendocrinology. 2009;90:349–63.
30. Sandor A. A retrospective analysis of 1570 appendiceal carcinoids. Am J Gastroenterol. 1998;93:422–8.
31. Stinner B. Neuroendocrine tumours (carcinoids) of the appendix. Best Pract Res Clin Gastroenterol. 2005;19:729–38.
32. O'Donnell ME. Malignant neoplasms of the appendix. Int J Colorectal Dis. 2007;22:1239–48.
33. Prommegger R. Retrospective evaluation of carcinoid tu- mors of the appendix in children. World J Surg. 2002;26:1489–92.
34. Parkes SE. Carcinoid tumours of the appendix in children 1957–1986: incidence, treatment and out- come. Br J Surg. 1993;80:502–4.
35. In't Hof KH. Carcinoid tumour of the appendix: an analysis of 1,485 consecutive emergency appendectomies. J Gastrointest Surg. 2008;12:1436–8.
36. Fornaio R. Appendectomy or right hemicolectomy in the treatment of appendiceal carcinoid tumors? Tumori. 2007;93:587–90.
37. Moertel CG. Carcinoid tumor of the appendix: treat- ment and prognosis. N Engl J Med. 1987;317:1699–701.
38. Bamboat ZM. Is right hemicolectomy for 2.0-cm appendiceal carcinoids justified? Arch Surg. 2006;141:349–52.
39. Alexandraki KI. Clinical value of right hemicolectomy for appendiceal carcinoids using pathologic criteria. J Endocrinol Invest. 2011;34:255–9.
40. Rossi G. Does mesoappendix infiltration predict a worse prognosis in incidental neuroendocrine tumors of the appendix? A clinicopathologic and immunohistochemical study of 15 cases. Am J Clin Pathol. 2003;120:706–11.
41. Dunn JP. Carcinoid tumours of the appendix: 21 cases, with a review of the literature. NZ Med J. 1982;95:73–6.
42. McGory ML. Malignancies of the appendix: beyond case series reports. Dis Colon Rectum. 2005;48:2264–71.
43. Landry CS. Analysis of 900 appendiceal carcinoid tumors for a proposed predictive staging system. Arch Surg. 2008;143:664–70.
44. O'Donnell ME. Surgical treatment of malignant carcinoid tumours of the appendix. Int J Clin Pract. 2007;61:431–7.
45. Toumpanakis C. Goblet cell carcinoid tumors (adeno- carcinoid) of the appendix. Dis Colon Rectum. 2006;50:315–22.
46. Pahlavan PS. Goblet cell carcinoid of the appendix. World J Surg Oncol. 2005;3:36.
47. Roy P. Goblet cell carcinoid tumors of the appendix: an overview. World J Gastrointest Oncol. 2010;2(6):251–8.
48. Tang LH. Pathologic classification and clinical behavior of the spectrum of goblet cell carcinoid tumors of the appendix. Am J Surg Pathol. 2008;32:1429–43.
49. Chang P. Adenocarcinoma of the appendix. Dis Colon Rectum. 1981;24:176–80.
50. Cortina R. Management and prognosis of adenocarcinoma of the appendix. Dis Colon Rectum. 1995;38:848–52.
51. Deans GT. Neoplastic lesions of the appendix. Br J Surg. 1995;82:299–306.
52. Gustafsson B. Uncommon cancers of the small intes- tine, appendix and colon: an analysis of SEER 1973–2004, and current diagnosis and therapy. Int J Oncol. 2008;33:1121–31.
53. Ronnett BM. Disseminated peritoneal adenomucinosis and peritoneal mucinous carcinomatosis. A clinicopathologic analysis of 109 cases with emphasis on distinguishing pathologic features, site of origin, prognosis, and relationship to "pseudomyxoma peritonei". Am J Surg Pathol. 1995;19(12):1390–408.
54. Panarelli NC. Mucinous neoplasms of the appendix and peritoneum. Arch Pathol Lab Med. 2011;135:1261–8.
55. Yantiss RK. Prognostic significance of localized extra-appendiceal mucin deposition in appendiceal mucinous neoplasms. Am J Surg Pathol. 2009;33(2):248–55.
56. Carr NJ. Tumours of the appendix. In: Bosman FT, Carneiro F, Hruban RH, Theise ND, editors. WHO classification of tumours of the digestive system, vol. 3. 4th ed. Lyon: IARC Press; 2010. p. 122–5. World Health Organization Classification of Tumours.
57. Edge SB. AJCC cancer staging manual. 7th ed. New York: Springer; 2010. p. 133–41.
58. Carr NJ. Epithelial noncarcinoid tumors and tumor-like lesions of the appendix: a clinicopathologic study of 184 patients with a multivariate analysis of prognostic factors. Cancer. 1995;75(3):757–68.
59. Miner TJ. Long-term survival following treatment of pseudomyxoma peritonei: an analysis of surgical therapy. Ann Surg. 2005;241(2):300–8.
60. Moran B. Consensus statement on the loco-regional treatment of appendiceal mucinous neoplasms with peritoneal dissemination (pseudomyxoma peritonei). J Surg Oncol. 2008;98(4):277–82.
61. Chua TC. Early- and long-term outcome data of patients with pseudomyxoma peritonei from appendiceal origin treated by a strategy of cytoreductive surgery and hyperthermic intraperitoneal chemotherapy. J Clin Oncol. 2012;30(20):2449–56.
62. Benedix F. Primary appendiceal carcinoma e Epidemiology, surgery and survival: Results of a German multi-center study. EJSO. 2010;36:763e771.
63. Nitecki SS. The natural history of surgically treated primary adenocarcinoma of the appendix. Ann Surg. 1994;219:51–7.
64. Lieu CH. Systemic chemotherapy and surgical cytoreduction for poorly differentiated and signet ring cell adenocarcinomas of the appendix. Ann Oncol. 2012;23:652–8.

23

Small bowel obstruction in the elderly: a plea for comprehensive acute geriatric care

Ekin Ozturk[1*], Marianne van Iersel[2], Martijn MWJ Stommel[1], Yvonne Schoon[2,3], Richard RPG ten Broek[1] and Harry van Goor[1]

Abstract

Small bowel obstruction is one of the most frequent emergencies in general surgery, commonly affecting elderly patients. Morbidity and mortality from small bowel obstruction in elderly is high. Significant progress has been made in the diagnosis and management of bowel obstruction in recent years. But little is known whether this progress has benefitted outcomes in elderly patients, particularly those who are frail or have a malignancy as cause of the obstruction, and when considering quality of life and functioning as outcomes. In this review, we discuss the specific challenges and needs of elderly in diagnosis and treatment of small bowel obstruction. We address quality of life aspects and explore how the concept of geriatric assessment can be utilized to improve decision-making and outcomes for elderly patients with a small bowel obstruction.

Keywords: Small bowel obstruction, Adhesions, Quality of life, Elderly patients

Background

Small bowel obstruction (SBO) is a common emergency diagnosis in elderly patients, which occurrence tends to increase parallel to the increasing number of elderly patients requiring acute medical care and emergency surgery [1, 2]. Approximately 10–12% of patients above 65 years presenting with abdominal pain at the emergency department (ED) is diagnosed with small bowel obstruction [2, 3]. Small bowel obstruction in general is one of the most frequent causes of general emergency surgery. In the UK, small bowel obstruction accounts for 51% of all emergency laparotomies [4]. Adhesiolysis and small bowel resection are two of seven main causes counting for 80% of morbidity and death related to emergency surgery [5]. Any emergency surgery in elderly is associated with high morbidity and mortality compared to elective operations [5–8].

Management of small bowel obstruction has advanced over recent years resulting in improved treatment results for small bowel obstruction in the general population [9]. Computed tomography (CT) has been a step forward in detecting different etiologies of bowel obstruction and of the completeness of the obstruction [10]. Adding water-soluble contrast can accurately predict completeness of obstruction and successful conservative treatment [11]. These diagnostic tools led to a more tailored approach and to a reduction of immediate operations. Today, more than 70% of small bowel obstructions are treated successfully by conservative approach, avoiding the risks of a potentially complicated operation [10, 12, 13]. Also, laparoscopic surgery of small bowel obstruction has been introduced as treatment option potentially reducing postoperative morbidity, although this minimal invasive approach is not suitable for every patient and harbours its own complications [14–16].

It is questionable if elderly patients with small bowel obstruction benefit from the progress in the management in small bowel obstruction because of specific challenges and demands in diagnosis and treatment in this patient population [17]. They represent a diverse group consisting of vital elderly patients who have enough resilience to cope with a 'second hit' like surgery compared to frail elderly patients with limited reserve capacity and high risk of complications even without surgery. Elderly patients often present with atypical clinical features, causing a delay in diagnosis and progressed disease at first presentation [18, 19]. Most elderly patients have reduced renal function increasing the risk of contrast nephropathy from contrast-enhanced CT [20].

* Correspondence: ekin-ozturk@live.nl
[1]Department of Surgery, Radboud University Medical Center, P.O. Box 9101, 6500 HB Nijmegen, The Netherlands

This risk is higher when fluid intake is diminished as in small bowel obstruction. The limited physiological reserves and frailty contribute to worse outcomes in the elderly patient in terms of functional decline, more complications and prolonged stay in hospital, regardless of treatment [6, 21, 22]. High age and common co-morbidities such as diabetes mellitus have been shown to be independent risk factors for mortality in small bowel obstruction [23]. Little is known about the interference of starvation treatment with necessity to continue medication for chronic disease and pre-existing nutritional deficiencies, which all seem a challenge in managing elderly patients with small bowel obstruction.

Regarding goal settings, frail elderly patients judge quality of life to be more important than prolongation of life, which implies a more balanced decision-making from the start (at the emergency department) taking into account psychosocial aspects of life in addition to clinical aspects. Conceivably, a standard approach based on guidelines may not suffice for appropriate decision-making in diagnosis and treatment of the elderly with small bowel obstruction [10, 24].

In this review, we will discuss the specific challenges and demands elderly patients have in diagnosis and treatment of small bowel obstruction and, if literature data are available, we compare these with younger patients. We will discuss quality of life aspects and explore how the concept of geriatric assessment can be utilized to improve decision-making and outcomes for elderly patients with small bowel obstruction. The results presented may contribute to the development of algorithms and guidelines for management of small bowel obstruction in elderly patients.

Methods

This is a narrative review with scoping aspects [25]. A formal systematic review and meta-analysis was not feasible due to paucity of studies addressing the relevant topics of small bowel obstruction in elderly patients mentioned above.

Search strategy

PubMed, the Cochrane database and EMBASE database were searched from inception to January 2018. The search strategy was verified by a senior medical librarian for completeness. PubMed studies were identified using Mesh terms 'intestinal obstruction', 'small intestine', 'ileum', 'jejunum' and 'aged' and free text 'small bowel obstruction', 'elderly', 'old', 'eldest' and 'geriatric'. A same search strategy was performed in Embase, after which duplicates were identified and deleted. Thereafter, the Cochrane database was searched for reviews concerning small bowel obstruction, resulting in three studies that focused on small bowel obstruction.

One hundred twenty studies from Embase and PubMed were eligible for full-text screening (Fig. 1). Thirteen studies were included for qualitative analysis, whereof two studies were specifically aimed at elderly patients. The Cochrane database search did not reveal a relevant paper. Main reasons for exclusion were as follows: studies did not include elderly patients and studies did not include small bowel obstruction. To ensure our review contained important geriatric themes/considerations that affect diagnosis and treatment of small bowel obstruction, we expanded our search after the systematic search by including more general studies on elderly patients.

This narrative review is divided in two sections; in the first more general section frailty and geriatric assessments are discussed, the second section encompasses the diagnosis and therapy for small bowel obstruction in elderly, decision-making and recommendations for practice or further research. For each section, we summarize and conclude the existing evidence in the literature on small bowel obstruction in the elderly followed by discussing the differences with small bowel obstruction management in the general population.

Frailty and geriatric assessments

Although different definitions exist, frailty is generally defined as the loss of reserves, after even small insults that lead to increased adverse outcomes [26, 27]. At

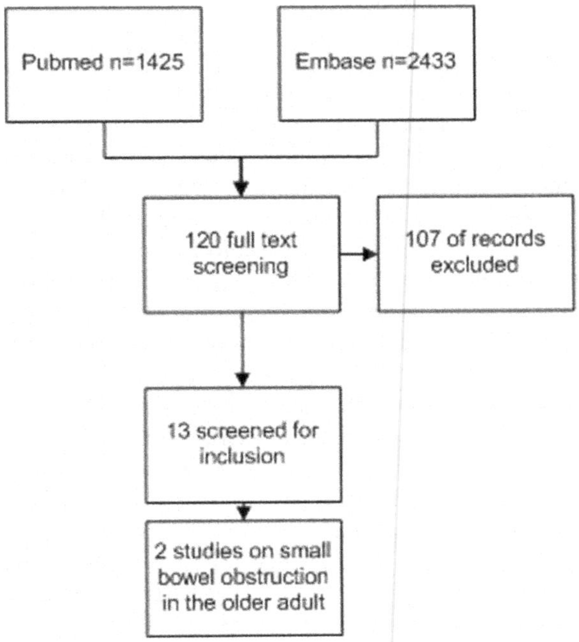

Fig. 1 Flow chart of search in PubMed and Embase databases; 120 studies were selected and searched with elderly patients as focus. Exclusion criteria: not focused on older adults, case reports, laparotomy vs laparoscopy, non-English/Dutch/German studies and studies focusing on phytobezoars

perioperative screening of elderly patients, frailty is a more important predictor for outcome than age. Frailty not only is independently associated with worse outcomes in terms of morbidity and mortality, but also gives higher risk for functional decline [28]. Around 70 different frailty tests exist, the majority of these tests are aimed at the elective situation, and walking speed is a frequent part of the test. The CSHA Clinical frailty scale by Rockwood et al. consists of 9 points to assess frailty and is relatively simple and quick to perform [29]. The scale correlates well with 5-year mortality and institutionalisation and can easily be used in the emergency situation.

There is only one study that describes frailty assessment in small bowel obstruction [30]. Fifty-three percent of patients in this observational study were mildly to severely frail and 25% were pre-frail, which indicates a high risk for progression to frailty. Unfortunately, frailty was not correlated to outcome, despite existing evidence that frailty negatively affects outcomes in patients undergoing emergency surgery [21].

Patients aged above 70 years with acute abdominal pain (and proven small bowel obstruction) could benefit from screening on frailty [21]. It seems that non-frail patients above 70 years old can be treated in the same way as other adult patients with small bowel obstruction. In frail patients, the higher risks of adverse outcomes and the patient specific goals in life should be added in the decision-making process.

Geriatric assessment

When patients are suspected or formally tested as being frail, a comprehensive geriatric assessment (CGA) should be performed prior to taking further steps in diagnosis and treatment. Such assessment demands considerable time and attention from geriatricians, but offers the most comprehensive information on frail patients and can help in choosing the treatment that optimally meets the demands and wishes of elderly. Reduced length of stay and lower percentage of change in discharge destination are reported after a CGA [31]. Although there are no data on a (shortened) CGA in small bowel obstruction patients, we believe that optimal care for frail elderly patients with small bowel obstruction will require a multidisciplinary approach from the start, at the ED. Similar to earlier reports on emergency surgery, management of polypharmacy and interactions between treatment of small bowel obstruction and co-morbidities can benefit from dedicated geriatric care and improve results for this frequent condition with high morbidity [4, 32].

There are several models for providing comprehensive geriatric care including geriatric consultation teams, interdisciplinary pathways, aged care consultation at nursing level and primary admittance to a geriatric ward [33, 34]. The optimal model for emergency care, e.g. small bowel obstruction remains undetermined and might vary with local expertise and resources. By all means, the model chosen should fulfil criteria of rapid availability of geriatric competence at the ED 24 h a day and a predefined multidisciplinary care path. We recently started a pilot at the ED of the Radboud University Medical Center (dually headed by a senior geriatrician and trauma surgeon), studying feasibility and short-term efficacy of a multidisciplinary team diagnosing and treating elderly patients with acute abdominal pain. Such a multidisciplinary team includes an emergency physician and nurse (coordinator), a surgeon, a radiologist and a geriatrician. We call this the 'Car Hood Deliberation' comparable with consultation between emergency services at the place of an accident.

Diagnosis

Most common causes of small bowel obstruction are adhesions, tumours and herniations, which are present in more than 90% of cases, with postoperative adhesions counting for approximately 60% [35–37]. Less frequent etiologies of bowel obstruction differ between older and younger adults in prevalence; Crohn's disease is rare in elderly patients while gallstone impaction is more frequent [36, 38, 39].

Symptom presentation of small bowel obstruction in elderly patients has not been studied in detail, but elderly patients seem to present later and with less profound symptoms at the ED compared to younger patients, resulting in a higher rate of misdiagnosis [3, 40, 41]. In a large cohort study, 52% of elderly patients presenting at the ED with abdominal pain had an incorrect initial diagnosis, compared to 45% of younger patients [40]. Medical staff should especially be aware that elderly patients with acute disease have less pronounced pain, leukocytosis and fever, signs that are relevant discriminating between uncomplicated and complicated small bowel obstruction [42]. There is an increase in pain threshold through lifespan, dependent of type of pain stimulus [43, 44]. Elderly have lower baseline temperatures and in 20–30% of cases show no fever at all in cases of serious infection [45]. Parker et al. studied the usefulness of leukocyte count and other laboratory screening test to distinguish elderly patients in need for acute care surgery from elderly patients with non-surgical emergencies. He found no difference in laboratory values, and 13% of patients in need for acute care surgery had complete normal test results [46]. If applicable to patients with small bowel obstruction, it might be more difficult to recognize strangulation or ischemic bowel in the elderly patient based on physical examination and laboratory screening.

The need for an oral and intravenous contrast-enhanced CT may be omitted in younger patients with high suspicion of adhesions as cause [10]. However, in elderly patients, it is a valuable diagnostic tool to identify patients with small bowel obstruction who require immediate surgery. A study in octogenarians and nonagenarians reported a significant change in small bowel obstruction diagnosis before and after CT [47]. A CT sensitivity and specificity between 90 and 98% for complete bowel obstruction was found in the elderly population [48, 49]. Millet et al. showed significant improvement in diagnosis and management after the use of unenhanced CT for acute abdominal pain in elderly patients [50]. Besides its value of facilitating diagnosis in older patients, unenhanced CT does not harbour the risk of contrast-induced nephropathy. Moreover, other causes or signs can be brought to light, such as unsuspected intra-abdominal neoplasm, intestinal pneumatosis or portal venous gas [47, 50, 51]. When patients have a history of (abdominal) malignancies, a CT may differentiate between malignant bowel obstruction and adhesive obstruction related to previous abdominal surgery [52]. Another, less often utilized imaging tool that is both diagnostic and therapeutic in adhesive small bowel obstruction is water-soluble contrast follow through abdominal film or CT. This has proven to be a reliable diagnostic tool to distinguish complete from incomplete obstruction [53]. Only one randomized study has been performed to assess the therapeutic effects of a water-soluble contrast follow through investigation in combination with somatostatin (analog) in patients with small bowel obstruction older than 65 years. The patients in the intervention group had less surgery, less pain, earlier start of oral intake and earlier stool passage [54, 55].

Treatment

The cornerstone of non-operative management of small bowel obstruction caused by adhesions is starvation, stomach decompression using a nasogastric tube and fluid resuscitation. This approach seems uniform for younger and older patients. Non-operative management should further include correction of electrolyte disturbances and nutritional support, especially in the frail older patient to avoid delirium, functional decline and complications as a result of starvation and malnutrition [36, 56, 57]. Non-operative management is effective in approximately 70–90% of patients with adhesive small bowel obstruction in general [35, 55, 58]. Though it has a significant failure rate, the nasogastric tube remains relevant in the conservative treatment of small bowel obstruction to initially relieve symptoms and avoid aspiration [10]. Triple-lumen long tubes have been claimed superior to nasogastric tubes in terms of failure [59]. A drawback of the triple-lumen tube is the frequent need for endoscopic placement with use of sedatives, which inherits a risk of pulmonary complications in the frail older patient. Additionally, elderly patients often have hyperactive delirium with a higher risk of accidental tube removal [60].

Starvation treatment can conflict with concurrent treatment of co-morbidities and multiple drug intake [61, 62]. There is surprisingly little evidence to support clinical decision-making on medication during starvation treatment. Clinicians have three options; discontinuing the medication, exempting medication from the starvation regimen, or administering the same or similar drug via other routes, e.g. intravenously. It is generally accepted that medication taken for long-term risk management can safely be discontinued during the course of treatment for small bowel obstruction [63]. Some oral medications can be administered safely with a short period clamping the tube; however, care should be taken in elderly patients with pre-existing dysphagia or neurologic conditions with risk of aspiration of medication. Even though oral ingestion or administering drugs via a tube is often feasible, the uptake of medication is questionable in small bowel obstruction [64]. There is marked paucity in data on complications that might arise from discontinuation or reduced uptake of oral medication in elderly patients with small bowel obstruction. For some medications, alternative routes show different pharmacokinetics with different clinical effects. Well-known examples are beta blockers and benzodiazepines, often prescribed to elderly patients [65, 66].

An ongoing debate in the management of small bowel obstruction is the duration of non-operative treatment that is deemed mandatory to resolve the bowel obstruction before the decision to operate. Most authors apply the 72-h safe-time rule for duration of initial non-operative therapy irrespective of age [10, 12, 55, 67]. It seems, however, that in the elderly, the non-operative treatment is chosen more often from the beginning and that the duration of non-operative treatment is longer compared to the younger population, arguing that the risks of complications and loss of quality of life associated with operation are then avoided [23, 68]. A more conservative approach in the elderly is questionable because the negative effects of delayed surgery seem more pronounced in the elderly patients [36, 55]. In a prospective study, Springer et al. reported a 14% mortality in elderly patients undergoing delayed surgery compared to 3% with early surgery [30]. Causes for increased deaths were not reported. A recent other study showed no difference in outcomes between younger and older patients with small bowel obstruction; however, these results should be interpreted with caution because of the retrospective design and risk selection bias with including the most fit elderly patients [69].

Table 1 Overview of known and unknown facts concerning small bowel obstruction in elderly patients

What this paper adds

- Adhesive small bowel obstruction (SBO) accounts for the largest group of SBO. Malignant small bowel obstruction, gall stone ileus and hernia incarceration are more prevalent in elderly patients
- Symptom presentation is otypical in elderly patients
- CT scan is highly sensitive and specific, and unenhanced CT is a safe method for diagnostics
- Frail elderly patients have more morbidity, mortality and functional decline
- A comprehensive geriatric approach, including patients' preference is preferable.
- Applied waiting period to surgery might be too long in older patients with SBO

What is not known?

- Functional outcomes of elderly patients after SBO
- Optimal 'safe' time to wait for resolution of SBO by conservative therapy
- Influence of frailty on outcomes in SBO

Although it has been recognized that treating elderly patients with small bowel obstruction is somewhat sailing between Scylla and Charybdis, we would make a plea for earlier decision-making for conservative or surgical treatment instead of following the 72-h non-operative treatment time. In this early phase, more comprehensive decision-making should be included in the decision-making process.

Malignant bowel obstruction

Small bowel obstruction due to malignancy is more common in elderly patients and has a different approach compared to other causes. It has a bad prognosis in the majority of patients, irrespective of age. Survival in general is circa 5 months. This is even lower in patients with gynecological cancers or peritoneal disease, who have a median survival of less than 3 months after

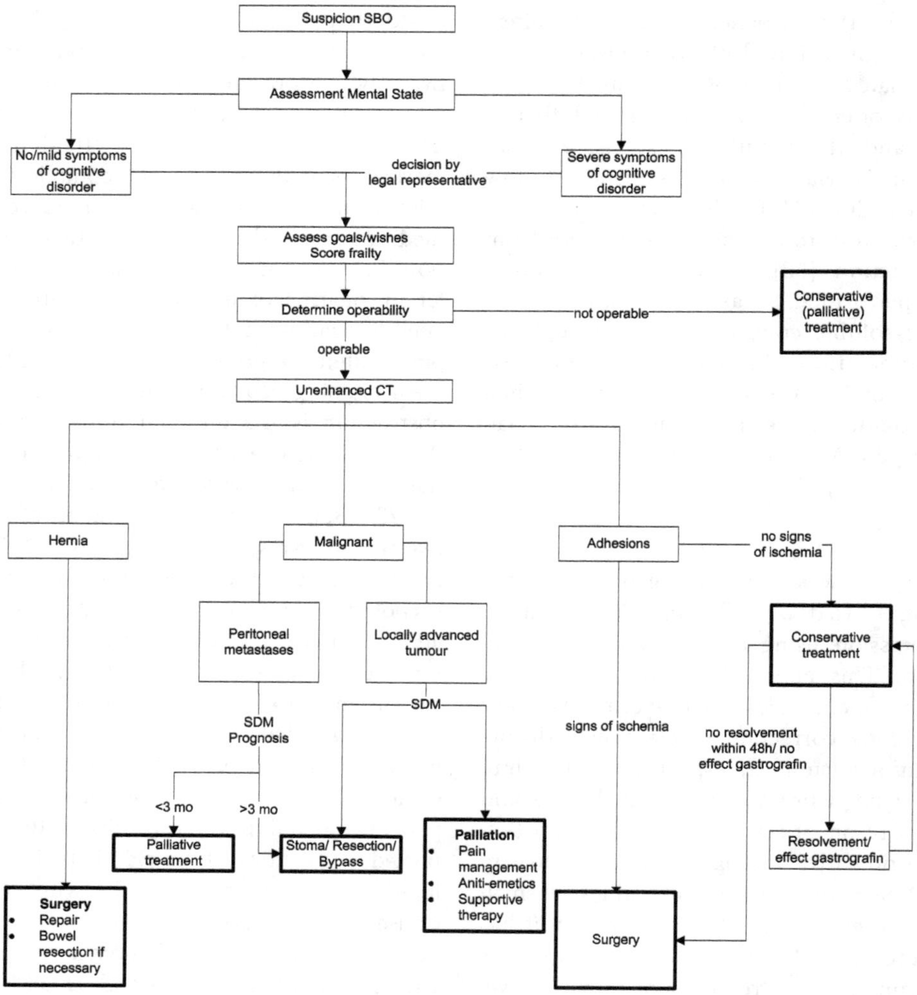

Fig. 2 Algorithm with suggested diagnostic and therapeutic steps for the elderly patient with small bowel obstruction. After assessing cognition, frailty and patient goals according to diagnosis, risks and benefits of surgical and conservative management should be weighed. SBO small bowel obstruction, SDM shared decision-making

surgery [52, 70–72]. Non-operative management shows high failure rates, although palliative treatment with percutaneous decompressing jejunostomy could be considered [73]. The results of palliative surgery in terms of mortality, morbidity and functional decline in the elderly population are not known in detail; however, increased age in general is a known risk factor for morbidity and mortality in malignant small bowel obstruction [71, 74]. In case of peritoneal carcinomatosis, surgery provides little to no relief. It will lead to high morbidity and prolonged hospitalization and very often to non-reparable re-obstruction [72, 75]. Therefore, surgery for malignant small bowel should be abandoned in frail elderly patients keeping in mind quality and not quantity of the remaining short life.

Quality of life, functioning and decision-making

In elderly patients quality of life considerations and functioning are important in decision-making, particularly regarding surgery. Focus should be laid on goals and wishes in their remaining life [76]. There is little information about the quality of life consequences of surgery for small bowel obstruction in the aged. Recommendations from guidelines on small bowel obstruction hardly help because these are largely based on studies with younger adults [76–78]. Jeppesen et al. surveyed the impact of small bowel obstruction surgery on pain and quality of life and functioning. They found that 19% of patients had pain-related functional impairments after surgery for small bowel obstruction. Patients with chronic postoperative pain had a significantly lower gastrointestinal quality of life score compared with those without postoperative pain (109 (IQR 39) vs. 127 (IQR 19), $P < 0.001$) [23]. Unfortunately, the authors excluded patients older than 75 years in their survey, but considering the relative high risk of complications, it can be assumed that surgery for small bowel obstruction in the elderly seriously impairs quality of life and functioning [6, 30, 79–82]. Scoring systems that predict outcomes in small bowel obstruction and include co-morbidities are currently being validated. These systems however do not include functional state, frailty, or age. Furthermore, they integrate the performed treatment in their score as a predictor of outcome, instead of being a predictor of optimal treatment [83]. Incorporating patient's preferences in decision-making regarding treatment for small bowel obstruction becomes increasingly important for older patients as they may 'run out of time' to overcome the physiological impact of treatment, particularly surgery. Dunn et al. pled for a different approach in old and frail patients with an indication for high-risk surgery. Instead of aiming at a prolonged life, the most relevant question for elderly patients is 'how he wants to live' [84]. This certainly applies for patients with a diagnosis of malignant small bowel obstruction.

Decision to refrain from palliative surgery for small bowel obstruction has drawbacks: signs and symptoms of small bowel obstruction remain with often the necessity for the patient to remain in hospital. Still, it would be worth exploring treatment preferences and incorporate them in the palliative approach, particularly in patients with poor quality of life from recurrent obstructions, when an advanced tumour is the cause of obstruction, and in patients with marginal pre-existing general condition.

Conclusion

There is few evidence regarding diagnosis and treatment of the elderly patient with small bowel obstruction. The scarce literature available demonstrates that elderly patients have an increased risk for complications and mortality and might benefit from earlier surgical intervention. It is important to take patients' preferences into account starting treatment in general and offering surgery specifically, because an operation may significantly affect quality of life. An assessment of frailty and a comprehensive geriatric approach to the elderly with small bowel obstruction with multidisciplinary specialist care is required from the start and preferably in the ED. More research on management of small bowel obstruction in elderly patients is urgently needed considering the rise in this age group (Table 1).

We conclude that management of small bowel obstruction requires more than just a 'copy and paste' of treatment recommendations and guidelines based on studies in younger adults. Based on current knowledge about frail elderly and small bowel obstruction, a flowchart has been developed that offers an approach to diagnosis and treatment of elderly patients with a small bowel obstruction (Fig. 2).

Abbreviations

CGA: Comprehensive Geriatric Assessment; CT: Computed tomography; ED: Emergency department; SBO: Small bowel obstruction

Authors' contributions

EO performed the search for relevant literature and wrote the first draft of the manuscript. MS, RtB and YS critically revised the manuscript. HvG and MvI made substantial contributions to the study conception, supervised the literature study, critically revised the manuscript and delivered essential geriatric and surgical information. HvG gave final approval of the manuscript. All authors read and approved the final manuscript.

Competing interests

The authors declare that they have no competing interests.

Author details
[1]Department of Surgery, Radboud University Medical Center, P.O. Box 9101, 6500 HB Nijmegen, The Netherlands. [2]Department of Geriatrics, Radboud University Medical Center, Nijmegen, The Netherlands. [3]Radboud Institute for Health Sciences, Radboud University Medical Center, Nijmegen, The Netherlands.

References

1. Cooper Z, Scott JW, Rosenthal RA, Mitchell SL. Emergency major abdominal surgical procedures in older adults: a systematic review of mortality and functional outcomes. J Am Geriatr Soc. 2015;63(12):2563–71.
2. Spangler R, Van Pham T, Khoujah D, Martinez JP. Abdominal emergencies in the geriatric patient. Int J Emerg Med. 2014;7:43.
3. Bugliosi TF, Meloy TD, Vukov LF. Acute abdominal pain in the elderly. Ann Emerg Med. 1990;19(12):1383–6.
4. Team NP. The second patient report of the National Emergency Laparotomy Audit (NELA). London: The Royal College of Anaesthetists; 2016.
5. Scott JW, Olufajo OA, Brat GA, Rose JA, Zogg CK, Haider AH, et al. Use of national burden to define operative emergency general surgery. JAMA surgery. 2016;151(6):e160480.
6. Arenal JJ, Bengoechea-Beeby M. Mortality associated with emergency abdominal surgery in the elderly. Canadian Journal of Surgery Journal Canadien De Chirurgie. 2003;46(2):111–6.
7. Davis P, Hayden J, Springer J, Bailey J, Molinari M, Johnson P. Prognostic factors for morbidity and mortality in elderly patients undergoing acute gastrointestinal surgery: a systematic review. Canadian Journal of Surgery Journal Canadien De Chirurgie. 2014;57(2):E44–52.
8. Tolstrup MB, Watt SK, Gogenur I. Morbidity and mortality rates after emergency abdominal surgery: an analysis of 4346 patients scheduled for emergency laparotomy or laparoscopy. Langenbeck's archives of surgery / Deutsche Gesellschaft fur Chirurgie 2016.
9. Zielinski MD, Bannon MP. Current management of small bowel obstruction. Adv Surg. 2011;45:1–29.
10. Di Saverio S, Coccolini F, Galati M, Smerieri N, Biffl WL, Ansaloni L, et al. Bologna guidelines for diagnosis and management of adhesive small bowel obstruction (ASBO): 2013 update of the evidence-based guidelines from the world society of emergency surgery ASBO working group. World Journal of Emergency Surgery. 2013;8(1):42.
11. Abbas S, Bissett IP, Parry BR. Oral water soluble contrast for the management of adhesive small bowel obstruction. Cochrane Database Syst Rev. 2007;3:CD004651.
12. Loftus T, Moore F, VanZant E, Bala T, Brakenridge S, Croft C, et al. A protocol for the management of adhesive small bowel obstruction. J Trauma Acute Care Surg. 2015;78(1):13–9.
13. ten Broek RP, Strik C, Issa Y, Bleichrodt RP, van Goor H. Adhesiolysis-related morbidity in abdominal surgery. Ann Surg. 2013;258(1):98–106.
14. Behman R, Nathens AB, Byrne JP, Mason S, Look Hong N, Karanicolas PJ. Laparoscopic surgery for adhesive small bowel obstruction is associated with a higher risk of bowel injury: a population-based analysis of 8584 patients. Ann Surg. 2017;266(3):489–98.
15. Sajid MS, Khawaja AH, Sains P, Singh KK, Baig MK. A systematic review comparing laparoscopic vs open adhesiolysis in patients with adhesional small bowel obstruction. Am J Surg. 2016;212(1):138–50.
16. ten Broek RPBKP, Di Saverio S. Bologna guidelines for diagnosis and management of adhesive small bowel obstruction (ASBO): 2017 update of the evidence-based guidelines from the world society of emergency surgery ASBO working group. World Journal of Emergency Surgery. 2018; Manuscript submitted for publication.
17. NCfHS. National hospital ambulatory medical care survey. Hyattsville: NCHS; 2004.
18. Ong M, Guang TY, Yang TK. Impact of surgical delay on outcomes in elderly patients undergoing emergency surgery: a single center experience. World Journal of Gastrointestinal Surgery. 2015;7(9):208–13.
19. Aminzadeh F, Dalziel WB. Older adults in the emergency department: a systematic review of patterns of use, adverse outcomes, and effectiveness of interventions. Ann Emerg Med. 2002;39(3):238–47.
20. Song W, Zhang T, Pu J, Shen L, He B. Incidence and risk of developing contrast-induced acute kidney injury following intravascular contrast administration in elderly patients. Clin Interv Aging. 2014;9:85–93.
21. Joseph B, Zangbar B, Pandit V, Fain M, Mohler MJ, Kulvatunyou N, et al. Emergency general surgery in the elderly: too old or too frail? J Am Coll Surg. 2016;222(5):805–13.
22. Clegg A, Young J, Iliffe S, Rikkert MO, Rockwood K. Frailty in elderly people. Lancet. 2013;381(9868):752–62.
23. Jeppesen M, Tolstrup MB, Gogenur I. Chronic pain, quality of life, and functional impairment after surgery due to small bowel obstruction. World J Surg. 2016; 40(9):2091–7.
24. Rubenstein LZ, Stuck AE, Siu AL, Wieland D. Impacts of geriatric evaluation and management programs on defined outcomes: overview of the evidence. J Am Geriatr Soc. 1991;39(9 Pt 2):8S–16S discussion 7S-8S.
25. Khalil H, Peters M, Godfrey CM, McInerney P, Soares CB, Parker D. An evidence-based approach to scoping reviews. Worldviews Evid-Based Nurs. 2016;13(2):118–23.
26. Robinson TN, Wu DS, Pointer L, Dunn CL, Cleveland JC Jr, Moss M. Simple frailty score predicts postoperative complications across surgical specialties. Am J Surg. 2013;206(4):544–50.
27. Le Maguet P, Roquilly A, Lasocki S, Asehnoune K, Carise E, Saint Martin M, et al. Prevalence and impact of frailty on mortality in elderly ICU patients: a prospective, multicenter, observational study. Intensive Care Med. 2014; 40(5):674–82.
28. Covinsky KE, Pierluissi E, Johnston CB. Hospitalization-associated disability: "she was probably able to ambulate, but I'm not sure". JAMA. 2011;306(16): 1782–93.
29. Rockwood K, Song X, MacKnight C, Bergman H, Hogan DB, McDowell I, et al. A global clinical measure of fitness and frailty in elderly people. CMAJ. 2005;173(5):489–95.
30. Springer JE, Bailey JG, Davis PJ, Johnson PM. Management and outcomes of small bowel obstruction in older adult patients: a prospective cohort study. Canadian Journal of Surgery Journal Canadien de Chirurgie. 2014;57(6):379–84.
31. Partridge JS, Harari D, Martin FC, Peacock JL, Bell R, Mohammed A, et al. Randomized clinical trial of comprehensive geriatric assessment and optimization in vascular surgery. Br J Surg. 2017;104(6):679–87.
32. Griffiths R, Beech F, Brown A, Dhesi J, Foo I, Goodall J, et al. Peri-operative care of the elderly 2014: Association of Anaesthetists of Great Britain and Ireland. Anaesthesia. 2014;69(Suppl 1):81–98.
33. Robinson A, Street A. Improving networks between acute care nurses and an aged care assessment team. J Clin Nurs. 2004;13(4):486–96.
34. Giusti A, Barone A, Razzano M, Pizzonia M, Pioli G. Optimal setting and care organization in the management of older adults with hip fracture. Eur J Phys Rehabil Med. 2011;47(2):281–96.
35. ten Broek RP, Issa Y, van Santbrink EJ, Bouvy ND, Kruitwagen RF, Jeekel J, et al. Burden of adhesions in abdominal and pelvic surgery: systematic review and met-analysis. BMJ. 2013;347:f5588.
36. Foster NM, McGory ML, Zingmond DS, Ko CY. Small bowel obstruction: a population-based appraisal. J Am Coll Surg. 2006;203(2):170–6.
37. Fevang BT, Fevang J, Lie SA, Soreide O, Svanes K, Viste A. Long-term prognosis after operation for adhesive small bowel obstruction. Ann Surg. 2004;240(2):193–201.
38. Miller G, Boman J, Shrier I, Gordon PH. Etiology of small bowel obstruction. Am J Surg. 2000;180(1):33–6.
39. Halabi WJ, Kang CY, Ketana N, Lafaro KJ, Nguyen VQ, Stamos MJ, et al. Surgery for gallstone ileus: a nationwide comparison of trends and outcomes. Ann Surg. 2014;259(2):329–35.
40. Laurell H, Hansson LE, Gunnarsson U. Acute abdominal pain among elderly patients. Gerontology. 2006;52(6):339–44.
41. Fenyo G. Acute abdominal disease in the elderly: experience from two series in Stockholm. Am J Surg. 1982;143(6):751–4.
42. Liang SY. Sepsis and other infectious disease emergencies in the elderly. Emerg Med Clin North Am. 2016;34(3):501–22.
43. Kaye AD, Baluch A, Scott JT. Pain management in the elderly population: a review. Ochsner J. 2010;10(3):179–87.
44. Lautenbacher S, Kunz M, Strate P, Nielsen J, Arendt-Nielsen L. Age effects on pain thresholds, temporal summation and spatial summation of heat and pressure pain. Pain. 2005;115(3):410–8.
45. Norman DC. Fever in the elderly. Clin Infect Dis. 2000;31(1):148–51.
46. Parker JS, Vukov LF, Wollan PC. Abdominal pain in the elderly: use of temperature and laboratory testing to screen for surgical disease. Fam Med. 1996;28(3):193–7.

47. Gardner CS, Jaffe TA, Nelson RC. Impact of CT in elderly patients presenting to the emergency department with acute abdominal pain. Abdom Imaging. 2015;40(7):2877–82.
48. Millet I, Alili C, Bouic-Pages E, Curros-Doyon F, Nagot N, Taourel P. Journal club: acute abdominal pain in elderly patients: effect of radiologist awareness of clinicobiologic information on CT accuracy. AJR Am J Roentgenol. 2013;201(6):1171–8 quiz 9.
49. Reginelli A, Russo A, Pinto A, Stanzione F, Martiniello C, Cappabianca S, et al. The role of computed tomography in the preoperative assessment of gastrointestinal causes of acute abdomen in elderly patients. Int J Surg. 2014;12(Suppl 2):S181–6.
50. Millet I, Sebbane M, Molinari N, Pages-Bouic E, Curros-Doyon F, Riou B, et al. Systematic unenhanced CT for acute abdominal symptoms in the elderly patients improves both emergency department diagnosis and prompt clinical management. Eur Radiol. 2017;27(2):868–77.
51. Lewis LM, Klippel AP, Bavolek RA, Ross LM, Scherer TM, Banet GA. Quantifying the usefulness of CT in evaluating seniors with abdominal pain. Eur J Radiol. 2007;61(2):290–6.
52. Butler JA, Cameron BL, Morrow M, Kahng K, Tom J. Small bowel obstruction in patients with a prior history of cancer. Am J Surg. 1991;162(6):624–8.
53. Biondo S, Pares D, Mora L, Marti Rague J, Kreisler E, Jaurrieta E. Randomized clinical study of Gastrografin administration in patients with adhesive small bowel obstruction. Br J Surg. 2003;90(5):542–6.
54. Zhang Y, Gao Y, Ma Q, Dang C, Wei W, De Antoni F, et al. Randomised clinical trial investigating the effects of combined administration of octreotide and methylglucamine diatrizoate in the older persons with adhesive small bowel obstruction. Dig Liver Dis. 2006;38(3):188–94.
55. Schraufnagel D, Rajaee S, Millham FH. How many sunsets? Timing of surgery in adhesive small bowel obstruction: a study of the nationwide inpatient sample. J Trauma Acute Care Surg. 2013;74(1):181–7 discussion 7-9.
56. Hu WH, Cajas-Monson LC, Eisenstein S, Parry L, Cosman B, Ramamoorthy S. Preoperative malnutrition assessments as predictors of postoperative mortality and morbidity in colorectal cancer: an analysis of ACS-NSQIP. Nutr J. 2015;14:91.
57. Thomas MN, Kufeldt J, Kisser U, Hornung HM, Hoffmann J, Andraschko M, et al. Effects of malnutrition on complication rates, length of hospital stay, and revenue in elective surgical patients in the G-DRG-system. Nutrition. 2016; 32(2):249–54.
58. Fazel MZ, Jamieson RW, Watson CJ. Long-term follow-up of the use of the Jones' intestinal tube in adhesive small bowel obstruction. Ann R Coll Surg Engl. 2009;91(1):50–4.
59. Chen XL, Ji F, Lin Q, Chen YP, Lin JJ, Ye F, et al. A prospective randomized trial of transnasal ileus tube vs nasogastric tube for adhesive small bowel obstruction. World J Gastroenterol. 2012;18(16):1968–74.
60. Young J, Murthy L, Westby M, Akunne A, O'Mahony R, Guideline Development G. Diagnosis, prevention, and management of delirium: summary of NICE guidance. BMJ. 2010;341:c3704.
61. Haider SI, Johnell K, Thorslund M, Fastbom J. Trends in polypharmacy and potential drug-drug interactions across educational groups in elderly patients in Sweden for the period 1992 - 2002. Int J Clin Pharmacol Ther. 2007;45(12):643–53.
62. Hovstadius B, Hovstadius K, Astrand B, Petersson G. Increasing polypharmacy - an individual-based study of the Swedish population 2005-2008. BMC Clin Pharmacol. 2010;10:16.
63. Leder SB, Lerner MZ. Nil per os except medications order in the dysphagic patient. QJM. 2013;106(1):71–5.
64. Gubbins PO, Bertch KE. Drug absorption in gastrointestinal disease and surgery. Clinical pharmacokinetic and therapeutic implications. Clin Pharmacokinet. 1991;21(6):431–47.
65. Shader RI, Greenblatt DJ. The use of benzodiazepines in clinical practice. Br J Clin Pharmacol. 1981;11(Suppl 1):5S–9S.
66. Mehvar R, Brocks DR. Stereospecific pharmacokinetics and pharmacodynamics of beta-adrenergic blockers in humans. J Pharm Pharm Sci. 2001;4(2):185–200.
67. Keenan JE, Turley RS, McCoy CC, Migaly J, Shapiro ML, Scarborough JE. Trials of nonoperative management exceeding 3 days are associated with increased morbidity in patients undergoing surgery for uncomplicated adhesive small bowel obstruction. J Trauma Acute Care Surg. 2014;76(6):1367–72.
68. Aldemir M, Yagnur Y, Tacyildir I. The predictive factors for the necessity of operative treatment in adhesive small bowel obstruction cases. Acta Chir Belg. 2004;104(1):76–80.
69. Krause WR, Webb T. Geriatric small bowel obstruction: an analysis of treatment and outcomes compared to a younger cohort. Geriatric small bowel obstruction: an analysis of treatment and outcomes compared with a younger cohort.Am J Surg. 2015;209(2):347–51.
70. Woolfson RG, Jennings K, Whalen GF. Management of bowel obstruction in patients with abdominal cancer. Archives of surgery (Chicago, Ill : 1960). 1997;132(10):1093–7.
71. Ripamonti C, Bruera E. Palliative management of malignant bowel obstruction. Int J Gynecol Cancer. 2002;12(2):135–43.
72. Blair SL, Chu DZ, Schwarz RE. Outcome of palliative operations for malignant bowel obstruction in patients with peritoneal carcinomatosis from nongynecological cancer. Ann Surg Oncol. 2001;8(8):632–7.
73. Kim YJ, Yoon CJ, Seong NJ, Kang SG, An SW, Woo YN. Safety and efficacy of radiological percutaneous jejunostomy for decompression of malignant small bowel obstruction. Eur Radiol. 2013;23(10):2747–53.
74. Wancata LM, Abdelsattar ZM, Suwanabol PA, Campbell DA Jr, Hendren S. Outcomes after surgery for benign and malignant small bowel obstruction. J Gastrointest Surg. 2017;21(2):363–71.
75. Paul Olson TJ, Pinkerton C, Brasel KJ, Schwarze ML. Palliative surgery for malignant bowel obstruction from carcinomatosis: a systematic review. JAMA Surgery. 2014;149(4):383–92.
76. van de Pol MH, Fluit CR, Lagro J, Slaats YH, Olde Rikkert MG, Lagro-Janssen AL. Expert and patient consensus on a dynamic model for shared decision-making in frail older patients. Patient Educ Couns. 2015.
77. Elwyn G, Laitner S, Coulter A, Walker E, Watson P, Thomson R. Implementing shared decision making in the NHS. BMJ. 2010;341:c5146.
78. Barry MJ, Edgman-Levitan S. Shared decision making--pinnacle of patient-centered care. N Engl J Med. 2012;366(9):780–1.
79. Law WP, Mackenzie E, Bhuta R, Lutton N. Umbilical metastasis (sister Mary Joseph nodule) from distal ileal carcinoid. Intern Med J. 2010;40:36.
80. Boyd CM, Landefeld CS, Counsell SR, Palmer RM, Fortinsky RH, Kresevic D, et al. Recovery of activities of daily living in older adults after hospitalization for acute medical illness. J Am Geriatr Soc. 2008;56(12):2171–9.
81. Bruce J, Krukowski ZH. Quality of life and chronic pain four years after gastrointestinal surgery. Dis Colon Rectum. 2006;49(9):1362–70.
82. Bakker FC, Persoon A, Bredie SJ, van Haren-Willems J, Leferink VJ, Noyez L, et al. The CareWell in hospital program to improve the quality of care for frail elderly inpatients: results of a before-after study with focus on surgical patients. Am J Surg. 2014;208(5):735–46.
83. Baghdadi YMK, Morris DS, Choudhry AJ, Thiels CA, Khasawneh MA, Polites SF, et al. Validation of the anatomic severity score developed by the American Association for the Surgery of Trauma in small bowel obstruction. J Surg Res. 2016;204(2):428–34.
84. Dunn GP. Shared decision-making for the elderly patient with a surgical condition. Br J Surg. 2016;103(2):e19–20.

24

Evaluation of capillary leakage after vasopressin resuscitation in a hemorrhagic shock model

Roberto Bini[1], Osvaldo Chiara[2], Stefania Cimbanassi[2], Giorgio Olivero[3], Antonella Trombetta[4] and Paolo Cotogni[5*]

Abstract

Background: Hemorrhagic shock (HS) is a major threat to patients with trauma and spontaneous bleeding. The aim of the study was to investigate early effects of vasopressin on metabolic and hemodynamic parameters and endothelium permeability by measuring capillary leakage compared to those of other resuscitation strategies in a HS model.

Methods: Forty-five Sprague-Dawley rats were randomized into five groups: S group ($n = 5$), sham-operated rats without shock or resuscitation; HS group ($n = 10$), HS and no resuscitation; RL group ($n = 10$), HS and resuscitation with Ringer's lactate (RL); RLB group ($n = 10$), HS and resuscitation with two-third shed blood plus RL; and vasopressin group ($n = 10$), HS and resuscitation with RL, followed by continuous infusion of 0.04 U/kg/min vasopressin. The effects of resuscitation on hemodynamic parameters [mean arterial pressure (MAP), superior mesenteric artery blood flow (MBF), and mesenteric vascular resistances (MVR)], arterial blood gases, bicarbonate, base deficit, and lactate levels as well as on capillary leakage in the lung, ileum, and kidney were investigated. Capillary leakage was evaluated with Evans blue dye extravasation.

Results: In the vasopressin group, the MAP was higher than in the RL and RLB groups ($p < 0.001$), while MBF was decreased ($p < 0.001$). MVR were increased only in the vasopressin group ($p < 0.001$). Capillary leakage was increased in the lungs of the animals in the vasopressin group compared to that in the lungs of animals in the RLB group ($p < 0.05$); this increase was associated with the lowest partial pressure of oxygen ($p < 0.05$). Conversely, decreased capillary leakage was observed with vasopressin in the ileum ($p < 0.05$). Increased capillary leakage was observed in the kidney in the RLB and vasopressin groups ($p < 0.05$). Lastly, vasopressin use was associated with higher base deficit and lactate levels when compared to the RL and RLB groups ($p < 0.001$).

Conclusion: Although vasopressin was proposed as a vasoactive drug for provisional hemodynamic optimization in the early phase of HS resuscitation, the overall findings of this experimental study focus on the possible critical side effects of vasopressin on metabolic parameters and endothelium permeability.

Keywords: Hemorrhage, Shock treatment, Arginine vasopressin, Vasopressors

* Correspondence: paolo.cotogni@unito.it
[5]Department of Anesthesia and Intensive Care, S. Giovanni Battista Hospital, University of Turin, Via Giovanni Giolitti 9, 10123 Turin, Italy
Full list of author information is available at the end of the article

Background

Hemorrhagic shock (HS) represents a major threat to trauma and spontaneous bleeding patients [1]. Organ dysfunction and/or failure may be consequences of HS and account for high mortality, despite adequate fluid resuscitation and subsequent restoration of normotension. There is an ongoing discussion on strategies used for resuscitation of trauma patients with HS [2]. Bleeding control and maintenance of tissue oxygenation with fluid resuscitation remain the mainstays of therapy for patients with HS. However, severe and protracted hypotension with decreased tissue perfusion induced by an ongoing hemorrhage may progress in a condition of profound shock, making the patient unresponsive to fluid resuscitation and catecholamines. Correction of hypovolemia does not resolve hypotension in these patients because of the occurrence of peripheral vasodilatation. Landry and Oliver [3] suggested the following three mechanisms that have been implicated in the pathogenesis of vasodilatory shock, which occurs during the late phase of HS: (a) activation of ATP-sensitive potassium channels in the plasma membrane of the vascular smooth muscles, (b) activation of the inducible form of nitric oxide synthase, and (c) deficiency of the hormone vasopressin. The last mechanism led to the investigation of the role of vasopressin in the treatment of advanced stages of HS [4].

Recent animal studies have shown that vasopressin treatment achieves hemodynamic optimization during the early phase of HS (mimicking the prehospital phase) while fluids and catecholamines showed neither improvement of hemodynamic parameters nor survival [5, 6]. However, vasopressin use has been associated with some adverse effects such as ischemic complications particularly in the splanchnic and skin circulation [7]. Moreover, a multicenter prospective cohort study suggested that the early use of vasopressors for hemodynamic improvement after HS when compared to aggressive volume resuscitation was deleterious and should be cautiously used, supporting the concept of "caution before constriction" [8]. Collier et al. found that vasopressin use was associated with increased mortality in trauma patients with shock [9].

It has been demonstrated that intense inflammatory response may develop after HS [10]. Massive blood loss and resuscitation cause a global ischemia-reperfusion effect with an upregulation of cytokine expression [11] and oxidative and nitrosative stresses [12] that may lead to organ damage and dysfunction. During advanced stages of HS, changes in capillary permeability with leak and plasma extravasation (i.e., capillary leakage) into the interstitial space contribute to microcirculatory disturbances and organ damage [13] with edema formation [14].

The aim of this study was to investigate the early effects of vasopressin on metabolic and hemodynamic parameters and endothelium permeability by measuring capillary leakage compared to those of other resuscitation strategies in a HS model.

Methods

Animal preparation and surgical procedure

All experiments were conducted in accordance with the requirements indicated in the guidelines of Institutional Animal Care and Use Committees (IACUC), after the approval from the Ethics Committee of the Piedmont Regulatory Agency for Care and Use of Laboratory Animals. Male Sprague-Dawley rats (weight range, 290–350 g; median weight, 325 g; age range, 50–65 days) were used (Charles River, Calco, Como, Italy). The animals were housed individually and allowed free access to food and water. The animal rooms were windowless with controlled temperature (22 ± 2 °C) and lighting (12-h light/dark cycle), where the rats were allowed to acclimatize for a minimum of 5 days after arrival at the laboratory. Subsequently, the animals were anesthetized with ketamine plus xylazine intramuscular (90 and 10 mg/kg body weight [b.w.], respectively) and restrained in a supine position. Body temperature was monitored by a rectal thermal probe and maintained at 37 °C with a heating pad. The left groin was shaved and prepped with povidone-iodine solution. The femoral artery was dissected using a minimal dissection technique, distally ligated and cannulated with a 22-gauge heparinized catheter. A blood pressure transducer (Isotec-Healthdyne Cardiovascular, Marietta, GA) and a monitor allowed for the continuous monitoring of mean arterial pressure (MAP). A midline laparotomy was performed, and superior mesenteric artery blood flow (MBF) was measured with a perivascular probe (T206, Transonic Systems, Ithaca, NY). Blood samples were collected from the arterial catheter. Mesenteric vascular resistances (MVR) were calculated as MAP/MBF. Arterial blood gases, bicarbonate, base deficit, and lactate levels were measured with a blood-gas analyzer (ABL System 500, Radiometer Medical, Copenhagen, Denmark).

Experimental protocol

Forty-five rats were randomized into the following five groups: S group ($n = 5$), sham-operated (S) without shock or resuscitation (anesthesia and artery cannulation only); HS group ($n = 10$), HS and no resuscitation; RL group ($n = 10$), HS and resuscitation with Ringer's lactate (RL) intravenously; RLB group ($n = 10$), HS and resuscitation with two-third shed blood (i.e., 2/3 the hemorrhage volume) plus RL; and vasopressin group ($n = 10$), HS and resuscitation with RL, followed by continuous infusion of 0.04 U/kg/min vasopressin via a syringe pump (5 ml/h). The experiment was carried out using a model with pressure-controlled hemorrhage previously described [15] (Fig. 1). Briefly, the experiment began by gradually bleeding

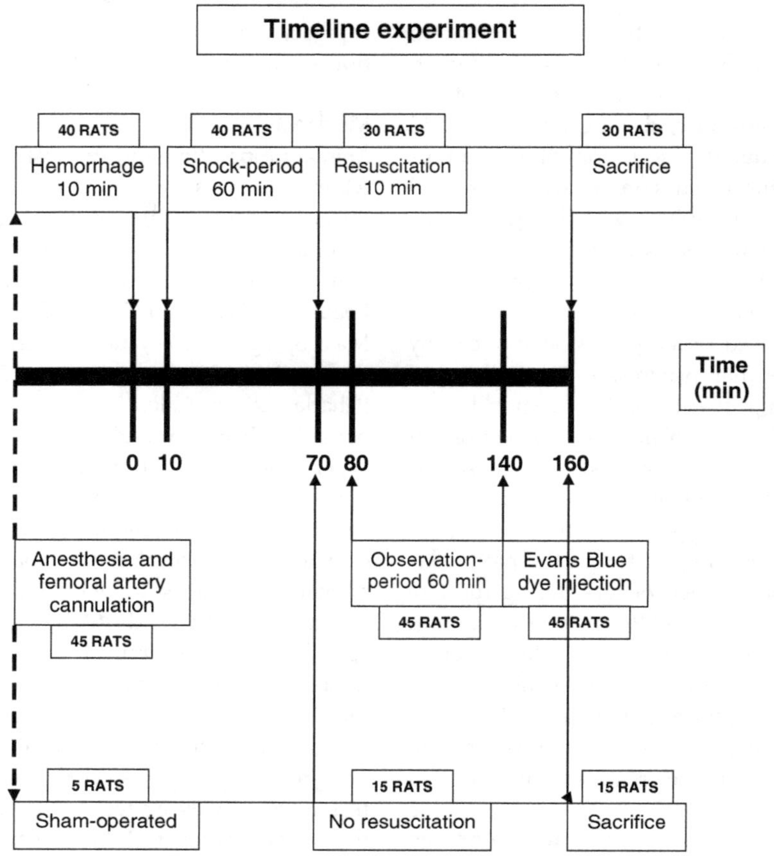

Fig. 1 Timeline experiment. Forty-five rats underwent anesthesia and artery cannulation. Forty rats were subjected to pressure-controlled hemorrhage over a 10-min period, while five rats were sham-operated. The target value of hemorrhagic shock was a reduction in mean arterial pressure (MAP) to 35–40 mmHg. The constant MAP was maintained for 60 min (shock period). After 1 h of shock, 30 hemorrhaged rats were resuscitated over a 10-min period according to the experimental protocol. One hour after the end of resuscitation (observation period), Evans blue dye was injected. Twenty minutes after Evans blue injection, all the rats were euthanized

each rat, except those in the S group, by withdrawing blood from a catheter inserted into the femoral artery over a 10-min period. The target value of HS was a reduction in MAP to 35–40 mmHg. The constant MAP was maintained for 60 min with further withdrawal or infusion of small amounts of shed blood. The blood was collected in a heparinized tube and incubated at 37 °C. After 1 h of shock, hemorrhaged rats, except those in the HS group, were resuscitated with the same volume of fluids or shed blood (11.3 ± 0.7 ml) over a 10-min period according to the experimental protocol. Afterward, all the rats underwent the same rate of fluid infusion (5 ml/h).

Monitoring after anesthesia recovery included attention to specific criteria for evaluating the signs of postoperative pain and distress. The rats were assessed clinically to judge the efficacy of the analgesia, and an analgesic was administered in the presence of behavioral signs of pain or distress (rapid breathing, abnormal movement or posture/positioning, twitching/trembling) according to our institutionally approved animal protocol developed through veterinary consultation. Postoperative analgesia (ketamine, 80 mg/kg b.w., intramuscular) was maintained throughout the experimental period until the animals were euthanized. In relation to the type and duration of surgical procedure, no animals showed any clinically apparent signs of pain or distress with a single postoperative dose of ketamine.

Effects of resuscitation on capillary leakage in the lung, ileum, and kidney were investigated in the three treatment groups and compared to the HS group. Capillary leakage was evaluated with Evans blue (EB) dye extravasation using the following method: 1 h after the end of resuscitation, 50 mg/kg b.w. of EB dye was injected as previously described by Schumacher et al. [16]. Twenty minutes after EB injection, the rats were euthanized with an overdose of sodium pentobarbital (intravenously; 150 mg/kg b.w.). The inferior vena cava was incised to exsanguinate the animals. An 18-gauge catheter was placed into the apex of the left ventricle with its tip inside the aorta in order to perfuse the circulatory system with 0.9% NaCl containing heparin (100 U/ml). The perfusion volume (at a perfusion pressure of 40 mmHg) was four times the calculated blood volume of rat (7.46 ml/100 g b.w.). This procedure allows the removal of excess intravascular dye following which the lungs, kidneys, and ileum were dissected and removed. The tissues were rinsed in saline, gently blotted, and weighed. Half of each tissue was dried by incubation at 60 °C for 48 h. EB was extracted from the remaining halves by incubation in formamide (4 ml/g tissue; 99.5%, F-7503, Sigma Aldrich Chemie, Germany) at room temperature for 48 h. The supernatant was removed from the tissues and read against a formamide blank at 620 nm (Spectrophotometer, Beckmann DU 7400, Germany). Absorbance was compared to a standard curve of 0.05–50 μg ml^{-1} EB in formamide. Extravasation was expressed as microgram EB per gram dry tissue. The blood samples and parameters (MAP, MBF, and MVR) were obtained at 0′ (at the start of the experiment), 10′ (end of shock period), and 140′ (at 1 h after the end of resuscitation). The collection of blood samples (hemoglobin, partial pressure of oxygen, bicarbonates, base deficit, and lactate) and tissue specimens (lung, ileum, and kidney) in the S and HS groups was time-matched to the resuscitation groups.

Statistical analysis

The hemodynamic and metabolic variables were expressed as mean ± standard deviation. Multiple comparisons between groups of parametric data were carried out using one-way ANOVA, followed by the Bonferroni post hoc test. The level of significance was defined as a p value < 0.05. Data were analyzed by R 3.3.2 (R Foundation for Statistical Computing, Vienna, Austria, http://www.r-project.org).

Results

Hemodynamic parameters

The amount of shed blood was 8.0 ± 0.7 ml (26 ± 3.1 ml/kg b.w.); no differences in total blood loss were observed between the groups. MAP decreased from 105 ± 10 to 40 ± 4 mmHg after blood withdrawal (10′) in the hemorrhaged rats. At 140′, the MAP was higher in the vasopressin group than in the RL and RLB groups (102 ± 12.9, 55.5 ± 8.0, and 68.5 ± 10.3 mmHg, respectively, $p < 0.001$) (Fig. 2a).

At 10′, there were no differences in MBF among the hemorrhaged groups. At 140′, the MBF was higher in the RL and RLB groups when compared to the vasopressin group (4.5 ± 0.5, 5.2 ± 0.6, and 2.7 ± 0.3 ml/min, respectively, $p < 0.001$) (Fig. 2b).

At 10′, no differences in MVR (i.e., MAB/MBF) among the hemorrhaged groups were noted. At 140′, the MVR were increased only in the vasopressin group (34.5 ± 4.2 mmHg ml^{-1} min, $p < 0.001$) and remained unmodified in the RLB (13.1 ± 1.0 mmHg ml^{-1} min) and RL groups (12.4 ± 1.4 mmHg ml^{-1} min) (Fig. 2c). No mortality occurred during the experimental period.

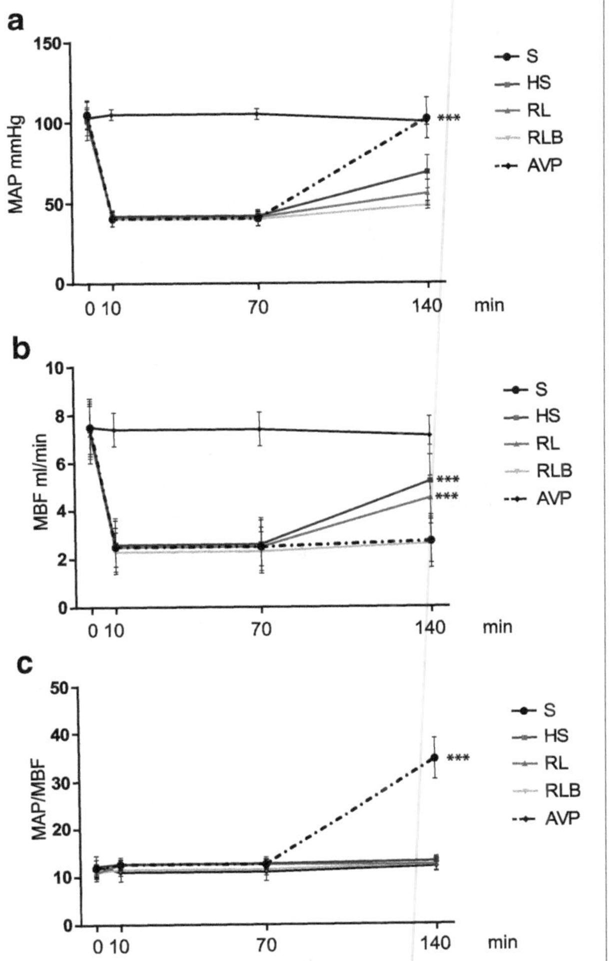

Fig. 2 Hemodynamic parameters. Data are represented as mean ± SD of mean arterial pressure (MAP) expressed as mmHg (**a**), mesenteric arterial blood flow (MBF) expressed as milliliters per minute (**b**), and MAP/MBF ratio (mmHg ml^{-1} min) (**c**). S, sham-operated; HS, hemorrhagic shock; RL, resuscitation with Ringer's lactate; RLB, resuscitation with Ringer's lactate and blood; AVP, resuscitation with Ringer's lactate and vasopressin infusion. **a** ***$p < 0.001$ AVP vs RL and RLB; **b** ***$p < 0.001$ RL and RLB vs AVP; **c** ***$p < 0.001$ AVP vs all

Laboratory data

Hemoglobin was decreased after hemorrhage and partially recovered at 140′ only in the RLB group ($p < 0.05$) (Fig. 3a). Likewise, the partial pressure of oxygen (pO_2) was partially recovered at 140′ in the RLB group only ($p < 0.05$). The pO_2 was significantly lowest in the vasopressin group when compared to the other groups ($p < 0.05$) (Fig. 3b).

At 10′, bicarbonate levels were decreased in all the groups (Fig. 4a), while base deficit (Fig. 4b) and lactate levels (Fig. 4c) were increased ($p < 0.001$). At 140′, bicarbonate levels were

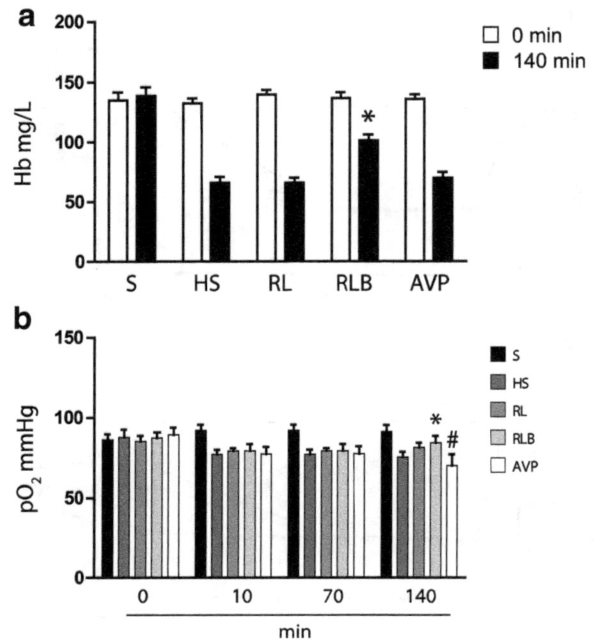

Fig. 3 Hemoglobin and partial pressure of oxygen. Data are represented as mean ± SD of hemoglobin (Hb) concentration expressed as milligrams per liter (**a**) and partial pressure of oxygen (pO_2) expressed as mmHg (**b**). S, sham-operated; HS, hemorrhagic shock; RL, resuscitation with Ringer's lactate; RLB, resuscitation with Ringer's lactate and blood; AVP, resuscitation with Ringer's lactate and vasopressin infusion. **a** *$p < 0.05$ RLB vs HS, RL, and AVP; **b** *$p < 0.05$ RLB vs HS and RL, #$p < 0.05$ AVP vs all

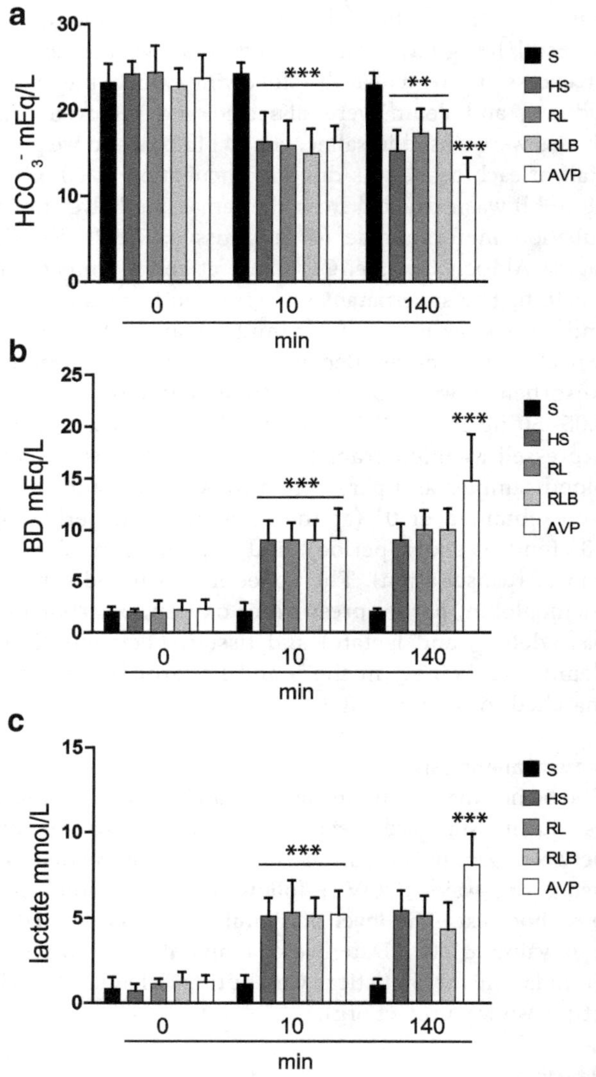

Fig. 4 Bicarbonates, base deficit, and lactate. Data are represented as mean ± SD of bicarbonate (HCO_3^-) levels expressed as milliequivalents per liter (**a**), base deficit (BD) levels expressed as mEq/l (**b**), and lactate levels expressed as millimoles per liter (**c**). S, sham-operated; HS, hemorrhagic shock; RL, resuscitation with Ringer's lactate; RLB, resuscitation with Ringer's lactate and blood; AVP, resuscitation with Ringer's lactate and vasopressin infusion. **a** ***$p < 0.001$ S vs all at 10′, **$p < 0.01$ HS, RL, and RLB vs S at 140′, ***$p < 0.001$ AVP vs all at 140′; **b** ***$p < 0.001$ S vs all at 10′, ***$p < 0.001$ AVP vs all at 140′; **c** ***$p < 0.001$ S vs all at 10′, ***$p < 0.001$ AVP vs all at 140′

persistently decreased in the HS, RL, and RLB groups ($p < 0.01$), and the vasopressin group ($p < 0.001$). A significant increase in base deficit was observed in the vasopressin group at 140′ when compared to the RL and RLB groups ($p < 0.001$). Furthermore, lactate levels were higher in the vasopressin group when compared to the RL and RLB groups at 140′ ($p < 0.001$).

Capillary leakage

Capillary leakage, evaluated as EB extravasation, was increased in the lung, ileum, and kidney in the HS group when compared to the S group ($p < 0.05$). In the lung, increased capillary leakage was observed in the RLB group when compared to the HS and RL groups ($p < 0.05$) and in the vasopressin group when compared to the HS and RL ($p < 0.01$) and RLB ($p < 0.05$) groups (Fig. 5a). In the ileum, increased capillary leakage was noted in the RLB group ($p < 0.05$) when compared to the HS and RL groups, whereas in the vasopressin group, the leakage was decreased when compared to the HS and RL ($p < 0.05$) and RLB ($p < 0.01$) groups (Fig. 5b). Increased capillary leakage was observed in the kidney in the RLB and vasopressin groups when compared to the HS and RL groups ($p < 0.05$) (Fig. 5c).

Discussion

Bleeding control, maintenance of tissue oxygenation with fluid resuscitation, coagulation support, and maintenance of normothermia remain the mainstays of therapy for patients with HS [2]. Maintenance of adequate perfusion pressure assists tissue oxygenation and reduces the risk of short- and long-term organ failure and sepsis. This practice has been challenged in both clinical trials and experimental

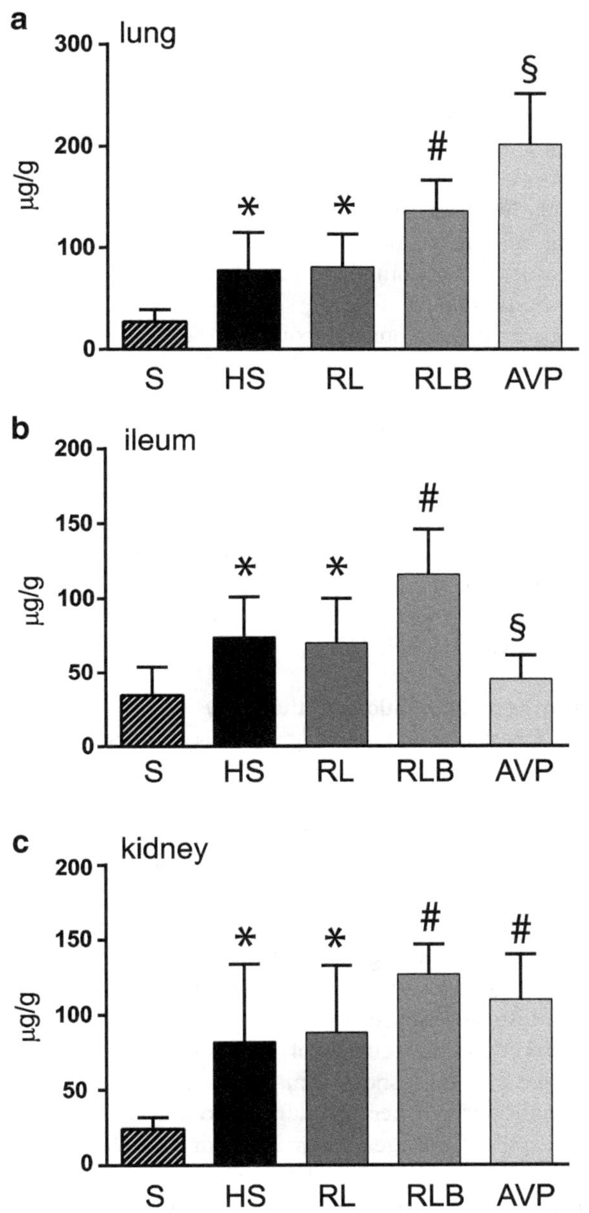

Fig. 5 Capillary leakage in the lung (**a**), ileum (**b**), and kidney (**c**). Data are expressed as mean ± SD of micrograms of Evans blue (EB) per gram of dried tissue. HS, hemorrhagic shock; RL, resuscitation with Ringer's lactate; RLB, resuscitation with Ringer's lactate and blood; AVP, resuscitation with Ringer's lactate and vasopressin infusion. **a** $^{*}p < 0.05$ HS and RL vs S; $^{\#}p < 0.05$ RLB vs HS and RL; $^{\S}p < 0.01$ AVP vs HS and RL and $p < 0.05$ AVP vs RLB; **b** $^{*}p < 0.05$ HS and RL vs S; $^{\#}p < 0.05$ RLB vs HS and RL; $^{\S}p < 0.05$ AVP vs HS and RL and $p < 0.01$ AVP vs RLB; **c** $^{*}p < 0.05$ HS and RL vs S; $^{\#}p < 0.05$ RLB and AVP vs HS and RL

models [17, 18]. After trauma, fluid infusion of large-volume normal saline or small-volume hypertonic saline solutions may result in side effects, such as tissue edema and re-bleeding with hemodynamic deterioration and increased mortality [19, 20].

The use of a vasopressor in case of vasodilatation or insufficient vasoconstriction is effective in restoring the hemodynamic parameters with adequate vital organ infusion, thereby reducing the need for continuous fluid infusion [21, 22]. Indeed, previous studies demonstrated increased survival when a small-volume fluid hypotensive resuscitation concept was used for penetrating trauma [23]. Several vasopressors including vasopressin have been studied in HS. Vasopressin acts via a number of receptors that are different from those of catecholamines. It exerts a direct vasoconstrictor effect on the systemic vascular smooth muscle by means of the vasopressin V1 receptors.

In our study, MAP was restored to baseline values only in the vasopressin group; administration of RL solution with or without blood did not obtain this effect. In the vasopressin group, we observed consistent vasoconstriction of the sub-diaphragmatic vascular bed, as demonstrated by the absence of improvement in MBF, leading to a significant increase in MVR. These results are consistent with those reported by Stadlbauer et al. [24].

In this study, we used an infusion rate of 0.04 U/kg/min which is much lower than the dose of vasopressin commonly used (i.e., 0.04 U/min) considering the rat median weight (i.e., 325 g). High amounts of vasopressin infusion were reported to be associated with detrimental side effects [8, 25].

Capillary permeability increases when there is damage or death of the endothelial cells and change in the intercellular space, rendering the endothelial cells and basement membrane less effective barriers to large molecules. Damage to the endothelial cells is initiated by an ischemia-reperfusion phenomenon, which promotes neutrophil activation and the release of proteases, oxygen radicals, and other toxic substances [26–28]. Various organs reveal different sensitivities to hypoxic-ischemic insult resulting in increased or decreased diffusion of macromolecules from the circulation into the interstitial space [29]. The initial phase of HS resuscitation comprises infusions of fluids, often leading to rapid tissue swelling, that may result in organ damage and dysfunction due to fluid and protein extravasation [30].

In the current study, HS alone was able to determine significant capillary leakage in the lung, ileum, and kidney, which was established by the albumin-bound EB extravasation in these organ tissues. Schumacher et al. also demonstrated significant capillary leakage in the lung and kidney in a similar HS experimental model [16]. In the vasopressin group, an increased capillary leakage, markedly higher than that in the group resuscitated with RL plus blood, was observed in the lung. This finding was also associated with a significant decrease in pO_2 in this group.

According to the equation by Starling, increase in vasopressin-induced capillary hydrostatic pressure determines the increase in capillary leakage, in the presence of a drop in plasma oncotic pressure owing to dilution of circulatory volume, protein loss, and extravascular leakage [30]. This is consistent with the results of the study by Stadlbauer et al., which asserts that one of the effects of vasopressin may be the shifting of blood away from below the diaphragm to above it with increased extravascular lung water [24].

Contrarily, Lee et al. [31] showed that the vasopressin group had lower pulmonary edema than the group resuscitated with RL and blood; however, the different experimental protocol (pulmonary edema formation was investigated 3 days after HS) used may account for this inconsistency. Feinstein et al., in an animal model of thoracic trauma and HS, showed that the early use of vasopressin improves lung function when compared to animals treated with fluids only [32]. This finding is not in conflict with our data because in that study, the animals were mechanically ventilated, whereas the rats in our study maintained spontaneous breathing throughout the experimental procedure. Actually, the positive pressure may have exerted a reduction in alveolar edema.

Interestingly, resuscitation with RLB was associated with increased capillary leakage in the ileum, whereas vasopressin use was accompanied by a decrease in leakage. However, the consistent vasoconstriction of mesenteric blood flow induced by vasopressin observed in our study may impair the gut mucosal perfusion. Stadlbauer et al. showed that infusion of vasopressin was followed by transient non-bloody diarrhea 3 h after stabilization, suggesting a potential gut ischemia [33].

In the present study, a similar increase in capillary leakage was noted in the kidney in the RLB and vasopressin groups. In the extracerebral tissues, vasopressin works primarily on the arterioles with less constriction on the coronary and renal vessels, thereby having vasodilatory effects on cerebral and pulmonary flow [34]. Besides, preservation of renal blood flow by vasopressin has been demonstrated in an experimental model of HS [35, 36].

In experimental models, early administration of vasopressors was able to restore a quasi-normal hemodynamic status by mobilizing non-constraint venous blood volume and thus normalizing hemodynamic parameters (arterial blood pressure, cardiac output, and pulse pressure variations) [37]. This masked hypovolemia was associated with deleterious effects of vasopressor use in experimental hemorrhage models, due to the worsening of tissue hypoperfusion leading to metabolic disturbances, such as metabolic acidosis [38, 39].

Interestingly, in the present study, we found significantly higher base deficit and lactate levels in the vasopressin group when compared to the other groups. This finding recognizes a multifactorial etiology. Recently, in a swine model of HS, Soller et al. [40] found that lactate is a predictor of mortality with an area under the ROC curve of 0.87. Besides, several studies have already identified worsening base deficit as an indicator of increased transfusion requirement [41, 42]. Furthermore, base deficit has been associated with increased mortality and intensive care unit and in-hospital lengths of stay, with a higher incidence of shock-related complications such as acute respiratory distress syndrome, renal failure, hemocoagulative disorders, and multiorgan failure [43]. Monitoring of base deficit has also been suggested as an indicator and a monitoring parameter for the success of resuscitation efforts [44].

On a final note, our controlled hemorrhage and resuscitation model does a good job of mimicking clinical reality, but we should make a strong case for translation of this research to humans. According to a very recent review [45], in HS, a successful resuscitation requires to stanch all sources of hemorrhage and rapidly restore the intravascular volume by a resuscitation approach that emphasizes the use of all blood products. However, vasopressin supplementation is considered a therapy that may reduce blood product and fluid requirements in patients with HS [45, 46].

Strengths and limitations of the study

To the best of our knowledge, this is the first study investigating the early effects of vasopressin on metabolic and hemodynamic parameters and endothelium permeability by measuring the capillary leakage in different organ tissues compared to those of other resuscitation strategies in a HS model.

This study has several limitations. First, we used a controlled hemorrhage model, not the same as free hemorrhage following injury. Second, we used a relatively small dose of vasopressin, less than is generally used in humans. Also, the effects of vasopressin infusion were observed only for a short-term period. Thus, the true clinical applicability is perhaps difficult to precise. Finally, we used capillary leakage as a marker for endothelium dysfunction in the experimental model; however, capillary leakage is not a "synonym" of organ dysfunction or damage. Indeed, histopathological and immunohistochemical analyses should be performed to evaluate the effects of vasopressin on organ damage or dysfunction.

Conclusions

Vasopressin was proposed as a vasoactive drug for provisional hemodynamic optimization in the early phase of HS resuscitation. In this study, vasopressin restored the MAP while causing a significant decrease in the mesenteric blood flow. In the vasopressin group, increased capillary leakage was observed in the lung, which was markedly higher than that in the group resuscitated with RL plus blood; this increase was also associated with a significant decrease in pO_2. Conversely, a decrease in capillary leakage was observed with vasopressin in the ileum. Lastly, we found that vasopressin use was associated with significantly higher base deficit and lactate levels when compared to the other groups.

In conclusion, vasopressin may be used as a bridge to definitive treatment for HS, but the overall findings of this experimental study focus on the possible critical side effects of vasopressin on metabolic parameters and endothelium permeability. Based on the available information and due to the small number of human studies on this issue, it is still controversial whether the use of vasopressin may positively impact on outcomes in uncontrolled bleeding patients. Thus, randomized controlled trials are needed to clarify the effects of vasopressin in HS [39, 47].

Abbreviations

b.w.: Body weight; EB: Evans blue; HS: Hemorrhagic shock; MAP: Mean arterial pressure; MBF: Mesenteric artery blood flow; MVR: Mesenteric vascular resistance; pO_2: Partial pressure of oxygen; RL: Ringer's lactate; RLB: Ringer's lactate and blood; S: Sham-operated

Acknowledgements

The authors would like to thank Enago (https://www.enago.com/) for the English language review.

Funding

None.

Authors' contributions

RB and PC designed and carried out the study and drafted the manuscript. AT performed the statistical analysis and drafted the figures. OC, SC, and GO participated in the study design and revised it critically for important intellectual content. All authors read and approved the final manuscript.

Competing interests

The authors declare that they have no competing interests.

Author details

[1]Department of Surgery, S. Giovanni Bosco Hospital, Turin, Italy. [2]Trauma Center and Metropolitan Trauma Network Department, Niguarda Hospital, Milan, Italy. [3]Department of Surgical Sciences, S. Giovanni Battista Hospital, University of Turin, Turin, Italy. [4]Department of Medical Sciences, University of Turin, Turin, Italy. [5]Department of Anesthesia and Intensive Care, S. Giovanni Battista Hospital, University of Turin, Via Giovanni Giolitti 9, 10123 Turin, Italy.

References

1. Kauvar DS, Lefering R, Wade CE. Impact of hemorrhage on trauma outcome: an overview of epidemiology, clinical presentations, and therapeutic considerations. J Trauma. 2006;60(6 Suppl):S3–11.
2. Rossaint R, Bouillon B, Cerny V, Coats TJ, Duranteau J, Fernández-Mondéjar E, et al. The European guideline on management of major bleeding and coagulopathy following trauma: fourth edition. Crit Care. 2016;20:100.
3. Landry DW, Oliver JA. The pathogenesis of vasodilatory shock. N Engl J Med. 2001;345:588–95.
4. Morales D, Madigan J, Cullinane S, Chen J, Heath M, Oz M, et al. Reversal by vasopressin of intractable hypotension in the late phase of hemorrhagic shock. Circulation. 1999;100:226–9.
5. Voelckel WG, Raedler C, Wenzel V, Lindner KH, Krismer AC, Schmittinger CA, et al. Arginine vasopressin, but not epinephrine, improves survival in uncontrolled hemorrhagic shock after liver trauma in pigs. Crit Care Med. 2003;31:1286–7.
6. Stadlbauer KH, Wagner-Berger HG, Raedler C, Voelckel WG, Wenzel V, Krismer AC, et al. Vasopressin, but not fluid resuscitation, enhances survival in a liver trauma model with uncontrolled and otherwise lethal hemorrhagic shock in pigs. Anesthesiology. 2003;98:699–704.
7. Dünser MW, Mayr AJ, Tür A, Pajk W, Barbara F, Knotzer H, et al. Ischemic skin lesions as complication of continuous vasopressin infusion in catecholamine-resistant vasodilatory shock: incidence and risk factors. Crit Care Med. 2003;31:1394–8.
8. Sperry JL, Minei JP, Frankel HL, West MA, Harbrecht BG, Moore EE, et al. Early use of vasopressors after injury: caution before constriction. J Trauma. 2008;64:9–14.
9. Collier B, Dossett L, Mann M, Cotton B, Guillamondegui O, Diaz J, et al. Vasopressin use is associated with death in acute trauma patients with shock. J Crit Care. 2010;25:173.e9–e14.
10. Brøchner AC, Toft P. Pathophysiology of the systemic inflammatory response after major accidental trauma. Scand J Trauma Resusc Emerg Med. 2009;17:43.
11. Shenkar R, Coulson WF, Abraham E. Hemorrhage and resuscitation induce alterations in cytokine expression and the development of acute lung injury. Am J Respir Cell Mol Biol. 1994;10:290–7.
12. Douzinas EE, Livaditi O, Tasoulis MK, Prigouris P, Bakos D, Goutas N, et al. Nitrosative and oxidative stresses contribute to post-ischemic liver injury following severe hemorrhagic shock: the role of hypoxemic resuscitation. PLoS One. 2012;7:e32968.
13. Oda M, Han JY, Nakamura M. Endothelial cell dysfunction in microvasculature: relevance to disease processes. Clin Hemorheol Microcirc. 2000;23:199–211.
14. Fishel RS, Are C, Barbul A. Vessel injury and capillary leak. Crit Care Med. 2003;31(8Suppl):S502–11.
15. Bini R, Cursio R, Belhacene N, Giudicelli J, Ferruà B, Olivero G, et al. Effect of caspase inhibition on thymic apoptosis in hemorrhagic shock. J Investig Surg. 2007;20:97–103.
16. Schumacher J, Binkowski K, Dendorfer A, Klotz KF. Organ-specific extravasation of albumin-bound Evans blue during nonresuscitated hemorrhagic shock in rats. Shock. 2003;20:565–8.
17. Mapstone J, Roberts I, Evans P. Fluid resuscitation strategies: a systematic review of animal trials. J Trauma. 2003;55:571–89.
18. Rhee P, Koustova E, Alam HB. Searching for the optimal resuscitation method: recommendations for the initial fluid resuscitation of combat casualties. J Trauma. 2003;54(5 Suppl):S52–62.
19. Solomonov E, Hirsh M, Yahiya A, Krausz M. The effect of vigorous fluid resuscitation in uncontrolled hemorrhagic shock after massive splenic injury. Crit Care Med. 2000;28:749–54.
20. Lucas CE, Ledgerwood AM. Physiology of colloid-supplemented resuscitation from shock. J Trauma. 2003;54(5 Suppl):S75–81.
21. Liu L, Tian K, Xue M, Zhu Y, Lan D, Peng X, et al. Small doses of arginine vasopressin in combination with norepinephrine "buy" time for definitive treatment for uncontrolled hemorrhagic shock in rat. Shock. 2013;40:398–406.
22. Dutton RP, Mackenzie CF, Scalea TM. Hypotensive resuscitation during active hemorrhage: impact on in-hospital mortality. J Trauma. 2002;52:1141–6.
23. Bickell WH, Wall MJ Jr, Pepe PE, Martin RR, Ginger VF, Allen MK, et al. Immediate versus delayed fluid resuscitation for hypotensive patients with penetrating torso injuries. N Engl J Med. 1994;331:1105–9.
24. Stadlbauer KH, Wenzel V, Krismer AC, Voelckel WG, Lindner KH. Vasopressin during uncontrolled hemorrhagic shock: less bleeding below the diaphragm, more perfusion above. Anesth Analg. 2005;101:830–2.
25. Malay MB, Ashton JL, Dahl K, Savage EB, Burchell SA, Ashton RC Jr, et al. Heterogeneity of the vasoconstrictor effect of vasopressin in septic shock. Crit Care Med. 2004;32:1327–31.
26. Reinhart K, Bayer O, Brunkhorst F, Meisner M. Markers of endothelial damage in organ dysfunction and sepsis. Crit Care Med. 2002;30(5 Suppl): S302–12.
27. Arumugam TV, Shiels IA, Woodruff TM, Granger DN, Taylor SM. The role of the complement system in ischemia-reperfusion injury. Shock. 2004; 21:401–9.

28. van Meurs M, Wulfert FM, Jongman RM, Schipper M, Houwertjes MC, Vaneker M, et al. Hemorrhagic shock-induced endothelial cell activation in a spontaneous breathing and a mechanical ventilation hemorrhagic shock model is induced by a proinflammatory response and not by hypoxia. Anesthesiology. 2011;115:474–82.
29. van Meurs M, Wulfert FM, Knol AJ, De Haes A, Houwertjes M, Aarts LP, et al. Early organ-specific endothelial activation during hemorrhagic shock and resuscitation. Shock. 2008;29:291–9.
30. Farand P, Hamel M, Lauzier F, Plante GE, Lesur O. Review article: organ perfusion/permeability related effects of norepinephrine and vasopressin in sepsis. Can J Anesth. 2006;53:934–46.
31. Lee CC, Lee MT, Chang SS, Lee SH, Huang YC, Yo CH, et al. A comparison of vasopressin, terlipressin, and lactated ringers for resuscitation of uncontrolled hemorrhagic shock in an animal model. PLoS One. 2014;9:e95821.
32. Feinstein AJ, Cohn SM, King DR, Sanui M, Proctor KG. Early vasopressin improves short-term survival after pulmonary contusion. J Trauma. 2005; 59:876–82.
33. Stadlbauer KH, Wenzel V, Wagner-Berger HG, Krismer AC, Konigsrainer A, Voelckel WG, et al. An observational study of vasopressin infusion during uncontrolled haemorrhagic shock in a porcine trauma model: effects on bowel function. Resuscitation. 2007;72:145–8.
34. Cossu AP, Mura P, De Giudici LM, Puddu D, Pasin L, Evangelista M, et al. Vasopressin in hemorrhagic shock: a systematic review and meta-analysis of randomized animal trials. Biomed Res Int. 2014;2014:421291.
35. Raedler C, Voelckel WG, Wenzel V, Krismer AC, Schmittinger CA, Herff H, et al. Treatment of uncontrolled hemorrhagic shock after liver trauma: fatal effects of fluid resuscitation versus improved outcome after vasopressin. Anesth Analg. 2004;98:1759–66.
36. Voelckel WG, Lindner KH, Wenzel V, Bonatti J, Hangler H, Frimmel C, et al. Effects of vasopressin and epinephrine on splanchnic blood flow and renal function during and after cardiopulmonary resuscitation in pigs. Crit Care Med. 2000;28:1083–8.
37. Hinder F, Stubbe HD, Van Aken H, Baba HA, Jahn UR, Brodner G, et al. Early multiple organ failure after recurrent endotoxemia in the presence of vasoconstrictor-masked hypovolemia. Crit Care Med. 2003; 31:903–9.
38. Johnson KB, Pearce FJ, Jeffreys N, McJames SW, Cluff M. Impact of vasopressin on hemodynamic and metabolic function in the decompensatory phase of hemorrhagic shock. J Cardiothorac Vasc Anesth. 2006;20:167–72.
39. Beloncle F, Mezia F, Lerolle N, Radermacher P, Asfar P. Does vasopressor therapy have an indication in hemorrhagic shock? Ann Intensive Care. 2013;3:13.
40. Soller B, Zou F, Prince MD, Dubick MA, Sondeen JL. Comparison of noninvasive pH and blood lactate as predictors of mortality in a swine hemorrhagic shock with restricted volume resuscitation model. Shock. 2015; 44(Suppl 1):90–5.
41. Davis JW, Parks SN, Kaups KL, Gladen HE, O'Donnell-Nicol S. Admission base deficit predicts transfusion requirements and risk of complications. J Trauma. 1996;41:769–74.
42. Rixen D, Raum M, Bouillon B, Lefering R, Neugebauer E. Base deficit development and its prognostic significance in posttrauma critical illness: an analysis by the trauma registry of the Deutsche Gesellschaft für Unfallchirurgie. Shock. 2001;15:83–9.
43. Rixen D, Siegel JH. Bench-to-bedside review: oxygen debt and its metabolic correlates as quantifiers of the severity of hemorrhagic and post-traumatic shock. Crit Care. 2005;9:441–53.
44. Mutschler M, Nienaber U, Brockamp T, Wafaisade A, Fabian T, Paffrath T, et al. Renaissance of base deficit for the initial assessment of trauma patients: a base deficit-based classification for hypovolemic shock developed on data from 16,305 patients derived from the Trauma Register DGU®. Crit Care. 2013;17:R42.
45. Cannon JW. Hemorrhagic shock. N Engl J Med. 2018;378(4):370–9.
46. Cohn SM, McCarthy J, Stewart RM, Jonas RB, Dent DL, Michalek JE. Impact of low-dose vasopressin on trauma outcome: prospective randomized study. World J Surg. 2011;35:430–9.
47. Gupta B, Garg N, Ramachandran R. Vasopressors: do they have any role in hemorrhagic shock? J Anaesthesiol Clin Pharmacol. 2017;33:3–8.

Three cases of resuscitative endovascular balloon occlusion of the aorta (REBOA) in austere pre-hospital environment—technical and methodological aspects

J. C. de Schoutheete[1,2*], I. Fourneau[3], F. Waroquier[1], L. De Cupere[1], M. O'Connor[4], K. Van Cleynenbreugel[1], J. C. Ceccaldi[1] and S. Nijs[2]

Abstract

Background: The present paper describes three cases where ER-REBOA® was used with partial aorta occlusion (AO), by performing a partial resuscitative endovascular balloon occlusion of the aorta or pREBOA, in an austere pre-hospital military environment.

In addition, because no specific REBOA algorithm for pre-hospital environment exists yet, this paper seeks to fill this gap, proposing a new pragmatic REBOA algorithm.

Methods: Belgian Special Operations Surgical Team applied REBOA in three patients according to a decisional algorithm, based on the MIST acronym used for trauma patients. Only 3 ml, in the first instance, was inflated in the balloon to get AO. The balloon was then progressively deflated, and reperfusion was tracked through changes of end-tidal carbon dioxide ($EtCO_2$).

Results: Systolic blood pressure (SBP) before ER-REBOA® placement was not higher than 60 mmHg. However, within the first 5 min after AO, SBP improved in all three cases. Due to the aortic compliance, a self-made pREBOA was progressively achieved while proximal SBP was raising with intravenous fluid infusion. Afterwards, during deflation, a steep inflection point was observed in SBP and $EtCO_2$.

Conclusions: ER-REBOA® is suitable for use in an austere pre-hospital environment. The MIST acronym can be helpful to select the patients for which it could be beneficial. REBOA can also be performed with pREBOA in a dynamic approach, inflating only 3 mL in the balloon and using the aortic compliance. Furthermore, while proximal SBP can be convenient to follow the occlusion, $EtCO_2$ can be seen as an easy and interesting marker to follow the reperfusion.

Keywords: Resuscitative endovascular balloon occlusion of the aorta, REBOA, Partial REBOA, Shock, Trauma, Pre-hospital, Austere surgery

* Correspondence: deschoutheete@outlook.com
[1]Burn Unit, Queen Astrid Military Hospital, B-1120 Brussels, Belgium
[2]Department of Trauma Surgery, University Hospitals Leuven, B-3000 Leuven, Belgium
Full list of author information is available at the end of the article

Background

Unlike the Combat Application Tourniquet which is now considered a gold standard in both military and civilian medicine as a proximal control for limb exsanguination in an austere environment or combat environment [1], there is currently no equivalent to control a massive non-compressible truncal bleeding until the patient gets surgical treatment.

The ER-REBOA® catheter [2] has recently been developed with the US department of Defense to fill this void [3]. The rationale is to temporary control the bleeding in the abdomen or pelvis using a resuscitative endovascular balloon occlusion of the aorta (REBOA) technique. This technique consists of placing a flexible catheter into the common femoral artery (CFA) rapidly, and maneuvering it into the aorta without using fluoroscopy and inflating a balloon at its tip. This stops blood flow beyond the balloon and thus arterial bleeding in the distal territory and, at the same time, increases afterload and thus coronary and cerebral perfusion. The balloon can either be placed into zone I or into zone III. Zone I extends from the origin of the left subclavian artery to the celiac artery. The balloon can be inflated there in case of intra-abdominal bleeding, e.g., a liver or splenic injury. Zone II extends from the celiac artery to the lowest renal artery. Zone III extends from the lowest renal artery to the aortic bifurcation [4]. A proximal control of a bleeding caused by a pelvic fracture can be achieved with balloon inflation in this zone.

Because of the ischemia in the distal tissues, this occlusion can only be a temporary maneuver. Total occlusion time is still debated but Irahara et al. [5] and Tsurukiri et al. [6] both described a significantly shorter total occlusion time in the survivor group than in the non-survivor group with 46.2 ± 15.0 vs. 224.1 ± 52.1 min ($p = .002$) and 54 ± 10 vs. 90 ± 27 min, respectively.

Nevertheless, it has recently been shown that REBOA can successfully be applied even in the case of an abdominal venous bleeding in a swine model. REBOA improves hemodynamics and lengthens survival time. Blood loss is similar between groups but the rate of bleeding is markedly decreased with REBOA. REBOA appears effective for central venous injuries and provides a sustained period of stabilization and an extended window for surgical intervention [7].

However, even if the REBOA is used in a variety of clinical settings to successfully elevate central blood pressure in the setting of shock [8–10], the evidence base is weak in trauma, with no demonstrated reduction in hemorrhage-related mortality [11]. Moreover, literature shows a mortality of 65% [12]. The cause of such a high mortality rate, even if not described, can potentially come from multiple organ failure, caused by ischemia-reperfusion injury of more than half the body, in particular in visceral organs, if the balloon is placed in zone I [13, 14].

Therefore, in order to reduce this mortality rate, it has recently been suggested to use a partial aorta occlusion (AO) with partial REBOA (pREBOA) to maintain the proximal systolic blood pressure (SBP) higher than 90 mmHg [15, 16]. Partial REBOA results in maintenance of near-baseline carotid blood flow and central mean arterial pressure, while complete REBOA (cREBOA) generates extreme central mean arterial pressure and prolonged supraphysiologic carotid blood flow, as Russo et al. [17] showed. Moreover, less rebound hypotension after balloon deflation is seen in the pREBOA compared with cREBOA groups. Complete REBOA resulted in higher serum lactate than both pREBOA and controls ($p < .01$). Histology reveals early necrosis and disruption of duodenal mucosa in all cREBOA animals, but none in pREBOA animals [8]. In another paper by Matsumura et al. [18], pREBOA results in a better hemodynamic response than cREBOA (improvement in hemodynamics, 92% vs 70%, $p = .004$; achievement of stability, 78% vs 51%, $p = .007$) and allows for longer occlusion duration (median 58 vs 33 min, $p = .041$).

Nevertheless, if Russo defines pREBOA as a partially inflated balloon until a 50% proximal to distal aortic pressure gradient is achieved (this aortic pressure gradient is measured and maintained continuously by manual adjustment of balloon inflation volume), Matsumura gives another definition (a gradual deflation of the balloon in small steps of 1–3 mL, after confirmation of hemodynamic stabilization, aiming to keep SBP at > 90 mmHg).

However, even if the definition of pREBOA varies between authors, it seems to give better results than a cREBOA. In addition to the better hemodynamic response, a pREBOA allows hemostasis through coagulation factors as well. This cannot be achieved if the flow is stopped due to a total AO.

As patients getting REBOA are intubated and ventilated, end-tidal carbon dioxide ($EtCO_2$) can be monitored, as already described in the swine model [19]. $EtCO_2$ is indeed the partial pressure of carbon dioxide (CO_2) in respiratory gases at the completion of an exhaled breath. Normal values vary from 35 to 40 mmHg. These values reflect cardiac output, production of CO_2 and alveolar function. When cardiac output is reduced, CO_2 delivery to the lungs decreases and $EtCO_2$ decreases as well [20]. Moreover, there is a correlation between $EtCO_2$ and lactic acidosis [21]. And there is also a strong positive correlation between total occlusion time with REBOA and lactate concentration ($p = .02$) [6]. In this emergency configuration, when intubated, the alveolar function of the patient is defined by the respiratory machine. If the settings of the respirator are not modified, only changes in cardiac output and production of CO_2 are influencing the $EtCO_2$. However, during balloon deflation, changes in cardiac output are visible on the monitoring following the SBP. So, reperfusion can be tracked through changes of $EtCO_2$.

Besides this, from a technical point of view, a 7-French sheath compatible REBOA catheter is commercialized in the USA since 2015, which needs only manual compression as closing technique and no closing device due to the diameter. Before that, only minimum 12-French sheath systems existed, and a surgical closure or the use of a closure device was required. Even if the surgeon still has to be able to deal with potential complications, like ongoing bleeding from the puncture point, false aneurysm, artery dissection, thrombo-embolism, or limb-threatening ischemia, the use of this 7-French sheath facilitates the use of REBOA in less technical environments. Moreover, as shown previously by Stensaeth et al. [22], it is possible to use this REBOA catheter without fluoroscopy. Another specific feature of this catheter, which makes it particularly suitable for use in an austere pre-hospital environment, is its self-guiding property in the aorta with its atraumatic tip, hence avoiding the need for a guide wire. Members of a US Air Force Special Operations Surgical Team (SOST) have recently used the ER-REBOA® in an austere military setting [23]. They used a hand-held ultrasound to diagnose hemoperitoneum performing a focused abdominal sonography for trauma (FAST) examination and to facilitate a 7-French femoral sheath access in the CFA. They obtained good results with no access- or REBOA-related complications and with all of their four patients surviving transport to the next echelon of care in stable condition. Besides that paper, Northern et al. described the use of 20 REBOAs in an austere pre-hospital environment by the US Air Force SOSTs [24]. They concluded that REBOA can be used as a pro-active resuscitation strategy and that the proficiency of non-surgeon physicians in the placement of REBOA is a force multiplier. To our knowledge, these are the only pre-hospital experience with the one of the London's Air Ambulance, although limited to one blind positioning in zone III only [25].

Taking that into consideration, the present paper describes three cases where ER-REBOA® was used in an austere pre-hospital military environment. A dynamic approach, doing on the one hand a pREBOA by inflating or deflating the balloon to keep the SBP not higher than 90 mmHg as well as using on the other hand the aortic compliance, defined as the ability of a vessel to distend and increase volume with increasing transmural pressure or the tendency of a vessel to resist recoil toward its original dimensions on application of a distending or compressing force, was chosen here.

Methods

Belgian SOST

Our SOST is a specialized team (comprising a trauma surgeon, an anesthetist, a scrub nurse, an emergency anesthesia and critical care registered nurse, and a paramedic as well as a special force combat medic) providing triage, damage control resuscitation (DCR), and damage control surgery (DCS) in an austere military environment. The team members are trained to deal with forward surgical care. Patients included in the present case series were treated in a casualty collection point (CCP), close to the front line where triage, DCR, and DCS could be performed, in accordance to the NATO doctrine about forward surgical element [26]. Neither X-ray nor laboratory tests were available. The only available technical investigation was ultrasound. The goal of deploying a SOST is to diminish the evacuation time until surgery and to allow a rapid stabilization of unstable patients, which would otherwise die during evacuation to a conventional medical treatment facility (MTF) [26]. On average, about 90 casualties were treated weekly at the location of the SOST. DCS proved necessary for an average of eight cases a week. Three patients were treated with a REBOA according to the decisional algorithm detailed in the next paragraph.

Treatment rationale using REBOA

Due to the lack of diagnostic devices, the high inflow of patients and the limited capacity of the surgical team, a pragmatic approach was required to use REBOA in the right patient. Therefore, ER-REBOA® was placed according to the following algorithm, depicted in Fig. 1 and based on the MIST acronym [27].

- Mechanism of injury: high-energy trauma (potentially causing penetration)
- Injury: following wounds localization and FAST examination in order to exclude any bleeding injury above the diaphragm
- Signs: shock, traditionally defined as SBP < 90 mmHg [28]

Afterwards, for the algorithm-elected patients, a pREBOA strategy following Matsumura et al. [18] was used. That means a gradual deflation of the balloon in small steps of 1–3 mL, after confirmation of hemodynamic stabilization, aiming to keep SBP at > 90 mmHg.

However, the first inflation of the balloon to get AO was smaller in our experience than that described by the ER-REBOA® company [2]. Instead of inflating height milliliters and then checking the effect on SBP, only 3 mL were used here in the first instance to get AO. Doing this, it was possible to use the vasoconstriction/vasodilatation of the aorta to perform a pREBOA. At the beginning, AO was achieved flushing 3 mL in the balloon because the hypovolemic patient was in vasoconstriction. At the same time, intravenous (IV) fluids and blood products were given, increasing the intravascular volume above the balloon. When the proximal SBP had increased, the balloon

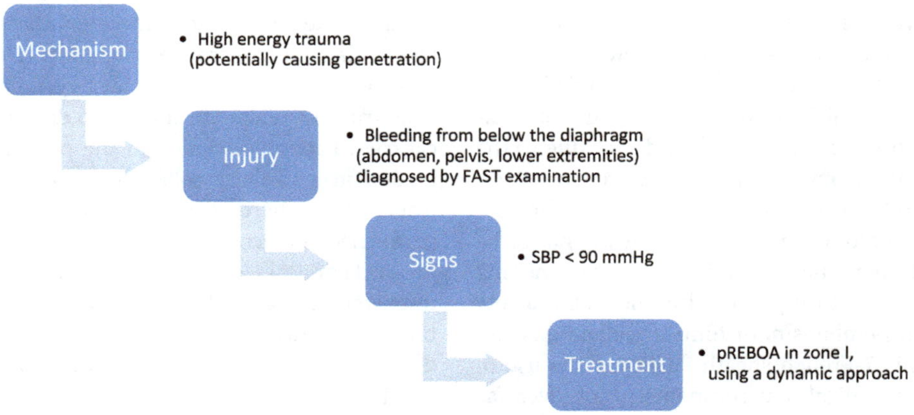

Fig. 1 Proposed algorithm for the placement of REBOA catheters in pre-hospital. Due to a lack of diagnostic devices in pre-hospital settings, in-hospital algorithms [45] are impossible to implement. Nevertheless, a pragmatic approach is required to use REBOA in the right patient. Therefore, REBOA catheters can be placed according to this algorithm based on the MIST acronym, widely accepted in pre-hospital care, and quickly useable by any medical provider, regardless of his training level

inflation was insufficient to keep a total AO and permitted some leakage, hence creating a self-made pREBOA through aortic compliance.

The pREBOA, obtained by a combination of small inflation and aortic compliance, brought about a dynamic approach.

Technique

First of all, it was essential to exclude cardiac tamponade and tension pneumothorax during the primary survey, prior to initiating a REBOA therapy. After that, an ER-REBOA® was inserted in all patients with SBP < 90 mmHg due to high-energy trauma below the diaphragm. Procedure was performed by the surgeon, helped by the scrub nurse. If blind percutaneous arterial access could not be achieved in 30 s, a cut-down procedure at the level of the CFA was performed. The idea was to avoid wasting time with only one technique—the percutaneous one—if it was not immediately successful. A super Arrow-Flex sheath introducer, 7-French (CP-07711), was systematically used. After sheath placement, only external anatomic landmarks [29] were used to position the REBOA catheter. Because the ER-REBOA ® balloon is not positioned at the end of the catheter, it is recommended to place the proximal edge of the balloon at the xiphoid level when measuring for positioning in zone I and to place the proximal edge of the balloon just above the umbilicus when measuring for positioning in zone III [30]. Fixation of the sheath in soft tissues and of the catheter on the skin was performed using Ethilon ® 2/0 sutures. After positioning of the catheter in the aorta, the balloon was inflated with 3 mL to cause total AO but permitting a dynamic approach as described earlier. The right effect of the REBOA balloon was controlled by direct view and/or palpation (depending on the access technique) of the gradual loose of pulsation in the CFA during inflation of the balloon. Later during surgery, the right position of the REBOA balloon was checked by manual palpation of a pulseless aorta just under the diaphragm, the balloon being placed in zone I. Because full deflation of the balloon at once may result in reperfusion injury, causing washout of metabolic byproducts and acidosis, saline was progressively (over 30 min) removed from the balloon as soon as possible during surgery to keep a SBP around 90 mmHg. Effects of balloon deflation on patients were constantly followed by heart rate (HR), SBP, and $EtCO_2$. After full deflation, the catheter was removed. Hence, the sheath was withdrawn under visual control, and the artery was closed using one or two Prolene® 5/0 sutures. Indeed, considering the unknown delay to transport the patient to the next MTF, in which circumstances the transport would happen, and if a vascular surgeon would be available at the next local MTF, it was decided not to use a manual compression to close the CFA.

Results

REBOA insertion procedure and technique (resumed in Table 1)

Percutaneous access was started in all cases but was only successful for one case under the first 30 s. A cut-down procedure was thus used in the two other cases. Total time needed to get AO varied between 5 min in the fastest case and 9 min in the slowest case. For the first patient, 8 min were needed because it was the first time the team, surgeon excepted, performed the procedure. The slowest ER-REBOA® placement, for the second patient, took 9 min because the surgical instruments were at that time in the autoclave for sterilization, slowing the cut-down procedure. Five minutes were needed for the third patient. No balloon migration was observed after inflation. Due probably to hypovolemia, a balloon inflation of 3 mL was

Table 1 REBOA procedures for the patients who required it following the presented algorithm

REBOA procedure	Patient 1	Patient 2	Patient 3
Technique for arterial access	Percutaneous	Cut-down	Cut-down
Volume inflated in balloon to get total AO	3 mL	3 mL	3 mL
Landing zone	Zone I	Zone I	Zone I
Duration of AO with 3 ml	30 min	30 min	34 min
Duration of balloon deflation	35 min	28 min	25 min
Site closure	Stitch	Stitch	Patch
Site complication	None	Thrombosis	Thrombosis

sufficient to get a total AO. The AO was maintained during approximately 30 min with a balloon inflated with 3 ml, and after that, the balloon was gradually deflated over approximately 30 min in all three cases. During the time the balloon was in place, DCR and DCS more particularly were performed.

Clinical evolution

All three patients had a high-velocity penetrating trauma, due to an improvised explosive device or gunshot wound. For so far known, they did not have prior history of peripheral vascular disease. The patients were brought to the SOST location directly from the point of injury by non-governmental organization ambulances. Transport time was about 20 min. Cardio-pulmonary resuscitation was not needed during transport. When arriving at the CCP, SBP before ER-REBOA® placement was not measurable and neither was carotid pulse felt in two patients. For the third one, SBP was 60 mmHg. However, within the first 5 min after AO, SBP improved in all cases but it was not higher than 90 mmHg in this first occlusion period. The SBP reached 90 mmHg after a maximum of 34 min after AO. IV fluids and blood products given varied from 3 to 4 L and from 1 to 2 L, respectively. Additionally, vasopressors were also required for two patients to keep SBP high enough, as depicted in Table 2. Surgical hemorrhage control delay varied from 26 to 135 min after AO, depending on the procedures performed: either liver packing and pelvic packing or pelvic packing and contralateral CFA shunting. The abbreviated injury scale (AIS) [31], the injury severity score (ISS) [32], the new ISS (NISS) [33], and the trauma injury severity score (TRISS) [34] were calculated and are detailed in Fig. 2. After sheath removal, two patients developed a thrombosis at the site of sheath placement. One developed it during DCS, when the sheath was in place (patient 3); the other one developed it 1 day later (patient 2). Regarding patient 2, the thrombosis was due to a technical error: the artery had to be closed in quick and dirty circumstances during an evacuation. That limb-threatening, but not life-threatening, complication was managed during the DCS procedure for patient 3 and at the Role 3 MTF for patient 2. Overall, the time at CCP was about 2 h for two patients; the third one stayed about 4 h and 30 min before transfer to the next MTF. Timelines are summarized in Table 3.

Evolution in SBP and $EtCO_2$ over time

Three parameters were followed during the intervention: HR, SBP, and $EtCO_2$. Looking at HR evolution, as in Fig. 3, no trend can be observed. However, the two other parameters can be described.

a. SBP (evolution resumed in Fig. 4)

SBP rose in all cases after balloon inflation. Then, after deflation, SBP further rose in two cases but not in the third one (patient 2). In that one, SBP before starting REBOA was 60 mmHg. Even if SBP rose to 90 mmHg after inflation, it dropped to 60 mmHg afterwards when the balloon was deflated. This happened because surgery had to be interrupted and the catheter had to be removed because the medical evacuation helicopter was coming. Epinephrine 1 mg was then given twice in the next minutes after full deflation to keep SBP as high as possible. Besides the role of ER-REBOA® to maintain an

Table 2 Damage control resuscitation regarding the patients who got a REBOA

Damage control resuscitation	Patient 1	Patient 2	Patient 3
Mechanism of injury	Mounted improvised explosive device	Dismounted improvised explosive device	Gunshot wound
Tranexamic acid	1 g	1 g	1 g
Antibiotics	Cefazolin 2 g Metronidazole 500 mg	Cefazolin 1 g Metronidazole 500 mg	Cefazolin 2 g Metronidazole 500 mg
Vasopressors	None	Epinephrin 1 mg × 2 Phenylephrin 100 μg × 4	Phenylephrin 100 μg × 10
Crystalloids	3 L	3.5 L	4 L
Blood products	2 FWB	4 FWB	2 FWB 3 PRBC
Estimated blood loss	2 L	3 L	4 L

Patient 1
male, 25 years
ISS: 21 - NISS: 29
TRISS: 81.76%

- FACE: Skin : 1 (laceration, minor)
- THORAX: Pneumothorax : 2
- ABDOMEN: Spleen : 4 (major devascularization) + Omentum : 2 (minor laceration) + Colon : 3 (full thickness laceration >50 of circumference without transection) + Mesentery: 2 (laceration, minor)
- EXTREMITIES: Penetrating injury shoulder: 1 + Penetrating injury above knee and below hip: 1

Patient 2
female, 54 years
ISS: 66 - NISS: 66
TRISS: 15.21%

- NECK: Thyroid artery : 2 (laceration, blood loss <20% by volume)
- THORAX: Pneumothorax : 2
- ABDOMEN: Jejunum-Ileum: 4 (transections) + Liver: 3 (>3cm parenchymal depth) + Colon: 3 (perforation, multiple) + Bladder: 3 (rupture) + Rectum: 5 (massive laceration)
- EXTREMITIES: Pelvic ring: 5 (incomplete disruption of posterior arch, large pelvic hematoma)
- EXTERNAL: Whole Body (explosion-type) injury: 4 (major (>25% TBSA) to skin, subcutaneous tissue and muscle with multiple fractures and multiple organ injuries

Patient 3
male, 40 years
ISS: 20 - NISS: 29
TRISS: 78.19%

- ABDOMEN: Retroperitoneum hematoma: 2
- EXTREMITIES: Femoral artery: 4 (transection with segmental loss, blood loss >20% by volume) + Penetrating injury above knee, below hip: 3 (blood loss >20% by volume) + Pelvic ring fracture: 2

Fig. 2 Abbreviated Injury Scale, Injury Severity Score, New Injury Severity Score, and Trauma Injury Severity Score (% of survival) of the three patients. Due to a lack of diagnostic devices, some lesions were missed. The calculated scores are therefore most probably underestimated

acceptable SBP, other adjuncts were simultaneously used as illustrated in patient 3. Because in that case, SBP was still less than 90 mmHg 30 min after full AO, fluids, blood transfusion, and phenylephrine were given and the deflation process was started. Direct proximal arterial control was achieved 5 min later by clamping the contralateral CFA just above a traumatic transection of that vessel. The balloon was then deflated to 1 mL and not fully deflated because SBP was only 90 mmHg at that time, and blood flow was coming back in the leg where the sheath was placed, causing more hypotension. The idea was to deal with reperfusion gradually. Twenty-five minutes later, full deflation occurred. The consequent dropping SBP was here again compensated giving phenylephrine.

Table 3 Timelines at CCP. Times are noted in minutes from the time at admission

Events	Patient 1	Patient 2	Patient 3
Start of AO procedure	71	15	9
Successful AO	79	24	14
Start of surgery	94	26	41
Hemodynamic stability (90 mmHg)	109	24	48
Definitive hemorrhage control	104	50	183
End of surgery	174	105	243
Evacuation	184	115	263

b. $EtCO_2$ (evolution resumed in Fig. 5)

$EtCO_2$ has not yet been used as parameter to follow reperfusion when the balloon is progressively deflated. Three different curves were observed for the three patients.

For patient 1, $EtCO_2$ rose from 36 to 46 after the first deflation. Then, it took 45 min to go back from 46 to 36. The last $EtCO_2$ of 39 cannot be correlated to the other ones because the patient was waking up. He was then not on the respiratory machine anymore, and the respiration rate was influencing the $EtCO_2$ at that moment.

On another side, for patient 2, it is important to notice that the first $EtCO_2$ measured was 28, which is quite low, potentially because the patient was hypothermic and hypovolemic at that moment. A deflation from 3 to 2 mL did not affect $EtCO_2$ so much, the other ones did affect, rising from 29 to 35 and then to 42.

However, for patient 3, $EtCO_2$ was relatively stable, varying from 32 to 39.

Discussion

When to place the REBOA catheter in pre-hospital?

Due to the austere environment, prioritization to allow for the most adequate resource allocation is key. For example, the time between admission at CCP and start of AO procedure was 71 min for patient 1. This is quite a long time, but it is because the SOST was operating on

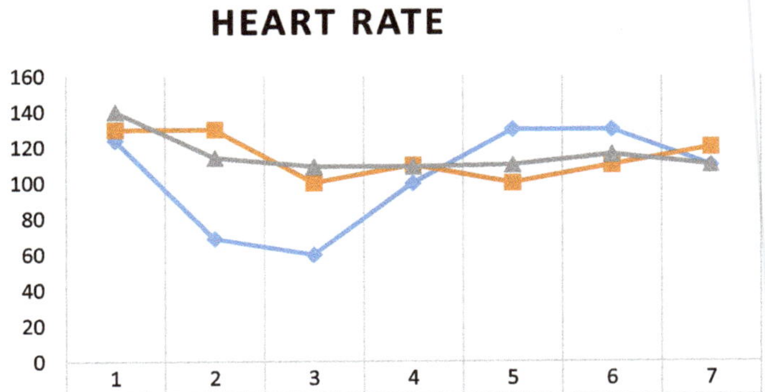

	1	2	3	4	5	6	7
Patient 1	124	69	60	100	130	130	110
Patient 2	130	130	100	110	100	110	120
Patient 3	140	114	109	/	110	116	110

Fig. 3 Heart rate during REBOA procedure. 1—at admission, 2—before REBOA, 3—within the first 5 min after AO, 4—after deflation of 1 cc (2 cc were directly deflated for patient 3), 5—after deflation of 2 cc, 6—after full deflation, and 7—at the end of the surgery

another patient when patient 1 arrived. As already suggested [24], the placement by someone else than the surgeon could have speeded up the treatment of the patient.

Due to a lack of diagnostic devices, usual in-hospital algorithms [4, 35] are impossible to implement. Nevertheless, a pragmatic approach is required to apply REBOA to the right patient. Therefore, ER-REBOA® was placed according to the algorithm depicted in Fig. 1 and based on the MIST acronym [27]. In a pre-hospital setting, the tactical combat casualty care guidelines [1] are required to stop a massive external bleeding at the level of the limbs or REBOA for massive non-compressible truncal bleeding below the diaphragm. Thereby, limited resources like blood can be spared and the patient can reach a conventional MTF where more diagnostic options exist and where further treatment can be given using more resources. Therefore, to be able to act quickly and to make it understandable to all medical care providers, no matter what their training level is, the idea of following the MIST acronym allows for a fast decision-making tool. Here, we used only three packed red blood cells (PRBC) and eight fresh whole blood (FWB) to keep the three patients alive, even with an ISS score between 20 and 66. This highlights the importance of the availability of FWB, as also by the US Air Force observed [24].

Percutaneous placement or cut-down procedure?

Data from the American Association for the Surgery of Trauma showed that a cut-down procedure is performed in 50% of cases, a percutaneous placement without

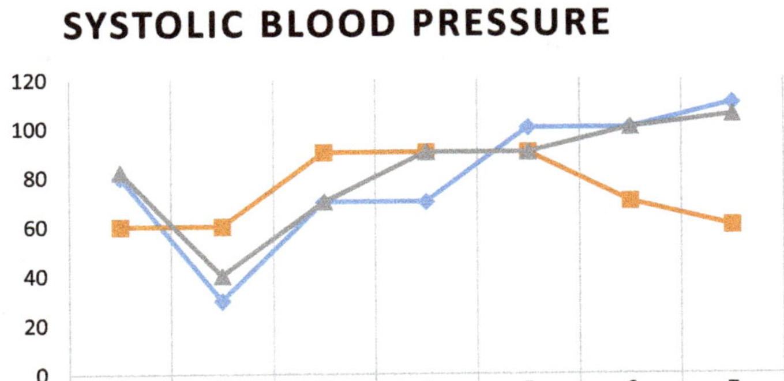

	1	2	3	4	5	6	7
Patient 1	80	NM	70	70	100	100	110
Patient 2	60	60	90	90	90	70	60
Patient 3	82	NM	70	/	90	100	105

Fig. 4 Systolic blood pressure during REBOA procedure. 1—at admission, 2—before REBOA (NM = not measurable for patients 1 and 3), 3—within the first 5 min after AO, 4—after deflation of 1 cc (2 cc were directly deflated for patient 3), 5—after deflation of 2 cc, 6—after full deflation, and 7—at the end of the surgery

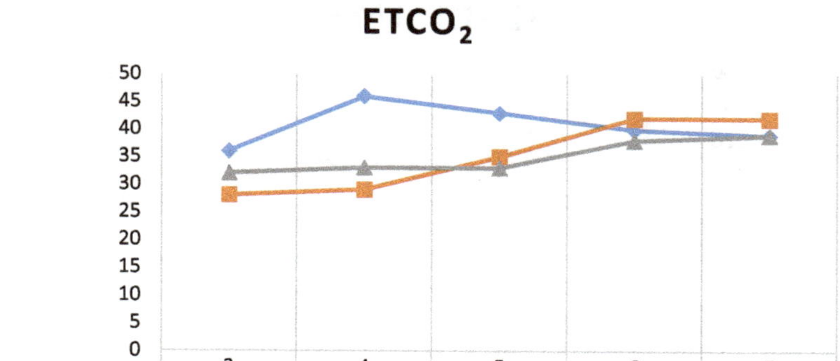

	3	4	5	6	7
Patient 1	36	46	43	40	39
Patient 2	28	29	35	42	42
Patient 3	32	/	33	38	39

Fig. 5 End-tidal carbon dioxide during REBOA procedure. Values at admission and before REBOA were not measured. 3—within the first 5 min after AO, 4—after deflation of 1 cc (2 cc were directly deflated for patient 3), 5—after deflation of 2 cc, 6—after full deflation, 7—at the end of the surgery. A steep inflection point can be observed in 4 for patient 1 and in 6 for the other patients

imaging in 28.3% of cases, and finally, 10.9% of cases are ultrasound guided [36]. This last option was used by the US Air Force SOST [23] to facilitate the femoral sheath access. We used another strategy because ultrasound control was seen as a time-consuming adjunct. If blind percutaneous arterial access could not be achieved in 30 s, then a cut-down procedure at the level of the CFA was performed. This "30-s" window was actually decided to let the surgeon already start with the percutaneous procedure and in parallel let the paramedic find and prepare the instruments for a cut-down procedure, hence avoiding preparation delays. Moreover, cut-down procedure was not seen as a failed procedure because open CFA closure was anyway planned in all cases. So, cut-down procedures were here seen as a helpful way to visualize the loose of pulsation in CFA when inflating the balloon. In addition, the placing of catheters by cut-down procedure was not very time-consuming. The same range of time in a pre-hospital configuration was described by the US team [23] using hand-held ultrasound. Romagnoli et al. [37] performed a resuscitative thoracotomy in a median time of 5.28 min and a REBOA in a median time of 7.9 min, but in a hospital.

Steep inflection point?

The biggest impact of AO on SBP for patient 2 was noticed when the last milliliter was removed from the balloon, suggesting first an important role of partial AO on the stability of the patient and second a nonlinear correlation between AO and SBP. This observation has actually been described by Davidson et al. [38] in a swine model where a steep inflection point occurs during balloon deflation that results in an abrupt increase in aortic flow and a concomitant decrease in mean arterial pressure. Furthermore, the onset of distal aortic flow was inconsistent across study animals and did not correlate with initial balloon volume or relative deflation volume.

Because HR and $EtCO_2$ were recorded here, measurements can be matched with SBP at the same moment. Thus, for patient 1, a deflation from 3 to 2 mL did affect HR and $EtCO_2$ much more than the other deflations. This observation suggests that the steep inflection point described for SBP could be followed by HR and $EtCO_2$ as well. For patient 2, even if a deflation from 3 to 2 mL did not affect $EtCO_2$ so much, the other ones did affect, raising from 29 to 35 and then to 42. The steep inflection point was then seen when deflating the last milliliter from the balloon, as written here above. Here, only a minimal raise of HR was observed at the same moment. For patient 3, even if $EtCO_2$ was relatively stable, varying from 32 to 39, a steep inflection point could be seen again when full deflation occurred. Identically, HR was stable but rose a bit at the moment of full deflation as well. However, this was less marked than for the two other patients.

Manual compression or surgical closure?

When a cut-down procedure is performed to place the sheath, there is no other choice than to surgically close the CFA. However, for the third patient, both options were available. Even if the ER-REBOA® is placed using a 7-French sheath, which allows for manual compression instead of a closing device, the surgical team is confronted to some important questions about the continuum of care in austere circumstances. Who will take care of the patient at a next local MTF? When will the patient arrive at the next local MTF? Do they have ultrasound at the next local MTF? What will happen if the CFA is bleeding during a difficult transport? Will the local ambulance team be able to deal with a bleeding? Will the patient not bleed due to trauma-related coagulopathy?

However, we observed a thrombosis in two of our patients, one before surgical closure and one after. The latter was due to a technical error, and no clear cause was identified for the former. This can perhaps be linked to a mix of a hypercoagulation status due to stress, fresh whole blood transfusion, vasopressors, and tranexamic acid.

But our data, although limited, are in contradiction with other authors who observed no complication related to sheath insertion or removal, including dissection, pseudoaneurysm, retroperitoneal hematoma, leg ischemia, or distal embolism [9, 39].

To leave the material in place for transport to next MTF?

One patient (patient 2) was transported to a NATO Role 2 MTF. There, the patient was reanimated. During reanimation, the surgeon removed the abdominal temporary closure device and compressed directly with his hand the aorta just under the diaphragm. The patient could recover and was then transported to a Role 3 MTF where further surgery and medical treatment was given until transport to a Role 4 MTF at day 4 post injury. This situation raises some considerations.

It would have been easier to monitor SBP if the sheath was left in place for transport. Moreover, it would have been easier to keep the patient stable with the catheter in place, still allowing some perfusion of distal tissue doing pREBOA. This could potentially have permitted a straight evacuation to the Role 3 MTF without any stop at the Role 2 MTF. This means that the patient has been brought faster to an MTF with a higher level of care. However, personnel need first to be confident with REBOA, being then able to take care of the catheter during transport. Second, if short transport is not possible, the evacuation team needs to be comfortable with flushing the sheath with saline on the 20 min to avoid thrombosis. Third, the transport team needs to be trained for potential massive CFA bleeding if there is any movement on the sheath causing a leak.

Which training and for whom?

Eastridge et al. [40] showed in a study about battlefield fatalities that 87.3% of all injury mortality occurred in the pre-MTF environment and that 24.3% were deemed potentially survivable. The injury/physiologic focus of potentially survivable acute mortality was largely associated with hemorrhage (90.9%). Furthermore, the site of lethal hemorrhage was truncal (67.3%), followed by junctional (19.2%) and peripheral-extremity (13.5%) hemorrhage. This means that it could be interesting to train pre-MTF personnel (e.g., SOST) to REBOA skills to reduce that potentially survivable acute mortality.

Virtual reality simulation showed good results in learning damage control endovascular procedures to doctors without any REBOA experience [41], reducing procedural task times (the task began when the guide wire entered the femoral arterial catheter and ended with the inflation of the balloon) from more than 4 min the first time to 2 min the sixth time. Besides this simulation, other possibilities exist as well like the endovascular skills for trauma and resuscitative surgery curriculum [42] or the endovascular and hybrid trauma and bleeding management workshop [43]. However, nothing about the skill decay in time has been described yet.

In our experience, REBOA procedure was reduced from 8 min at the beginning to 5 min after two times. Nevertheless, because, in an austere environment with only a few resources, coordination among team members is paramount, we would encourage the whole SOST to follow a simulation course. We saw indeed that the skills of the scrub nurse and paramedic were the time limitation factor in our series.

Limitations

The dynamic approach, obtained by combination of balloon small inflation and aortic compliance, was based on a physical rationale and not on any measurement. Therefore, measuring this on an animal model in the future would better define this physical rationale.

Another limitation of this report is its retrospective nature and the fact that it describes only a series of three cases.

Additionally, it was not possible to keep long-term data for the patients due to the transfer in local MTF for further treatment.

Conclusions

ER-REBOA® in pre-hospital austere environment

Due to his feature, this catheter is particularly suitable for use in an austere pre-hospital environment, as shown by Manley et al. [23] and here. Moreover, as described in Fig. 1, it is efficient to use it following the MIST acronym. This means that when (1) the patient sustained a high-energy trauma, (2) a lower limb external bleeding could not be controlled by manual compression nor a tourniquet or an internal bleeding from the abdomen or pelvis was diagnosed with the hand-held ultrasound, and (3) SBP was below 90 mmHg during the triage and resuscitation. The catheter is then used to buy time to get the patient alive on the operation table. From that moment, DCS can be performed, the source of the bleeding can be located, and the balloon can be gradually deflated. Furthermore, in an austere environment where resources are limited, temporary blocking inflow of blood below the diaphragm improves the surgical performance by facilitating perioperative view as well as reducing the need for blood transfusion. This, thus, saves the limited blood supply, and it reduces trauma coagulopathy. Finally, even a patient with an as low as non-measurable and not felt SBP can still be resuscitated out of a hospital if temporary AO is obtained.

Dynamic approach using pREBOA

In our opinion, REBOA should not be approached as an "ON-OFF" technique. As shown here, REBOA can also be used with a partial AO or pREBOA in a dynamic approach. With 3-mL inflation in the balloon, enough proximal control of the bleeding can be reached to raise the SBP, using simultaneously other resuscitation ways like IV fluids, blood products, vasopressors, and light anesthesia. Furthermore, while SBP can be used to follow the occlusion, HR but especially $EtCO_2$ can both be seen as easy and interesting markers to follow the reperfusion and the steep inflection point.

From our experience, further considerations can arise, and we mention three of them. First, because patients can become hemodynamically unstable at the onset of sedation, would it then be better to already place the sheath using local anesthetic before sedating the patient, perhaps already during the primary survey? Second, because the surgeon is focused on his surgery during DCS, would it not then be better to let the anesthetist inflate and deflate the balloon of the REBOA and follow adequately the inflation time? Third, because pREBOA in a dynamic approach is an adjunct for resuscitation, would it then be helpful to use REBOA during transport between two MTF as suggested by Reva [44]? For such a usage, more people in the whole chain of evacuation, also from the transport team, would definitely need to comprehend this relatively new paradigm and to be confident with the material. However, some initiatives already exist in this sense [41–43].

Abbreviations

AIS: Abbreviated Injury Scale; AO: Aorta occlusion; CCP: Casualty collection point; CFA: Common femoral artery; CO_2: Carbon dioxide; cREBOA: Complete resuscitative endovascular balloon occlusion of the aorta; DCR: Damage control r; DCS: Damage control surgery; $EtCO_2$: End-tidal carbon dioxide; FAST: Focused abdominal sonography for trauma; FWB: Fresh whole blood; HR: Heart rate; ISS: Injury severity score; IV: Intra-venous; MTF: Medical treatment facility; NISS: New injury severity score; PRBC: Packed red blood cells; pREBOA: Partial resuscitative endovascular balloon occlusion of the aorta; REBOA: Resuscitative endovascular balloon occlusion of the aorta; SBP: Systolic blood pressure; SOST: Special Operations Surgical Team; TRISS: Trauma injury severity score

Acknowledgements

The authors would like to express their sincere gratitude to Major Nathalie Pattyn, MD, MPsy, PhD, for her valued assistance in the preparation of this manuscript.

Funding

The authors would like to express their sincere gratitude to Prytime Medical Company for sponsoring the material they used.

Authors' contributions

JCdS analyzed and interpreted the data. He also wrote this paper. SN and IF reviewed and interpreted the data. FW and LDC collected and analyzed the data. MOC collected and reviewed the data. KVC and JCC collected the data. All authors have read and approved the final manuscript.

Competing interests

The authors declare that they have no competing interests.

Author details

[1]Burn Unit, Queen Astrid Military Hospital, B-1120 Brussels, Belgium. [2]Department of Trauma Surgery, University Hospitals Leuven, B-3000 Leuven, Belgium. [3]Department of Vascular Surgery, University Hospitals Leuven, B-3000 Leuven, Belgium. [4]175th Surgical Detachment, US Army, Fort Campbell, Kentucky, USA.

References

1. NAEMT. Tactical Combat Casualty Care Guidelines for All Combatants. https://www.naemt.org/docs/default-source/education-documents/tccc/tccc-ac/updates-1708/00-tccc-ac-guidelines-1708/tccc-guidelines-for-all-combatants-1708.pdf?sfvrsn=7559ca92_2. Accessed 5 Aug 2018.
2. Prytime Medical™. ER-REBOA™. http://prytimemedical.com/product/#er-reboa. Accessed 5 Aug 2018.
3. Med Device Online. Pryor Medical Devices Receives 510(k) Clearance For Distribution Of ER-REBOA Catheter. https://www.meddeviceonline.com/doc/pryor-medical-devices-receives-k-clearance-for-distribution-of-er-reboa-catheter-0001. Accessed 5 Aug 2018.
4. Stannard A, Eliason JL, Rasmussen TE. Resuscitative endovascular balloon occlusion of the aorta (REBOA) as an adjunct for hemorrhagic shock. J Trauma. 2011;71(6):1869–72. https://doi.org/10.1097/TA.0b013e31823fe90c.
5. Irahara T, Sato N, Moroe Y, Fukuda R, Iwai Y, Unemoto K. Retrospective study of the effectiveness of intra-aortic balloon occlusion (IABO) for traumatic haemorrhagic shock. World J Emerg Surg. 2015;10(1):1. https://doi.org/10.1186/1749-7922-10-1.
6. Tsurukiri J, Akamine I, Sato T, et al. Resuscitative endovascular balloon occlusion of the aorta for uncontrolled haemorrahgic shock as an adjunct to haemostatic procedures in the acute care setting. Scand J Trauma Resusc Emerg Med. 2016;24(1):13. https://doi.org/10.1186/s13049-016-0205-8.
7. Lallemand MS, Moe DM, McClellan JM, Smith JP, Daab L,Marko S, Tran N, Starnes B, Martin MJ. Resuscitative endovascular balloon occlusion of the aorta for major abdominal venous injury in a porcine hemorrhagic shock model. J Trauma Acute Care Surg. 2017;83(2):230–236.
8. Russo RM, Neff LP, Lamb CM, et al. Partial resuscitative endovascular balloon occlusion of the aorta in swine model of hemorrhagic shock. J Am Coll Surg. 2016;223(2):359–68. https://doi.org/10.1016/J.JAMCOLLSURG.2016.04.037.
9. Teeter WA, Matsumoto J, Idoguchi K, Kon Y, Orita T, Funabiki T, Brenner ML, Matsumura Y. Smaller introducer sheaths for REBOA may be associated with fewer complications. J Trauma Acute Care Surg. 2016;81(6):1039–45.
10. Brenner M, Teeter W, Hoehn M, Al E. Use of resuscitative endovascular balloon occlusion of the aorta for proximal aortic control in patients with severe hemorrhage and arrest. JAMA Surg. 2018;153(2):130–5.
11. Morrison JJ, Galgon RE, Jansen JO, Cannon JW, Rasmussen TE, Eliason JL. A systematic review of the use of resuscitative endovascular balloon occlusion of the aorta in the management of hemorrhagic shock. J Trauma Acute Care Surg. 2016;80(2):324.
12. Gamberini E, Coccolini F, Tamagnini B, et al. Resuscitative endovascular balloon occlusion of the aorta in trauma: a systematic review of the literature. World J Emerg Surg. 2017;12(1):42. https://doi.org/10.1186/s13017-017-0153-2.
13. Saito N, Matsumoto H, Yagi T, Hara Y, Hayashida K, Motomura T, Mashiko K, Iida H, Yokota H, Wagatsuma Y. Evaluation of the safety and feasibility of resuscitative endovascular balloon occlusion of the aorta. J Trauma Acute Care Surg. 2015;78(5):897–903.
14. Moore LJ, Brenner M, Kozar RA, Pasley J, Wade CE, Baraniuk MS, Scalea T, Holcomb JB. Implementation of resuscitative endovascular balloon occlusion of the aorta as an alternative to resuscitative thoracotomy for noncompressible truncal hemorrhage. J Trauma Acute Care Surg. 2015;79(4):523.
15. Hörer TM, Cajander P, Jans A, Nilsson KF. A case of partial aortic balloon occlusion in an unstable multi-trauma patient. Trauma. 2016;18(2):150–4. https://doi.org/10.1177/1460408615624727.

16. Johnson MA, Neff LP, Williams TK, DuBose JJ; EVAC Study Group. Partial resuscitative balloon occlusion of the aorta (P-REBOA): Clinical technique and rationale. J Trauma Acute Care Surg. 2016;81(5 Suppl 2 Proceedings of the 2015 Military Health System Research Symposium):S133–S137.
17. Russo RM, Williams TK, Grayson JK, Lamb CM, Cannon JW, Clement NF, Galante JM, Neff LP. Extending the golden hour: Partial resuscitative endovascular balloon occlusion of the aorta in a highly lethal swine liver injury model. J Trauma Acute Care Surg. 2016;80(3):372–8.
18. Matsumura Y, Matsumoto J, Kondo H, Idoguchi K, Ishida T, Kon Y, et al. Fewer REBOA complications with smaller devices and partial occlusion: evidence from a multicentre registry in Japan. Emerg Med J. 2017;34(12): 793. https://doi.org/10.1136/emermed-2016-206383.
19. Sadeghi M, Hörer TM, Forsman D, et al. Blood pressure targeting by partial REBOA is possible in severe hemorrhagic shock in pigs and produces less circulatory, metabolic and inflammatory sequelae than total REBOA. Injury. 2018;0(0). doi:https://doi.org/10.1016/j.injury.2018.09.052
20. Courtney DM, Watts JA, Kline JA. End tidal CO2 is reduced during hypotension and cardiac arrest in a rat model of massive pulmonary embolism. Resuscitation. 2002;53(1):83–91. https://doi.org/10.1016/S0300-9572(01)00504-4.
21. McGillicuddy DC, Tang A, Cataldo L, Gusev J, Shapiro NI. Evaluation of end-tidal carbon dioxide role in predicting elevated SOFA scores and lactic acidosis. Intern Emerg Med. 2009. https://doi.org/10.1007/s11739-008-0153-z.
22. Stensaeth KH, Sovik E, Haig INY, Skomedal E, Jorgensen A. Fluoroscopy-free resuscitative endovascular balloon occlusion of the aorta (REBOA) for controlling life threatening postpartum hemorrhage. PLoS One. 2017. https://doi.org/10.1371/journal.pone.0174520.
23. Manley JD, Mitchell BJ, DuBose JJ, Rasmussen TE. A modern case series of resuscitative endovascular balloon occlusion of the aorta (REBOA) in an out-of-hospital, combat casualty care setting. J Spec Oper Med. 2017;17(1):1–8.
24. Northern DM, Manley JD, Lyon R, et al. Recent advances in austere combat surgery: use of aortic balloon occlusion as well as blood challenges by special operations medical forces in recent combat operations. J Trauma Acute Care Surg. 2018. https://doi.org/10.1097/TA.0000000000001966.
25. Sadek S, Lockey DJ, Lendrum RA, Perkins Z, Price J, Davies GE. Resuscitative endovascular balloon occlusion of the aorta (REBOA) in the pre-hospital setting: an additional resuscitation option for uncontrolled catastrophic haemorrhage. Resuscitation. 2016. https://doi.org/10.1016/j.resuscitation.2016.06.029.
26. North Atlantic Treaty Organization. Allied Joint Doctrine for Medical Support. AJP-4.10. https://www.coemed.org/images/Courses_pdf/stanags/mmsop/2228_AJP-4.10%20EDB%20V1%20E.pdf EDB V1 E.pdf. Published 2015. Accessed 5 Aug 2018.
27. Hodgetts T, Deane S, Gunning K. Trauma rules. London: BMJ Publishing Group; 1997.
28. Centers for Disease Control and Prevention. Guidelines for field triage of injured patients. https://fems.dc.gov/sites/default/files/dc/sites/fems/publication/attachments/CDC%20Guidelines%20for%20Field%20Triage%20of%20Injured%20Patients.pdf. Published 2012. Accessed 5 Aug 2018.
29. Linnebur M, Inaba K, Haltmeier T, et al. Emergent non-image-guided resuscitative endovascular balloon occlusion of the aorta (REBOA) catheter placement: a cadaver-based study. J Trauma Acute Care Surg. 2016. https://doi.org/10.1097/TA.0000000000001106.
30. EMCrit RACC. Podcast 170 – the ER REBOA Catheter with Joe DuBose. https://emcrit.org/emcrit/er-reboa/. Accessed 5 Aug 2018.
31. Gennarelli TA, Wodzin E. AIS 2005: a contemporary injury scale. Injury. 2006. https://doi.org/10.1016/j.injury.2006.07.009.
32. Baker SP, O'Neill B, Haddon W Jr, Long WB. The injury severity score: a method for describing patients with multiple injuries and evaluating emergency care. J Trauma Acute Care Surg. 1974;14(3):187–96.
33. Osler T, Baker SP, Long W. A modification of the injury severity score that both improves accuracy and simplifies scoring. J Trauma Acute Care Surg. 1997;43(6):922–5.
34. Boyd CR, Tolson MA, Copes WS. Evaluating trauma care: the TRISS method. Trauma score and the injury severity score. J Trauma. 1987;27(4):370–8.
35. Biffl WL, Fox CJ, Moore EE. The role of REBOA in the control of exsanguinating torso hemorrhage. J Trauma Acute Care Surg. 2015;78(5):1054–8.
36. DuBose JJ, Scalea TM, Brenner M, Skiada D, Inaba K, Cannon J, Moore L, Holcomb J, Turay D, Arbabi CN, Kirkpatrick A, Xiao J, Skarupa D, Poulin N; AAST AORTA Study Group. The AAST prospective Aortic Occlusion for Resuscitation in Trauma and Acute Care Surgery (AORTA) registry: Data on contemporary utilization and outcomes of aortic occlusion and resuscitative balloon occlusion of the aorta (REBOA). J Trauma Acute Care Surg. 2016; 81(3):409–19.
37. Romagnoli A, Teeter W, Pasley J, Hu P, Hoehn M, Stein D, Scalea T, Brenner M. Time to aortic occlusion: It's all about access. J Trauma Acute Care Surg. 2017;83(6):1161–1164.
38. Davidson AJ, Russo RM, Ferencz SE, Cannon JW, Rasmussen TE, Neff LP, Johnson MA, Williams TK. Incremental balloon deflation following complete resuscitative endovascular balloon occlusion of the aorta results in steep inflection of flow and rapid reperfusion in a large animal model of hemorrhagic shock. J Trauma Acute Care Surg. 2017;83(1):139–143.
39. Taylor JRIII, Harvin JA, Martin C, Holcomb JB, Moore LJ. Vascular complications from resuscitative endovascular balloon occlusion of the aorta: Life over limb? J Trauma Acute Care Surg. 2017;83(1 Suppl 1):S120–S123.
40. Eastridge BJ, Mabry RL, Seguin P, et al. Death on the battlefield (2001–2011): implications for the future of combat casualty care. J Trauma Acute Care Surg. 2012;73(6).
41. Brenner M, Hoehn M, Pasley J, Dubose J, Stein D, Scalea T. Basic endovascular skills for trauma course: Bridging the gap between endovascular techniques and the acute care surgeon. J Trauma Acute Care Surg. 2014;77(2):286–91.
42. Villamaria CY, Eliason JL, Napolitano LM, Stansfield RB, Spencer JR, Rasmussen TE. Endovascular Skills for Trauma and Resuscitative Surgery (ESTARS) course: Curriculum development, content validation, and program assessment. J Trauma Acute Care Surg. 2014;76(4):929–35.
43. Endovascular Resuscitation and Trauma Management. EVTM Workshop. https://www.jevtm.com/workshop/. Accessed 5 Aug 2018.
44. Reva VA, Hörer TM, Makhnovskiy AI, Sokhranov M V, Samokhvalov IM, DuBose JJ. Field and en route resuscitative endovascular occlusion of the aorta: A feasible military reality? J Trauma Acute Care Surg. 2017;83(1 Suppl 1):S170–S176.
45. Napolitano LM. Resuscitative endovascular balloon occlusion of the aorta. Crit Care Clin. 2017;33(1):55–70. https://doi.org/10.1016/j.ccc.2016.08.011.

Permissions

All chapters in this book were first published in WJES, by BioMed Central; hereby published with permission under the Creative Commons Attribution License or equivalent. Every chapter published in this book has been scrutinized by our experts. Their significance has been extensively debated. The topics covered herein carry significant findings which will fuel the growth of the discipline. They may even be implemented as practical applications or may be referred to as a beginning point for another development.

The contributors of this book come from diverse backgrounds, making this book a truly international effort. This book will bring forth new frontiers with its revolutionizing research information and detailed analysis of the nascent developments around the world.

We would like to thank all the contributing authors for lending their expertise to make the book truly unique. They have played a crucial role in the development of this book. Without their invaluable contributions this book wouldn't have been possible. They have made vital efforts to compile up to date information on the varied aspects of this subject to make this book a valuable addition to the collection of many professionals and students.

This book was conceptualized with the vision of imparting up-to-date information and advanced data in this field. To ensure the same, a matchless editorial board was set up. Every individual on the board went through rigorous rounds of assessment to prove their worth. After which they invested a large part of their time researching and compiling the most relevant data for our readers.

The editorial board has been involved in producing this book since its inception. They have spent rigorous hours researching and exploring the diverse topics which have resulted in the successful publishing of this book. They have passed on their knowledge of decades through this book. To expedite this challenging task, the publisher supported the team at every step. A small team of assistant editors was also appointed to further simplify the editing procedure and attain best results for the readers.

Apart from the editorial board, the designing team has also invested a significant amount of their time in understanding the subject and creating the most relevant covers. They scrutinized every image to scout for the most suitable representation of the subject and create an appropriate cover for the book.

The publishing team has been an ardent support to the editorial, designing and production team. Their endless efforts to recruit the best for this project, has resulted in the accomplishment of this book. They are a veteran in the field of academics and their pool of knowledge is as vast as their experience in printing. Their expertise and guidance has proved useful at every step. Their uncompromising quality standards have made this book an exceptional effort. Their encouragement from time to time has been an inspiration for everyone.

The publisher and the editorial board hope that this book will prove to be a valuable piece of knowledge for researchers, students, practitioners and scholars across the globe.

List of Contributors

Ziyad Alharbi, Andrzej Piatkowski, Sven Reckort, Gerrit Grieb, Jens Kauczok and Norbert Pallua
Department of Plastic and Hand Surgery, Burn Centre Medical Faculty, RWTH Aachen University Hospital, Pauwelsstr 30, Aachen 52074, Germany

Andrzej Piatkowski
Department of Plastic and Reconstructive Surgery, azM University Hospital, Maastricht, Netherland

Rolf Dembinski
Department of Operative Intensive Care, Medical Faculty, RWTH Aachen University, Aachen, Germany

Sven Reckort
Department of Anaesthesia and Intensive Medicine, St. Elisabeth Hospital Geilenkirchen, Geilenkirchen, Germany

Giulia Montori, Federico Coccolini, Roberto Manfredi, Marco Ceresoli, Luca Campanati, Stefano Magnone, Michele Pisano, Elia Poiasina, Gabriela Nita and Luca Ansaloni
Unit of General and Emergency Surgery, Papa Giovanni XXIII Hospital, P.zza OMS 1, 24128 Bergamo, Italy

Fausto Catena
General surgery department, Ospedale Maggiore, Parma, Italy

Sayf Gazala, Yvonne Tul, Sandy L Widder and Rachel G Khadaroo
Department of Surgery, University of Alberta, 2D WMC, 8440-112 St NW, Edmonton, AB, Canada T6G 2B7

Adrian Wagg
Department of Medicine, University of Alberta, Edmonton, Alberta, Canada

Derya Ozturk, Bedriye Müge Sonmez, Ertugrul Altinbilek, Cemil Kavalci, Engin Deniz Arslan and Serhat Akay
Numune Training and Research Hospital, Emergency Department, Ankara, Turkey

Shaheed Merani and Judd Payne
Department of Surgery, Faculty of Medicine and Dentistry, University of Alberta, Edmonton, Alberta, Canada

Raj S Padwal
Department of Medicine, University of Alberta, Edmonton, Alberta, Canada

Darren Hudson, Sandy L Widder and Rachel G Khadaroo
Division of Critical Care Medicine, Faculty of Medicine and Dentistry, University of Alberta, Edmonton, Alberta Canada

Rachel G Khadaroo
Department of Surgery, University of Alberta, 2D Walter Mackenzie Center, 8440-112 St. NW, Edmonton, Alberta T6G 2B7, Canada

Dimitrios Symeonidis, Michail Spyridakis, Georgios Koukoulis, Grigorios Christodoulidis, Ioannis Mamaloudis and Konstantinos Tepetes
Department of General Surgery, University Hospital of Larissa, Mezourlo, 41110, Larissa, Greece

Bruno Monteiro T. Pereira, Guilherme Vieira Meirelles and Gustavo Pereira Fraga
Division of Trauma Surgery, Department of Surgery, School of Medical Sciences, University of Campinas (Unicamp), Campinas, SP, Brazil

Osvaldo Chiara and Stefania Cimbanassi
Trauma Team, Ospedale Niguarda Milano, Milan, Italy

Fabio Ramponi and Korana Musicki
Department of Cardiothoracic Surgery, John Hunter Hospital, Newcastle, NSW, Australia

Dieter G. Weber and Cino Bendinelli
Department of Traumatology, John Hunter Hospital, Newcastle, NSW, Australia

Belinda De Simone and Fausto Catena
Department of Emergency and Trauma Surgery of the University Hospital of Parma, Parma, Italy

Luca Ansaloni and Federico Coccolini
Department of general and emergency surgery, Papa Giovanni XIII Hospital, Bergamo, Italy

Massimo Sartelli
Department of surgery, Macerata Hospital, Macerata, Italy

Salomone Di Saverio
Department of surgery, Maggiore Hospital of Bologna, Bologna, Italy

Ram Venkatesh Anantha and Dave Paskar
Division of General Surgery, Department of Surgery, Schulich School of Medicine and Dentistry, Western University, London, ON, Canada

Kelly Vogt
Division of Trauma and Acute Care Surgery, Department of Surgery, Los Angeles County and University of Southern California Medical Center, Los Angeles, CA, USA

Silvie Crawford
Executive Leadership (Patient Centred Care), London Health Sciences Centre, London, ON, Canada

Neil Parry
Trauma Program, London Health Sciences Centre, London, ON, Canada
Division of Critical Care, Department of Medicine, Schulich School of Medicine and Dentistry, Western University, London, ON, Canada

Ken Leslie
Victoria Hospital, London Health Sciences Centre, Room E2-217, 800 Commissioners Road East, London, ON N6A 5W9, Canada

Job Kuteesa, Olivia Kituuka, Dan Namuguzi, Samuel Kirunda and Moses Galukande
Department of Surgery, College of Health Sciences, Makerere University, Mulago Hill road, Kampala, Uganda, East Africa

Cynthia Ndikuno
Department of Nursing, College of Health Sciences, Makerere University, Kampala, Uganda

David Mukunya
Department of Paediatrics, College of Health Sciences, Makerere University, Kampala, Uganda

Job Kuteesa
Department of Surgery, School of Medicine, College of Health Sciences, Makerere University, Kampala, Uganda

David Czeiger and Gad Shaked
Department of General Surgery and Trauma Unit, Soroka University Medical Center and Ben-Gurion University, Beer Sheva, Israel

Anton Osyntsov and Gad Shaked
Department of General Surgery, Soroka University Medical Center and Ben-Gurion University, Beer Sheva 84101, Israel

Lidia Osyntsov
Pathology Institute, Soroka University Medical Center and Ben- Gurion University, Beer Sheva, Israel

Chad G Ball
Department of Surgery, University of Calgary, Calgary, Alberta, Canada

Roy Gigi
Department of Orthopedics, Tel Aviv Sourasky Medical Center, Tel Aviv, Israel

James Bailey, Janeen Jordan and Ernest E. Moore
Department of Orthopaedics, Naval Medical Center, San Diego, CA 92134, USA

Todd VanderHeiden, Sarah Pinski-Sibbel and Philip F. Stahel
Department of Orthopaedics, Denver Health Medical Center, University of Colorado School of Medicine, 777 Bannock Street, Denver, CO 80204, USA

Clay Cothren Burlew
Department of Surgery, Denver Health Medical Center, University of Colorado School of Medicine, 777 Bannock Street, Denver, CO 80204, USA

Massimo Sartelli
Department of Surgery, Macerata Hospital, Via Santa Lucia 2, 62019 Macerata, Italy

Fausto Catena
Department of Surgery, Maggiore Hospital, Parma, Italy

Luca Ansaloni
General Surgery Department, Papa Giovanni XXIII Hospital, Bergamo, Italy

Aleksandar Karamarkovic
Clinic for Emergency Surgery, Faculty of Medicine, University of Belgrade, Belgrade, Serbia

Kenji Inaba
Department of Surgery, Division of Acute Care Surgery and Surgical Critical Care, Los Angeles County and University of Southern California Medical Center, Los Angeles, CA, USA

Carlos A. Ordonez
Department of Surgery, Fundación Valle del Lili, Hospital Universitario del Valle, Universidad del Valle, Cali, Colombia

Arda Isik
Department of Surgery, Mengucek Gazi Training Research Hospital, Erzincan, Turkey

Daniel Rios-Cruz
Department of Surgery, Hospital de Alta Especialidad de Veracruz, Veracruz, Mexico

Rodolfo Soto
Department of Emergency Surgery and Critical Care, Centro Medico Imbanaco, Cali, Colombia

Selim Yigit Yildiz, Ali Ciftci and Hamdi Taner Turgut
Department of General Surgery, Kocaeli Derince Training and Research Hospital, Kocaelı, Izmit, Turkey

Murat Kendirci
General Surgery, Edirne State Hospital, Edirne, Turkey

Serkan Akbulut
Department of Surgical Oncology, Ankara University Medical School, Ankara, Turkey

Suleyman Hengirmen
Department of General Surgery, Ankara Numune Training and Research Hospital, Ankara, Turkey

Shefki Xharra
Department of Surgery, Regional Hospital, Prizren, Kosovo

Lumturije Gashi-Luci
Institute of Pathology, Faculty of Medicine, University of Prishtina, Prishtina, Kosovo

Kumrije Xharra
Department of Microbiology, National Institute of Public Health of Kosovo, Prishtina, Kosovo

Fahredin Veselaj
Department of Urology, University Clinical Center of Kosovo, Prishtina, Kosovo

Besnik Bicaj and Avdyl Krasniqi
Department of Abdominal Surgery, University Clinical Center of Kosovo, Prishtina, Kosovo

Fatos Sada
Department of Anesthesiology, University Clinical Center of Kosovo, Prishtina, Kosovo

Cyrille Huchon and Arnaud Fauconnier
Service de gynécologie & obstétrique, CHI Poissy-St-Germain, 10 rue du champ Gaillard, BP 3082 78303, Poissy CEDEX, France

Alexandre Dumont
Equipe d'accueil EA 7285 "Risques, cliniques et sécurité en santé des femmes et en santé périnatale", Université Versailles-Saint-Quentin en Yvelines, 78000 Versailles, France
UMR 216, IRD Paris Descartes, 4 Avenue de l'Observatoire, Paris - Université, 75 006 Paris Descartes, France

Anne Chantrys
INSERM, UMR S953, Epidemiological Research Unit on Perinatal Health and Women's and Children's Health, Hôpital Cochin, Paris, Frances

Bruno Falissard
INSERM UMR S669, Université Paris Sud, Paris, France

Zuhoor K Al-gaithy
Department of Surgery, King Abdulaziz University, Jeddah 21589, Saudi Arabia

Yoshimitsu Izawa, Shuji Hishikawa and Alan Kawarai Lefor
Center of Development for Advanced Medical Technology, Jichi Medical University, 3311-1 Yakushiji, Shimotsukeshi, Tochigiken 329-0498, Japan
Department of Digestive Surgery, Jichi Medical University, 3311-1 Yakushiji, Shimotsukeshi, Tochigiken 329-0498, Japan

Tomohiro Fausto Catena Muronoi, Keisuke Yamashita and Masayuki Suzukawa
Department of Emergency and Critical Care Medicine, Jichi Medical University, 3311-1 Yakushiji, Shimotsukeshi, Tochigiken 329-0498, Japan

Kate Sullivan
Physiotherapy Department, Launceston General Hospital, Charles St, Launceston, Tasmania 7250, Australia
School of Primary Health Care, Faculty of Nursing, Medicine and Health Science, Monash University, Frankston, Victoria 3199, Australia

Ianthe Boden
Department of Physiotherapy, The University of Melbourne, Melbourne, Victoria 3052, Australia
Physiotherapy Department, Launceston General Hospital, Charles St, Launceston, Tasmania 7250, Australia

Claire Hackett and Melissa McKinnon
Department of Physiotherapy, Princess Alexandra Hospital, Woolloongabba, Queensland 4102, Australia

Brooke Winzer
Physiotherapy Department, Northeast Health Wangaratta, Green Street, Wangaratta, Victoria 3677, Australia

Rebecca Lane
School of Physiotherapy, Faculty of Health Sciences, Australian Catholic University, Ballarat, Victoria 3350, Australia

Iain Robertson
Biostatistician, Clifford Craig Foundation, Launceston General Hospital, Charles Street, Launceston, Tasmania 7250, Australia
College of Health Sciences, University of Tasmania, Locked Bag 1320, Launceston, Tasmania 7250, Australia

Federico Coccolini, Giulia Montori and Marco Ceresoli
General, Emergency and Trauma Surgery Department, Papa Giovanni XXIII Hospital, Piazza OMS 1, 24127 Bergamo, Italy
Emergency Surgery Department, Parma University Hospital, Parma, Italy

Rao Ivatury
Virginia Commonwealth University, Richmond, VA, USA

Dimitrios Damaskos
John Radcliffe Hospital, Oxford, UK

Arda Isik
Erzincan University Faculty of Medicine Mengucek Gazi Training Research Hospital Erzincan, Erzincan, Turkey

Kuo-Ching Yuan
Chang Gung Memorial Hospital, Taoyuan, Taiwan

Miguel Leon Arellano
Hospital La Paz, Madrid, Spain

Sefa Ozyazici
Adana Numune Training and Research Hospital, Department of Surgery, Adana, Turkey

Gianluca Costa
Ospedale Sant' Andrea University Hospital Sapienza, Rome, Italy

Ramiro Manzano Nunez, Maria Paula Naranjo and Erika Rincon
Clinical Research Center, Fundación Valle del Lili, Cali, Colombia

Esteban Foianini
Clinical Foianini, Santa Cruz de La Sierra, Bolivia

Paula Ferrada
Virginia Commonwealth University, Richmon, VA, USA

Herney Andrés García-Perdomo, Alberto F. García and Carlos A. Ordoñez
Universidad del Valle, Cali, Colombia

Alberto F. García and Carlos A. Ordoñez
Division of Trauma and Acute Care Surgery, Fundación Valle del Lili, Cali, Colombia

Juan Pablo Herrera
Department of Surgery, Brigham and Women's Hospital, Boston, MA, USA

Paola Burbano
School of Medicine, Universidad Javeriana Cali, Cali, Valle del Cauca, Colombia

Nicola Tartaglia, Roberta Iadarola, Alessandra Di Lascia, Pasquale Cianci, Alberto Fersini and Antonio Ambrosi
Department of Surgery, University of Foggia, Luigi Pinto Street, No. 1, 71122 Foggia, Italy

Frederico José Ribeiro Teixeira Jr
Surgical Oncology Group from the III Surgical Clinic Division, Hospital das Clínicas of the University of São Paulo (USP), School of Medicine, Rua Dr. Ovídio Pires de Campos,
255, 8 th floor, room 8131, Cerqueira César 05403-010, São Paulo, Brazil

Sérgio Dias do Couto Netto
Surgical Oncology Group from the III Surgical Clinic Division, Hospital das Clínicas of the University of São Paulo (USP), School of Medicine, Rua Dr. Ovídio Pires de Campos, 255, 8 th floor, room 8131, Cerqueira César 05403-010, São Paulo, Brazil
6850, Francisco Matarazzo Avenue, apt 181, Bloco 2, Zip Code 05001-200 Perdizes, São Paulo, Brazil
Emergency Surgical Service, Hospital das Clínicas of the University of São Paulo (USP), School of Medicine, Rua Dr. Ovídio Pires de Campos, 255, 8 th floor, room 8131, Cerqueira César 05403-010, São Paulo, Brazil

Eduardo Hiroshi Akaishi
Sarcoma and Melanoma Surgery group - São Paulo Cancer Institute, University of São Paulo, School of Medicine, Cerqueira César, Brazil

Edivaldo Massazo Utiyama
General and Trauma Surgery - III Surgical Clinic Division, Hospital das Clínicas of the University of São Paulo (USP), School of Medicine, Rua Dr. Ovídio Pires de Campos, 255, 8 th floor, room 8131, Cerqueira César 05403-010, São Paulo, Brazil

Carlos Augusto Metidieri Menegozzo
General Surgery Senior Resident - III Surgical Clinic Division, Hospital das Clínicas of the University of São Paulo, School of Medicine, São Paulo, Brazil

Marcelo Cristiano Rocha
Chief of Staff of the Emergency Surgical Service - III Surgical Clinic Division, Hospital das Clínicas of the University of São Paulo, School of Medicine, São Paulo, Brazil

Ekin Ozturk, Martijn MWJ Stommel, Richard RPG ten Broek and Harry van Goor
Department of Surgery, Radboud University Medical Center, 6500 HB Nijmegen, The Netherlands

Marianne van Iersel
Department of Geriatrics, Radboud University Medical Center, Nijmegen, The Netherlands

Yvonne Schoon
Radboud Institute for Health Sciences, Radboud University Medical Center, Nijmegen, The Netherlands

Roberto Bini
Department of Surgery, S. Giovanni Bosco Hospital, Turin, Italy

Osvaldo Chiara and Stefania Cimbanassi
Trauma Center and Metropolitan Trauma Network Department, Niguarda Hospital, Milan, Italy

Giorgio Olivero
Department of Surgical Sciences, S. Giovanni Battista Hospital, University of Turin, Turin, Italy

Antonella Trombetta
Department of Medical Sciences, University of Turin, Turin, Italy

Paolo Cotogni
Department of Anesthesia and Intensive Care, S. Giovanni Battista Hospital, University of Turin, Via Giovanni Giolitti 9, 10123 Turin, Italy

J. C. de Schoutheete, I, F. Waroquier, L. De Cupere, K. Van Cleynenbreugel and J. C. Ceccaldi
Burn Unit, Queen Astrid Military Hospital, B-1120 Brussels, Belgium

S. Nijs
Department of Trauma Surgery, University Hospitals Leuven, B-3000 Leuven, Belgium

Fourneau
Department of Vascular Surgery, University Hospitals Leuven, B-3000 Leuven, Belgium

M. O'Connor
175th Surgical Detachment, US Army, Fort Campbell, Kentucky, USA

Index

www.ingramcontent.com/pod-product-compliance
Lightning Source LLC
LaVergne TN
LVHW080710210926
848485LV00003B/442
9781639274901